KNOW YOUR REMEDIES

Know Your Remedies

PHARMACY AND CULTURE IN
EARLY MODERN CHINA

HE BIAN

PRINCETON UNIVERSITY PRESS

PRINCETON & OXFORD

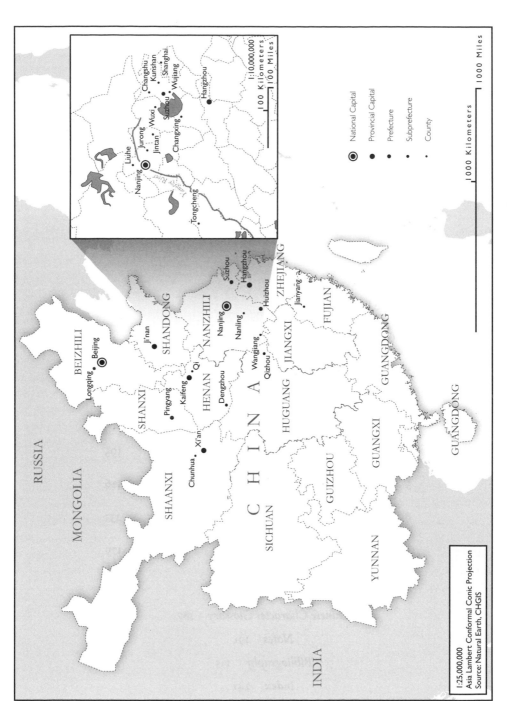

MAP 0.1. Ming provinces with Jiangnan inset

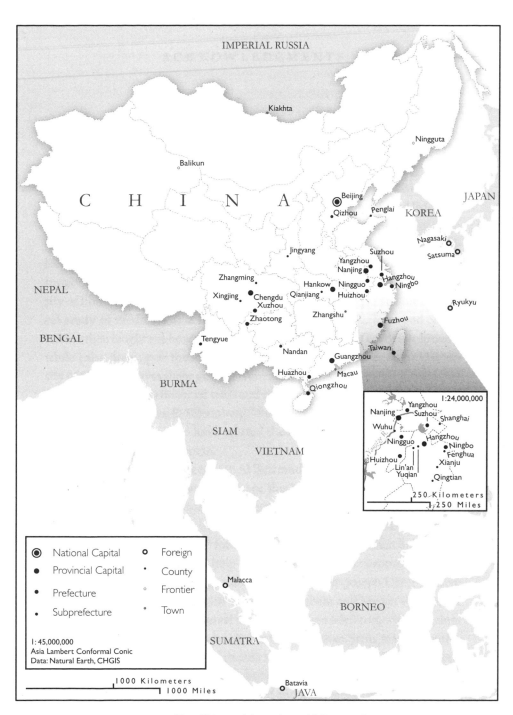

MAP 0.2. Qing China and the region, with Jiangnan inset

materia medica) gradually lost its commanding authority. Instead, a diverse range of pharmaceutical knowledge and practice emerged that sought to redefine the bencao tradition, motivated by new divisions of intellectual and professional labor that took shape under the Qing dynasty (1636–1912). This early modern transformation of pharmacy and pharmaceutical knowledge bears broad implications for China's modern scientific and medical developments, as can be seen from the prevalent practice of Traditional Chinese Medicine (TCM) around the world today.

The peculiar features of traditional Chinese pharmacy have fascinated many but offered few clues for a historical understanding. Back in the 1880s, the Pharmaceutical Society of Great Britain received a scale model of a Chinese pharmacy in the city of Canton (see figure 0.1). The carefully crafted shop front, peopled with figurines, exuded Oriental grandeur: the well-dressed owner, the pipe-smoking customer, and the clerks doing their jobs using rudimentary tools. The wares on display achieved a similar effect: conspicuous signs advertising ginseng, "jade cinnamon," deer horn, and monkey gallstones (*houzao*), with the pharmacist's neatly packed porcelain jars promising access to such exotic treasures. Should we, viewing the model today, take its facade of tradition at face value, seeing the pharmacy as a material manifestation of certain essential traits of Chinese civilization? Or can we see through the air of serenity and mystery shrouding the space, and imagine instead a recent past in which this kind of shop had not yet become a ubiquitous symbol of Chineseness? In other words, do pharmacies in China have a history, and, if so, where should we begin?

"There is no paradox or mystery in finding what is most human through what is most corporeal and palpable," writes Edward H. Schafer in his memorable study of medieval exotica in China.[3] No one, not even the emperor or the most enlightened philosopher of the day, could claim complete control over the pharmacist's cabinet; nor could they live without its offerings. Far from a timeless, monolithic tradition, pharmacy in China served as a dynamic meeting point of elite and popular culture, and is therefore subject to historical analysis. Pharmacies are also translocal enterprises, connecting the world of letters to that of the marketplace bridging nations and continents. Compared to the neat formulations of medical theory, the chaos, messiness, and contentions that inevitably arise during the therapeutic processes fascinate historians of medicine. Well into the early twentieth century, few governments around the world could exert effective regulations over the pharmaceutical trade, a global network in which Chinese actors played a pivotal role.[4] A pharmacy-

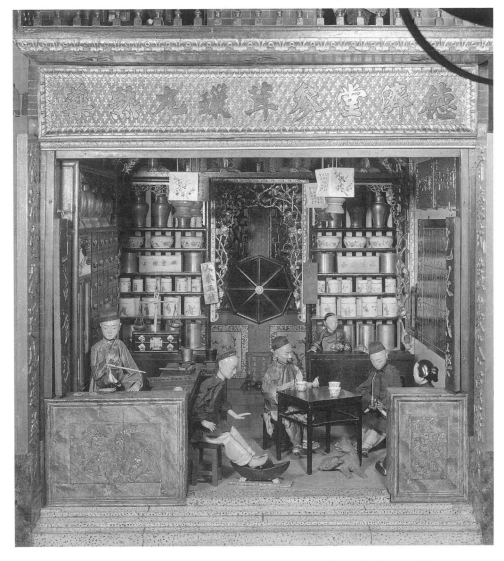

FIGURE 0.1. Model of Chinese pharmacy, nineteenth century. Credit: Wellcome Collection.

centered vantage point thus allows us to discern patterns of cultural change without necessarily prioritizing one group's knowledge over that of others.

The central historical question in this book is why the bencao pharmacopeia, a composite knowledge form that came under state patronage early on in Tang dynasty China (c. 659 CE; see more discussions below), ceased to claim

Having charted out the basic contours of my argument, I now turn to a brief overview of how the scientific tradition of bencao came to be entangled with state power in medieval times. The task of explaining the early modern discontinuity of this state-centered tradition posed great difficulties in the historiography of Chinese science. After a review of that literature, I then present ways in which an inclusive category of knowledge opens new venues for historical interpretation. Finally, I offer a quick guide to key themes and actors in the chapters.

Universalism and Territoriality: State-Commissioned Pharmacopeias in Tang-Song Times

Based on excavated manuscripts and artifacts, we now know that healers in early China used various medicinal substances along with various techniques of acupuncture, moxibustion, and massage. The term "bencao" first appeared in the historical record at the beginning of the Common Era, when rulers of the Han dynasty issued an edict to recruit capable individuals who could master the use of materia medica. Also around this period, a corpus of canonical texts took shape that would define the contours of classical medicine still recognized in the teaching of TCM today. In this core literature, pharmacy appeared to be a marginal subject in these early texts in contrast to lengthy discourses on human physiology and etiology, as well as instructions on acupuncture.[11]

The medical landscape of early medieval China mirrors the heterogeneity and confluence of ideas in the divided political and religious realms. In the fifth century, the Daoist master Tao Hongjing (456–536 CE) synthesized various teachings of pharmacy under one collected commentary (*jizhu*). Out of the various schools, Tao endorsed one particular tradition identifying with the ancient sage-king Divine Farmer (*Shennong*) who, according to legend, tasted one hundred herbs to distinguish medicine from poison. Combining a set of 365 drugs from the Divine Farmer tradition with another 365 from a different source, Tao Hongjing created a standardized format and organizing principle for the study of bencao.[12] Despite his status as a hermit who stayed away from court politics, Tao's medical and alchemical works received generous sponsorship from regional rulers of the south.

State involvement in the medical arts intensified following the unification of the northern and southern regimes under the Sui (581–618) and Tang (618–906) dynasties. In 658 CE, a group of officials and court physicians appointed by Emperor Gaozong completed a newly compiled (*xinxiu*) bencao based on Tao Hongjing's *Collected Commentary*, expanding the number of entries from 730 to 850. Following the Tang precedent, regional regimes in the tenth century, such as the Later Shu (934–65 CE), commissioned their own pharmacopeia in an effort to claim imperial legitimacy. The nascent Northern Song dynasty began compiling its first pharmacopeia in 973, even before its conquest of the south was completed. During 1057–61, the Song court issued another round of even more ambitious pharmacopeia projects, raising the number of entries to 1,083.[13]

It is important to note here that the Tang and Song bencao pharmacopeias were universalist in spirit and territorial in organization. At court, the emperor enabled medical experts and literati officials to work in collaboration, drawing both from reports and from specimens gathered from local administrations. On the one hand, the universalist character of state-commissioned pharmacopeias made a point of public interest transcending the proprietary practice of individual physicians. The pharmacopeia offered a stable, authoritative reference that encouraged, if not enforced, standardization in the sourcing, processing, and dispensing of simple and compound drugs. Taking pharmacy out of the esoteric realm of medical practitioners, the State harnessed their intimate knowledge of the potent substances while relying on the help of court literati to refine "vulgar language" into elegant prose.[14] In this sense, I use the term "pharmacopeia" to imply this normative task without suggesting that the legal infrastructure that surrounded the use of these texts in medieval China was identical to that introduced to European city guilds much later.[15] Once compiled, the bencao texts served as a basis for testing and selecting personnel to staff the imperial medical offices, but not for regulating the dispensing of cures by the average practitioner. If anything, the Chinese pharmacopeias were meant to counteract the anonymity and caprice of the marketplace of healing, not to set up rules for the marketplace per se.

The universalist outlook of Tang-Song pharmacopeias is also manifest in their scope of coverage. Aside from the immediate purpose of alleviating human suffering with drugs, these encyclopedic texts sought to name and describe all creatures and to designate them to their proper place in the world. On a symbolic level, they offered a framework of knowledge about the origin of all creatures that could be endlessly expanded. Su Song (1020–1101), chief compiler of one mid-eleventh-century bencao, announced in his preface that the emperor "nourishes and nurtures all living beings" (*hanyang shenglei*) with ultimate benevolence and virtue. The beneficiaries of this imperial compassion consisted not just of humans, but also minerals, plants, and animals. "He feels sorrowful," writes Su, "even if one thing loses its proper place."[16] The pharmacopeia, therefore, had to be universal in its coverage, so as to prove that the emperor was truly acting in accord with the Mandate of Heaven. The governance of all life—what historian TJ Hinrichs has called "transformative governance"—formed the ideological basis of the collaboration between Confucian officials and medical experts at court in producing a pharmacopeia.[17]

The territorial organization of the Tang-Song bencao is arguably the most conspicuous departure from earlier pharmaceutical texts. Medico-alchemical practitioners knew that the procurement of rare material resources was closely tied to the territorial control of the state. Tao Hongjing, writing at a time of north–south division, framed the disruption of pharmaceutical supplies in political terms in his *Collected Commentary*:

> Ever since [the Jin Dynasty] retreated to the south of the Yangzi River, small and miscellaneous drugs often come from places nearby, and their power and nature are inferior to those from their original places. . . . This must be the reason why medication is less efficacious than previous generations.[18]

Later, Tao's own statements started to look parochial in the eyes of the Tang courtiers. Kong Zhiyue, a descendant of Confucius and son of classicist Kong Yingda (574–648), played a central role in the compilation of the pharmacopeia. In his preface, Kong made the following remarks about Tao Hongjing:

> At that time, regional regimes confronted each other, and he could not have heard or seen much about the distant lands. Without the opportunity for deliberating with colleagues, his interpretation was preoccupied with his own learning. And so . . . he made mistakes in [describing] millet and rice's yellow and white colors . . . and could not tell lead from tin, or oranges from pomelo.[19]

By contrast, the Tang pharmacopeia commissioned reports from all commanderies and districts (*junxian*), changing place-names that marked natural sites into the standard administrative nomenclature under the unified regime. The tone of superiority over ordinary practitioners was very clear.

Overall, the Tang-Song state's appropriation of the bencao tradition resulted in a clear shift of priorities as expressed in its core terminologies. The *Divine Farmer's Classic*, quoted by Tao Hongjing, directed practitioners to specific sites, such as sacred mountains and caves, where plants, animals, and minerals "live/grow" (*sheng*). In the additional entries that Tao attached to the old text, he described sites where medicinal substances "exist" (*you*). In the mid-seventh century, the Tang bencao listed names of local administrations where valuable drugs "come forth/emerge" (*chu*). By Song times, we see the discourse of "products/production" (*chan*) entering the pharmacopeia, which carries a more explicit meaning of exploitation. In chapter 2, we will see how this formulation was also entangled with the means by which the state obtained critical resources for its own use.

It is beyond the scope of this book to give a full historical account of Tang-Song pharmacopeias, about which much exciting new research continues today. It suffices to note that the Tang-Song pharmacopeias were no monolithic tradition, but contingent products of the political, economic, and intellectual exigencies of their times. Nevertheless, the court's high-profile sponsorship of these monumental texts, which lasted for over five hundred years starting in the seventh century, became a conspicuous point of reference against which later developments were measured. We now turn to the major approaches to the placement of later bencao in larger narratives about Chinese science and civilization.

Bencao and the Periodization of Chinese Science

"There is no zoology in ancient India, only catalogs of meats," writes Francis Zimmermann in his study of ecological themes in Hindu medicine.[20] Someone examining the Chinese pharmacopeia might draw a similar conclusion, for even though the bencao recognizes minerals, plants, and animals as belonging to different kinds (*lei*), it approaches them all as pharmaceutical objects. Nonmedical approaches to flora and fauna (e.g., a lexicographical approach to the names of creatures) developed in parallel with bencao but never received comparable prestige or the fanfare associated with imperial patronage in Tang-Song times.[21]

When Emil Bretschneider, a Baltic German who served as a medical officer in the Russian embassy in Peking beginning in 1866, discovered the value of Chinese bencao for the modern discipline of botany, the main reference he used was *Bencao gangmu* (*Systematic Materia Medica*) by the sixteenth-century physician Li Shizhen. Containing 1,892 entries, Li Shizhen's bencao surpassed previous pharmacopeias in its breadth and sophistication. Through his writings, Bretschneider presented the first systematic description of the unique Chinese tradition of state-commissioned pharmacopeias, citing them as valuable sources for the study of botanical and cultural exchange throughout the ages.[22] For practical reasons also, physicians, missionaries, and foreign residents of the proliferating treaty ports found themselves urgently in need of an understanding of the native pharmacy. At the turn of the twentieth century, the Iowa-born G. A. Stuart (1858–1911) published an interpretive study of the Chinese pharmacopeia, preserving Chinese terminologies and adding notes from his observations on the bustling trade.[23] In the early decades of the twentieth century, Bernard E. Read (Chinese name Yi Bo-en, 1887–1949) taught pharmacology at the Rockefeller-sponsored Peking Union Medical College and later obtained his own PhD in pharmacology at Yale. Working with his Chinese colleagues, Read systematically studied Li Shizhen's *Bencao gangmu* and published studies of botanical, avian, fish, and other animal-derived drugs in the 1930s.[24]

Building on those early works, a verifiable field of research dedicated to the study of bencao and Chinese pharmacy emerged after the end of World War II. Scholars in Japan and Europe continued along their respective traditions of Sinological research with a focus on textual interpretation and bibliographical research. Motivated by the dominant ideological divide of the Cold War, historians in mainland China searched for a Marxist interpretation of premodern Chinese science, while publishing modern editions of bencao to facilitate the popular application of traditional therapies. Paul U. Unschuld, the preeminent scholar of Chinese medicine in Germany, built his own work on Japanese scholarship and collaboration with Chinese colleagues. Their meticulous research on bencao has provided a solid foundation for the present study.[25]

The postwar sentiments of national development and ideological rivalry came to be distilled in the so-called Needham question: based in Cambridge, the British embryologist-turned-historian Joseph Needham and his collaborators designed an ambitious publishing project known as the Science and Civilisation in China (SCC) series. The task of Needham's project was twofold: first, to document the awe-inspiring accomplishments of Chinese science and technology prior to the modern era; and second, to perform the "grand titration" of progress, so as to determine the point in time when Western civilization decisively surpassed that of China.[26] The case of bencao, which was translated as "pandects" of "pharmaceutical natural history" by Needham, presented excellent material for this task: on the one hand, the great Tang and Song pharmacopeias predated European efforts to implement medical administration by centuries, spurning the notion that already in the Song dynasty, China had undergone a sort of renaissance in science and assumed a modern outlook in its politics and society. On the other hand, Li Shizhen's *Bencao gangmu*, hailed as the crowning achievement for the "prince of pharmacists" by Needham, sparked no further pursuit along similar lines in Ming-Qing China. "Nothing was quite the same" after Li Shizhen's death in 1593, lamented Needham.[27] This again seemed clear proof that the rise of the West could be dated to the late sixteenth to early seventeenth century, conveniently contemporary to Newton and the Scientific Revolution in England, where Needham resided. The case of bencao fit the general consensus of the 1970s and 1980s that late imperial China was trapped in a sort of "high-level equilibrium" of productivity and cultural maturity.[28] Only external forces, imposed by the ascending West, could deliver China from its predicament.

However, we must not ignore the fact that Chinese authors in the seventeenth and eighteenth centuries did create a large number of bencao. They did not follow the "pandect" type of Li Shizhen and earlier pharmacopeias. Bibliographical research of extant Chinese medical texts indicates that more than 130 new titles can be dated to the seventeenth century and over 110 to the eighteenth century, compared to fewer than 20 in the fifteenth century and 50–60 in the sixteenth century.[29] Compelled to evaluate their significance by earlier standards, historians have largely dismissed the later titles as either "eclectic" monographs that merely rearranged earlier insights, or worse, atavistic attempts to return to the ancient nucleus of bencao, discarding by the wayside the progress made over centuries.[30] In any case, the Needham question has become a rhetorical device that invites the set answer of a race between civilizations for scientific dominance, which China lost circa 1600.

Today, the Needham question appears outdated to our multicultural sensibilities. Scholarly consensus has indeed moved from a search for priority of discovery and competitiveness in science toward interpreting science as practice and culture, malleable to political exigencies and constructible social norms.[31] It is thus most fitting to see the French sinologist Georges Métailié take over Needham's unfinished discussion of botany in China and reformulate the latter's questions along very different lines. Rejecting *The Grand Titration* and its presumption of cross-cultural commensurability, Métailié closely studied Li Shizhen's *Bencao gangmu*, along with the Song pharmacopeia in its textual and pictorial conventions, to explain how different they were from their European counterparts. Highlighting the interactive nature of pharmaceutical objecthood, Métailié rejected the applicability of terms such as "botany" to Chinese bencao, preferring "ethnobotany" instead to connect the study of plants with human affairs. Doing so allowed Métailié to cast his net widely across the seventeenth-century transition and see *continuities* in Ming-Qing approaches to the natural world. His work broke new ground and shed light on the confluence of the study of plants with Confucian natural and political philosophy in the later period. In the end, Métailié saw neither evidence nor necessity that traditional botany in China and the modern science of botany could have a "fusion point."[32]

Replacing Needham's concern with civilizations with a more flexible notion of epistemic cultures, the early 2000s saw a further diversification of interpretive strategies toward China's scientific past. In *The Monkey and the Inkpot*, Carla Nappi offers an intimate reading of Li Shizhen's epistemic and compositional strategies in *Bencao gangmu*, taking the readers on a panoramic tour of the world presented therein. Writing against the notion of irreducible cultural difference—and the tendency, therefore, to see non-Western culture as irrational—Nappi shows the ways in which the spontaneous transformation of matter informed Li's understanding of the world, as well as the myriad species that reside in it. Similarly, Dagmar Schäfer's study of Song Yingxing (1587–1666), another figure of the late Ming who was much discussed in isolation but rarely contextualized, sheds light on the debt Song owed to earlier advocates of materialistic ontology, which in turn allowed Song to formulate a powerful discourse on the cosmic efficacy of technology. These two works carry forward Nathan Sivin's earlier insight about the possibility of redefining revolutionary moments in Chinese science independent of Western-centered periodization. Both studies also go beyond cultural comparisons to emphasize the necessity of elucidating the epistemic premises and genealogy of ideas that motivated Chinese authors.[33]

Another important development since 2000 calls for a reexamination of regional and global scientific exchange, emphasizing the agency of Chinese actors who, in Benjamin Elman's words, reacted and engaged with Western learning "on their own terms." In so doing, we can now see the seventeenth century as a multidirectional reckoning of global connections and differences, in which Chinese science emerged as an object of intense interest *and* underwent deep transformations at the same time. Furthermore, Elman's account also serves to connect the early modern in a continuous arc with the nineteenth and early twentieth centuries, allowing us to see how Chinese reformers in the late Qing drew their inspiration not only from Western nations and Japan, but also from within the Chinese intellectual tradition.[34] In the regional context, Federico Marcon and Suyoung Suh's works shed light on the different dynamics in early modern Japan and Korea, where Chinese ideologies and artifacts informed, but by no means predetermined, local scientific cultures.

Exchanges of medical and pharmacological ideas, in addition to the more prominently discussed fields like astronomy and mathematics, inspired many new works and ongoing research.[35] Below, I turn to the ways in which this book makes a new contribution to this vibrant field.

The Ming-Qing Transition as a History of Knowledge: Three Themes

No singular pattern governs any period of Chinese history. The Tang-Song pharmacopeia celebrates a neat model of pharmaceutical knowledge that keeps expanding along with the state's power, and yet the processes of making such knowledge were fraught with digressions, deletions, and dissonances. Similarly, the end of the pharmacopeia tradition must be grasped as the gradual unraveling of multiple conditions that once sustained its legitimacy. Following historians Karine Chemla and Evelyn Fox Keller's call to examine science as "culture without culturalism," I treat the unruly corpus of Ming-Qing bencao as evidence of ongoing contention within the Chinese epistemic tradition.[36] Extraordinary individuals such as Li Shizhen and Song Yingxing, like trees in a forest, stood at the edges of the whole range of possible epistemic positions in their times. By following the changing contours of bencao across three hundred years, this book seeks to give a holistic sketch of the life of that forest.[37] Let me now introduce three consecutive themes that will guide my analysis in this book.

The Sixteenth Century: Reconstituting the Center

Historians of late imperial China often speak of the state in terms of the center versus the local. The literati elite used the civil service examination system to gain access to national politics, or, in adversarial times, retreat to a "localist" stage of leadership. The Mandate of Heaven (*tianming*), which bestowed supreme power on the emperor to govern all lives, also bound him to adhere to a set of moral codes that was considered natural. Prefects and magistrates, appointed by the emperor through an intricate process of bureaucratic assignment, administered the locality and formed, in Sarah Schneewind's words, a sort of "Minor Mandate" vis-à-vis the populace they directly governed. Thus constituted, the State sought to monopolize the field of political action and mold the fabric of society according to its own image, notwithstanding the reality that commoners could always find ways of resistance, evasion, and subversion.[38]

Seen from a different perspective, the State also mediated the relationship between human society and the larger world. We have discussed how the universalist outlook of the Tang-Song pharmacopeia equipped the emperor with knowledge of all things, so as to better perform his duties in a kind of "transformative governance" that mimicked the nurturing (and punitive) powers of heaven. Seen thus, medicine, along with astrology, became an essential technology that upheld the imperial state's promise to fulfill Heaven's Mandate. Along with productive technologies that also, in Dagmar Schäfer's words, fostered the "inception of things" (*kaiwu*), medical and astrological experts claimed their rightful place in central and local government.

Beginning in the fifteenth century, we see a steady atrophy of what Angela K. C. Leung has called "organized medicine" in government, replaced by a more aggressively human-centered theory of governance that emphasized the welfare of human society above all else. The advocates of this humanist politics were, unsurprisingly, also vocal teachers and preachers of neo-Confucianism. Empowered by a righteous conviction deduced from their fervent belief in cosmic unity, these scholar-officials pushed for a decisive shift in Ming policy on all fronts. Francesca Bray's study of agricultural treatises vividly captures the scholar-official elite's ambition to dominate the technical sphere of governance, while at the same time criticizing state involvement in other kinds of technology such as industry, seafaring, and trade.[39] The process of reconstituting the center, replete with strife and uncertainty, took place over the fifteenth and sixteenth centuries and would become keenly felt in all corners of the Ming world. The reason why this process has not yet received much scholarly attention lies in the fact that the historiography of Ming China, which itself stemmed from these policy debates, was dominated by sympathizers and descendants of activist scholar-officials.[40] We still live in the shadow of this ideologically charged historiographical stance that sought to impose moral judgment on its subjects, offering caricatures of powerful eunuchs and technicians at court in particular. The corpus of bencao and the pharmacist's cabinet offered a good vantage point from which to see a different aspect of the changing nature of the Ming state.

The Seventeenth Century: Literati Amateurism and Its Discontent

In his influential trilogy on Confucianism and China's "modern fate," historian Joseph Levenson chose to open the entire study with two short chapters on the "tone of early-modern Chinese intellectual culture." Back in the 1960s when Levenson wrote, it was radical of him to see an intellectual continuity between Ming-Qing times and the twentieth century by speaking of an "early modern" moment. In his analysis, however, Levenson considered the subject of science only to claim that empiricism in early Qing thought was "abortive" and nowhere close to becoming truly scientific (we now have, among others, Elman's account of Qing philology that refutes Levenson's claim on this point). For Levenson, the modern transformation of Chinese intellectual culture was synonymous with the "corrosion of the amateur ideal," in which the Confucian literati, whether serving in central offices or living a local gentry's life, possessed the authority to be the cultural arbiter of all trades. Using literati painting as his primary example, Levenson observed that "the Ming style was the amateur style; Ming culture was the apotheosis of the amateur."[41]

Was amateurism, or a kind of "epistemic promiscuity" in our terms today, truly a hallmark of premodern Chinese elite culture? To say so risks essentializing Levenson's observation of Ming China as an *ahistorical* explanatory framework. In the *Analects*, we can, in fact, find a famous passage in which Confucius demonstrates the utmost humility by conceding expertise over farming and planting to experienced farmers and gardeners.[42] It is more historically accurate to see statements of Confucian amateurism as aspirational, contentious, and always in competition with other claims to technical expertise. For instance, the Han dynasty scholar Yang Xiong (53 BCE–18 CE) defined a Confucian (*ru*) as "someone who thoroughly comprehends heaven, earth, and human beings," as opposed to a technician (*ji*) who "comprehends heaven and earth, but *not* people."[43] While acknowledging the technician's mastery over the external world, Yang reaffirms the humanistic core of Confucianism as not only compatible with technical learning, but also capable of transcending "mere technicians" in forging a holistic understanding of both inner and outer worlds. Yang's flamboyant statement became a point of reference for like-minded Confucians in later times, yet it by no means indicated that their polymath ambitions were necessarily fulfilled in social life.

Seen in this light, the emergence of the bencao pharmacopeia in Tang-Song times rather proved the tenacity of medical expertise in the face of rising Confucian interest in the art of medicine for a range of ethical, intellectual, and political reasons (more on this in chapter 3). The literati elite became more generally inclined to claim medical expertise during the Northern Song, at the very moment when their privileged access to politics was cemented in the regularization of civil examinations.[44] Confucian amateurism in medicine served, in other words, almost always as a metaphor of their command over politics on the national stage, and this remained true also for literati medicine in Ming-Qing times.[45] The heightened sense of amateurism in late Ming culture should thus be read as a symptom of politics at that time, not as an unchanging feature of Chinese elite culture. Nevertheless, we will see that Confucian amateurism did play a crucial role in the transformation of bencao throughout the seventeenth century.

Compared with previous high points of Confucian amateurism, the impact of certain iconic cultural figures became much more amplified by the flourishing print culture. The effectiveness of print, however, also lowered the barriers to access, inviting heretofore marginal cultural actors to claim their own voice in published words. Historian Kai-Wing Chow sees publishing as a crucial venue for the emergence of the so-called *shishang* (literati and merchant) culture, one that was capable of forging a "public domain" of expression distinct from the State.[46] Elite women also gained access to published authorship during this time; so did a large number of middling literati who were kept out of official careers and ended up as professional writers.[47] The diversification and commodification of culture continued after the wars of Qing conquest concluded following the 1680s. By that time, however, it had turned out that the widened venues of publishing had become an equally effective means for opponents of Confucian amateurs to rebuild orthodoxy in their areas of expertise.[48] Again, we can see the convulsions of war and conquest leave a clear mark on the diverse corpus of bencao compiled during the seventeenth century.

The Eighteenth Century: A Triangle of Knowledge-Wealth-Power

By the time the Ming fell in the 1640s, the previous model of transformative governance, and its manifestation in state-commissioned pharmacopeias, had become outdated and contorted beyond recognition. Therefore, the succeeding Qing dynasty faced the challenge of redefining the State vis-à-vis human society as well as the larger world. The Long Eighteenth Century, also known as the High Qing era, witnessed the consolidation of Qing responses to both questions under the leadership of three Manchu emperors and their court officials. In social administration, the Qing state strengthened monarchical leadership over the civil bureaucracy, compressing the local administrator's autonomy in performing the "Minor Mandate." Instead, the Qing government, staffed by elite officials who vowed absolute loyalty to the emperor alone, used its administrative muscle to manage society in areas such as hydraulic engineering and famine relief. To fund governmental initiatives without raising agricultural taxes, the Qing state also entered into an informal alliance with mercantile interests, both encouraging, and later on directly investing in, commerce and various industries.[49]

There began to emerge "luxurious networks," as Yulian Wu put it, which entangled the political and mercantile elite in Qing times and decisively shaped the outlook of culture in eighteenth-century China. The Qing rulers relished their command over the material realm and made a point of asserting the *technical* sophistication of the administration on all fronts, including the directed production of highly valued objects such as porcelain, jade, and certain fashions of attire. The imprint of Manchu rule was visible on dresses, shoes, every adult man's shaved forehead and braided queue, food, and collectibles such as fancy carved inkstone. The Qing was, in Dorothy Ko's words, a "material empire" in a different sense from the Ming.[50] Whereas historians are hard-pressed to locate many records of the Ming state's equally extraordinary material ventures (such as the early fifteenth-century expeditions that reached the shores of Africa), scholars of Qing China can use the abundant archival records generated by the growing bureaucratic management of material resources, coupled with a rich collection of extant artifacts. The existence of such records has not only enabled the reconstruction of the "social lives" of individual commodities but also reflects the changing cultural priorities throughout the eighteenth century. The commodification of pharmaceuticals offers a distinct yet related example vis-à-vis other bulk commodities, such as grains, timber, and salt for the domestic market, and porcelain, tea, and silk for the export-oriented economy during this period. While much scholarship has focused on ginseng, the wonder drug of China's early modernity and the only medicinal herb monopolized under the Qing administration, we still do not have a good account of how pharmaceutical trade as a whole evolved with relatively little formal intervention from the State.[51]

The question of knowledge inevitably comes up to form the third leg of a triangle, adding to the nexus of power and wealth. Just as in social administration, the Qing state took a much more active role in reshaping the world of letters than its Ming predecessor, achieving nothing short of a complete reclassification of knowledge in numerous monumental projects conducted at court. Instead of ceding cultural authority to the elite literati, the Qing state co-opted them and patronized their scholarship so long as their pursuit remained within regulated boundaries of propriety.[52] Yet it would be wrong to see the various moments of alliance and antagonism between the Qing state and scholars in isolation from the widening disparity of status. Classically educated men in Qing China, whose numbers had greatly increased compared to earlier periods, had a much slimmer chance of entering governmental positions through the civil examination than their Ming predecessors. As a result, they no longer acted in concert politically as a "literati" class, but assumed a variety of statuses, priorities, and, for that matter, intellectual orientations. As a result, the holistic ideals of Ming neo-Confucian philosophy gave rise not only to High Qing philology but also to many other subfields that came to be redefined during the eighteenth century. Among them was a new type of bencao that reflected primarily orthodox medical interests, and a new trend of encyclopedic documentation of minerals, plants, and animals that became demedicalized, resembling natural history (see chapter 4).

The triangular relationship among power, wealth, and knowledge was by no means stable. Toward the end of the eighteenth century, pharmacy had achieved a similar transition from the emblem of literati culture to part of what Evelyn Rawski and Susan Naquin have described as an emergent "national culture with a broad urban base."[53] Largely excluded from elite sources, the popular culture among laborers, peddlers, and other increasingly volatile sectors of society generated its own clandestine codes of expression and channels of communication.[54] The harvest, preparation, and consumption of pharmaceutical objects provided a meeting point between elite consciousness and popular culture, opening up questions of epistemic power among plebeians and its political implications.[55] The question of pharmaceutical objecthood persisted long after the disintegration of the bencao pharmacopeia and the diversification of knowledge forms that derived from it.

Chapter Outlines

Chapter 1 traces the decentralization of prestige associated with the state-commissioned pharmacopeia up until the end of the sixteenth century. Chapter 2 tells a parallel story of the State's retreat from directly procuring materia medica from localities as tribute, resorting instead to collecting a monetized surtax. Chapter 3 zooms in on the early decades of the seventeenth century to examine the amateurization of bencao in certain literati circles. The division of parts one and two at the juncture of dynastic transition is intended not as a marker of absolute discontinuity, but a deliberate pause for the reader to consider the multiplicity of actors covered so far, as well as their future trajectories under a new regime.

Chapter 4 picks up the transformation of bencao in post-Conquest Jiang-nan to highlight the vocal critics of amateur authors and consider the ways in which the Qing state's cultural policy over the eighteenth century shaped the now-marginalized field. Chapter 5 describes the commodification of the wholesale and retail trades of pharmaceuticals since late Ming times and as-sesses the contribution of mercantile actors to the overall discourse of phar-macy. Chapter 6 ends the book by considering the marginal literati authors whose knowledge of exotica drew from both official sources and the market-place. Qing China entered the nineteenth century with not one but many competing claims to knowledge that would trigger a new round of negotiation over pharmaceutical objecthood in the modern era.

One last note before we proceed to the chapters. The writer Katherine White (1892–1977, married to E. B. White) reviewed mail-order gardening catalogs for the *New Yorker* in the 1950s and 1960s. Like her, I found myself more inter-ested in the human actors responsible for creating catalogs of pharmaceuticals than in how to use the pharmaceuticals themselves.[56] It is not my purpose here to vouch for the efficacy of the substances deployed by my historical actors, nor am I qualified to evaluate their pharmacological mechanisms. I do hope that the historical analysis presented in this book might shed new light on protracted debates over TCM, and I offer some preliminary thoughts in the epilogue.

In this book, I refer to pharmaceutical materials by their common names in English wherever possible (e.g., ginseng [*renshen*], rhubarb [*dahuang*], aco-nite [*fuzi*]), in consultation with Shiu-ying Hu's guide to Chinese materia medica. In doing so, I hope both to minimize cluttering of the prose and also to offer leads for readers interested in the technical details. Dates for Chinese dynasties discussed in this book and Ming-Qing reign eras, as well as a table of conversion for Chinese units, are provided in the appendix for reference. Unless otherwise noted, Chinese names are mentioned with family names preceding given names. Authors of secondary sources in Chinese or Japanese are mentioned in the notes with their full names, and in the bibliography with original characters.

PART I

1

The Last Pharmacopeia

IN THE SUMMER OF 1505, Zhu Youcheng, the emperor of Ming China under the reign name of *Hongzhi* (Grand Governance), became ill and died at thirty-five. Leading officials attributed the young emperor's premature death to hot-natured drugs that should never have been prescribed to treat diseases arising from summer heat. They blamed Liu Wentai, superintendent of the Imperial Academy of Medicine, and Zhang Yu, the chief palace eunuch, for the crime of regicide.[1]

The irony in this accusation lies in the fact that Liu and Zhang had only recently claimed a great accomplishment in the field of pharmacy. The late Hongzhi emperor had always cherished the art of medicine, frequently donating medications to the poor.[2] In 1503, the emperor asked Liu and Zhang to compile a new bencao pharmacopeia with a team of palace physicians. Two years later, the team presented the throne with a beautifully illustrated manuscript that documented 1,815 kinds of materia medica, further adorned with a short preface by the emperor himself, under the title *Yuzhi Bencao pinhui jing-yao* (*Imperially Commissioned, Essentials of Assorted and Collected Materia Medica*; hereafter *Essentials*). A few months later, Liu and Zhang fell from grace following the sudden passing of Hongzhi. The pharmacopeia was sealed off and never distributed outside the palace.[3]

In scholar-official circles, stories about Liu Wentai lingered throughout the sixteenth century. One popular anecdote claimed that Liu was in fact also responsible for the death of the Chenghua emperor (Hongzhi's father) back in 1487. Having narrowly escaped severe punishment, so the story goes, Liu lashed out against his foes, forcing a well-respected minister to retire.[4] More stories portrayed the Hongzhi emperor on his deathbed begging for water, his nose bleeding from excessive heat, with Liu refusing to let him drink. Another questioned how Liu and Zhang managed to escape the death penalty—or, might it have been the emperor's widow, deceived by her trust in Liu and Zhang's long-time service, who intervened and exonerated them?[5] The making of the Hongzhi pharmacopeia, too, was replete with dissonance: when Liu Wentai requested the help of two Hanlin academicians to serve as "proofreaders," the grand secretariat took it as an insult. Arguing that a scholar's proper job was the "discussion and deliberation" (*lunsi*) of state policy, they refused to work with the palace physicians.[6]

This divisive battle over an emperor's death offers us a crucial context for understanding the rapid transformation of bencao as a field of knowledge during the sixteenth century. By casting Liu in an unholy light, the tales fit into the contentious mood stoked by later controversies over imperial succession during the long Jiajing (1522–66) and Wanli (1572–1620) reigns. Scholar-officials, seeking to rectify public affairs with their moral learning, felt compelled to weigh in on issues pertaining to the health and maintenance of the imperial family. The sensational anecdotes emerged out of their fear that it took only one incompetent physician—or even worse, an intentionally malignant person—to shake the "root of the State" (*guoben*).[7] Medical experts and eunuchs, meanwhile, were quick to punch back whenever they had a chance. In his preface to the Hongzhi pharmacopeia, Liu Wentai took a subtle jab at the scholar-official who would not deign to work with him. "The old bencao is intelligible only to virtuous gentlemen and erudite scholars," noted Liu, whereas his text would be "easy to understand by novices and mediocre persons without much hard thinking."[8] Hiding behind his self-deprecating tones is a defiance that is hard to miss.

In the short term, the fate of a state-commissioned pharmacopeia was doomed by the political impasse between scholar-officials and technical experts in the Ming polity. In this chapter, I offer a different narrative that examines instead the longer trajectory of textual transmission and reception for these "pandects" of pharmaceutical objecthood. I argue that the decentralization of authority had already been well under way since the eleventh century, when the Northern Song court did commission multiple bencao pharmacopeias. Proceeding chronologically, three trends stand out when we examine bencao as a field of inquiry. First, the Song state could not exert much control over these elaborate texts in transmission. A variety of authors, acting independently of the imperial court, made changes to the official edition and promoted their work through the manuscript or the newly available technology of printing.

Second, major medical innovations during the Jin-Yuan period (thirteenth through fourteenth centuries) inspired physicians to explain pharmacological action in cosmic, systematic terms. Turning away from the pharmacopeia's erudition, these authors aimed instead to create a practical curriculum of pharmacy informed by correlative cosmology. Their efforts were augmented by the rising influence of commercial publishers at that time. Lastly, regional official publishing—a hallmark of Ming book culture—made the elaborate Song pharmacopeia widely available in print from the mid-fifteenth century. As a result, an unprecedented number of texts emerged that attempted to *integrate* cosmic pharmacology with the pharmacopeia, creating new discourses and textual genres. Ming readers came to learn pharmacy by the book, creating *textual communities* among themselves that no longer depended on the imperial court.[9]

Armed with this insight drawn from book history, we can revisit Li Shizhen's *Bencao gangmu* as a peculiar product of sixteenth-century book culture. On the one hand, Li Shizhen benefited from the widespread availability of bencao texts and other important sources in print. On the other hand, we should also see how unusual it was for Li Shizhen to presume that he could make a new pharmacopeia that, as we have seen, fell short as a political project in the early sixteenth century. In the end, it was not imperial patronage that made Li Shizhen's magnum opus a lasting success, but the demands of learned readers.

The Persistence of Pharmacopeias during the Song-Yuan-Ming Transition

Even prior to the advent of printing, the content of early bencao was transmitted widely in manuscript copies. The original Tang pharmacopeia housed at the court archive, however, consisted of multiple parts divided by different kinds of analysis: commentaries, local reports, and illustrations. The pictorial component was hardly seen beyond the capital city, whereas fragments of text traveled much more freely. Both Tao Hongjing's fifth-century commentaries and the Tang bencao circulated as far as Dunhuang and Turfan to the west, and Hei'an Japan to the east.[10]

Come the eleventh century, Song courtiers followed the Tang precedent to create a two-part pharmacopeia: an expanded commentary and a compilation of local reports (*tujing*, or "map guides"). Headed by separate teams, the two parts were completed within five years (1057–61) and were much longer compared to the Tang version. Although the court commissioned each part to be reproduced in woodblock print and distributed to local offices, they proved unwieldy to use. Local readers soon started to compile their own digests and commentaries based on the official pharmacopeia. For example, a physician named Chen Cheng (fl. 1086–1110) produced a composite bencao by combining relevant sections in each part of the official text, which eventually earned him a desirable post in the imperial medical administration.[11] Similarly, Kou Zongshi (fl. 1111–17), a minor official stationed in later-day Hunan, compiled his own commentary to "propagate the meanings" (*yanyi*) of the official pharmacopeia. He was later promoted to the "purveyor and inspector of materia medica" (*bianyan yaocai*) in the capital city, and his relatives promoted his bencao commentaries in print as well.[12] From these examples, we see how bencao became a field of common interest in which physicians and scholar-officials could freely converse, and accomplishment in bencao scholarship could lead to promotions in officialdom.

In the early 1100s, the local administrator of Hangzhou sponsored the printing of a new bencao manuscript. No one in Hangzhou knew anything about the author, Tang Shenwei, and yet they were impressed by his work, which not only combined the two-part official pharmacopeia but also included five hundred new entries of materia medica culled from a wide range of medical and literary sources. This 1108 print edition, known as the *Daguan bencao* after the current reign title, thus surpassed the Song official pharmacopeia in many ways. Ever enthusiastic about medical matters, Emperor Huizong ordered court physicians to quickly produce a new edition with official revisions. The result was rebranded as the *Zhenghe bencao* (the reign name when the new edition was released in 1116). Following its appearance, the two-part Song official pharmacopeia gradually ceased to circulate, and only in the twentieth century did scholars reconstruct each part for historical research.[13] In 1127, the Song regime fell to Jurchen attacks from the north, and one prince retreated to the south, consolidating his rule in Hangzhou. The resulting hostility and blockade between the Jurchen Jin dynasty and the Southern Song resulted in the unintended separation of two slightly different editions of Tang Shenwei's bencao.

In both south and north, new information emerged to shed light on Tang Shenwei's identity. A southern source revealed that Tang Shenwei was a physician living and practicing in West China, and that a military official had recruited him to live in Chengdu.[14] In the north, Yuwen Xuzhong (1079–1146), a veteran Song official imprisoned by the Jurchens as a state emissary, wrote a short epigraph to the *Zhenghe bencao* during his captivity. In it, Yuwen claimed to have witnessed Tang Shenwei treat his father with miraculous efficacy during Tang's stay in Chengdu. Describing Tang as a man "ugly in appearance and slow in demeanor and speech," Yuwen explained that he treated literati not for money, but instead asked for texts with medical content. In so doing, Yuwen hinted, Tang was able to gather enough secret recipes and rare texts to compile a bencao that surpassed the official pharmacopeia in erudition. In this story, Tang Shenwei became an idealized symbol in Yuwen's melancholy reminiscence of literary culture in Song times.[15]

Publishing records suggest that the north-south cultural rivalry during much of the twelfth and thirteenth centuries in fact perpetuated the authority of bencao pharmacopeias. In the south, soon after installing himself in Hangzhou, the Gaozong emperor (r. 1127–62) commissioned a new pharmacopeia. In a pattern foreshadowing the Liu Wentai controversy 350 years later, the Southern Song bencao was completed but never gained public endorsement due to the bickering between officials and the chief palace physician.[16] Palace physicians continued to refer to the Song pharmacopeia to recruit new personnel. In written examinations, candidates were asked to identify certain kinds of materia medica and construct formulas based on the properties of each ingredient as documented in the bencao. Interestingly, court physicians complained that most qualifying candidates for the exams hailed from the vicinity of the capital, indicating that the circulation of these elaborate texts probably did not go very far.[17] Instead, "vulgar imprints" (*suke*) of the pharmacopeia, often greatly truncated from its original length of over 1,600 pages, appeared in the growing publishing sectors in Southeast China. In response, civil officials felt compelled to fund additional editions to correct these imprints' errors, a pattern that we shall also see repeat in the late fifteenth and early sixteenth centuries.[18]

In the north, an important edition of *Zhenghe bencao* came out in 1249 in the Pingyang Prefecture, a center of literary culture and publishing in southern Shanxi (see map 0.1). The publisher, Zhang Cunhui, recruited skillful artisans to produce beautiful woodcut illustrations that accompanied the description of every drug, including three full-page illustrations of sea salt and rock salt yards (the latter native to that part of Shanxi). Two prominent literati officials wrote prefaces for the text, stating the centrality of bencao as a cultural asset, at a time when the Jin regime in turn had just been conquered by the Mongols.[19] The Chinese literati were, however, not the only advocates for bencao: in the last decades of Jin rule, a slightly altered version of Tang Shenwei's pharmacopeia appeared in the *Daoist Canon*, a monumental undertaking fueled by the widespread popularity of Quanzhen Daoism. Bencao remained thereafter part of the Daoist corpus, and many readers later got access to them via Daoist connections.[20]

To sum up, for 150 years of divided rule after the Northern Song's demise, the bencao pharmacopeia retained its appeal and prestige in both the north and south. The multitude of actors involved in saving, transmitting, and appropriating bencao crossed political divisions and religious creeds. After the Mongol conquest of the Southern Song, the Yuan dynasty briefly entertained the idea of a new bencao under the rule of Kublai Khan, but the resulting text, if it ever existed, is long lost.[21] Contingencies aside, the shift of attention away from pharmacopeia-making may also have had to do with changing priorities in medical learning.

The Rise of Cosmic Pharmacology

Monumental in scale and eclectic in content, the Tang and Song pharmacopeias were not intended for the average medical practitioner of the day. During the twelfth century, when the extensive pharmacopeias remained visible among elite literati circles, a new type of pharmacology rose to prominence via the writing and teaching of a few master physicians. The so-called Masters of Jin-Yuan made their fame by articulating not *what* individual drugs could cure, but also *why* they did so, and in what ways medical practices could be invigorated by a thorough understanding of pharmacology. Their success also depended on inventing new textual genres that proved extremely successful in an expanding culture of print.[22]

One product of this new pharmacology is a short text titled *Pearl Pouch and Rhymes on the Nature of Drugs* (*Zhenzhu nang yaoxing fu*), attributed to Zhang Yuansu (1151–1234). In contrast to the Song pharmacopeia's coverage of more than 1,700 drugs, *Pearl Pouch* selects only 200–300 common drugs, and divides them into four groups by their "nature" (*xing*) as cold, hot, warm, or "flat." Although such descriptions existed in the bencao tradition, the Tang and Song pharmacopeias did not offer a systematic explanation of these properties, nor did they classify drugs by their pharmacological action. *Pearl Pouch* is also very easy to read: Each drug gets a one-sentence description with no reference to previous literature, and every two sentences form a couplet that rhymes with the next pair. This text belongs to the rising genre of primers and mnemonic guides—a phenomenon linked to the ascendance of the civil service examination in popular culture at the time. Various renditions of *Pearl Pouch* would remain popular as an introductory text on pharmacology well into the early twentieth century.[23]

Another short text, attributed to Li Gao (1180–1251), articulates a more specific theory of cosmic pharmacology. A well-educated physician whose practice emphasized the use of warming tonics, Li witnessed the Mongol conquest of northern China and taught medicine that emphasized alleviating diseases caused by hunger and distress. The short treatise on pharmacology proposes seeing cold, hot, warm, and flat (cool) as not mere sensations of pharmacological action, but "regular images" (*faxiang*) of the four seasons, or different yin/ yang configurations of heaven (historian Ulrike Unschuld translated this theory as describing a kind of "thermogenic nature").[24] Similarly, the taste of drugs, also described in pharmacopeias but not systematized, became standardized in order to match the five phases that constituted the Earth. A coherent picture of the cosmos, combining heaven and Earth, thus encompassed endless combinations of those variables that in turn mapped on to different seasonal cycles and pharmacological actions. Employing this model, the master physician's diagnosis and prescription thus became a complex process of reasoning that took everything into account: time, location, the site of the disease, the patient's bodily constitution, and the nature of individual drugs (see table 1.1). In other words, to be a good physician was to read the hidden mechanisms of the macro- and microcosms like a diviner.

Historians have written at length about the innovative aspects of this new cosmic medicine and its long-lasting legacy.[25] Since Zhang Yuansu, Li Gao, and their disciples all lived in the north under Jin rule, their cosmic pharmacy came to be remembered as a northern phenomenon. Yet contemporary to Zhang's time, we also find Zhu Xi (1130–1200), a leading figure in Southern Song Confucianism, taking an active interest in the nature of drugs. In the recorded conversations between Zhu and his disciples (who were, in general, not training to practice medicine), Zhu Xi repeatedly brought up the topic of materia medica to make two claims important to his doctrine. First, despite their "withered and dried" (*kugao*) appearance, drugs were no inert matter, but obviously potent. In this sense, Zhu discussed the "nature" of aconite being hot (causing the sensation of heat) and that of rhubarb being "cold." This, argued Zhu Xi, proves that human beings possess the invisible, but nevertheless potent, capacity of moral judgment in their "Nature" (*xing*). Through the nature of drugs, Zhu pointed to the existence of a greater coherence (*li*) of the world.[26]

TABLE 1.1. Cosmic Pharmacology in Jin-Yuan Medicine

Yin/Yang dyad	Yin of Yang	Yang of Yang	[Neutral]	Yang of Yin	Yin of Yin
Primary *qi*	Warm	Hot		Cool	Cold
Five phases	Wood	Fire	Earth	Metal	Water
Primary taste	Sour	Bitter	Sweet	Pungent	Salty
Bodily viscera	Liver	Heart	Spleen	Lung	Kidney
Season	Spring	Summer	(Long Summer)	Autumn	Winter
Pathogenic factor	Wind	Heat	Humidity	Dryness	Cold
Cosmic action	Rising	Floating	Transforming	Descending	Sinking
Physiological stage	Birth	Growth	Maturation	Harvest	Storage
Representative drug	Ephedra (*mahuang*)	Aconite (*fuzi*)	Ginseng	Fungus (*fuling*)	Rhubarb
Pharmacological action	Astringent	Dehydrating	Tonic	Moistening; dissipating	Purgative

Source: Prepared based on Li Shizhen's summary in *Bencao gangmu.*

A second point derives from the first one in seemingly contradictory ways. While the nature of drugs could illuminate the moral nature of humanity, Zhu Xi sought to uphold a strict hierarchy between the high and the low, the grand and the minuscule. He dismissed the idea that one could know perfect truth from mere appearances—for example, by examining the dried herbs in a pharmacy. Zhu took great pains to explain that perfect coherence existed in this imperfect material world like a "bright pearl dropped into turbid water."[27] For Zhu Xi, materiality prevented the full manifestation of this coherence, and he was only interested in the nature of drugs insofar as it helped him prove that coherence was indeed invisible and omnipresent. In chapter 3, we will revisit this influential doctrine and its critics in the seventeenth century.

The important point here is that there existed a confluence of interest in cosmic medicine in both north and south, and that the new theories received endorsement by both physicians and Confucian literati. A synthetic treatise along these lines emerged in the late thirteenth century, titled *Tangye bencao* (*Materia medica for decoctions*) and authored by Wang Haogu (fl. 1264), a disciple of both Zhang Yuansu and Li Gao. Whereas Zhang and Li made no attempt to replace the bencao pharmacopeia with their own teachings, Wang felt confident to claim the "orthodox learning" (*zhengxue*) of the Divine Farmer in his own teachings. In his preface, Wang rejected the Tang and Song pharmacopeias' classification system that sorted objects by the order of minerals, plants, and animals, proposing instead to discuss the 200–300 common drugs according to their nature and sites of pharmacological action.[28] Printed collections of Zhang, Li, and Wang remained popular under Mongol rule, after the latter vanquished the Southern Song in 1279. Arguably, during no other period in Chinese history had there been a closer, or more mutually beneficial, interaction between Confucian literati and medical experts.

How, then, should we understand this moment of triumph for medicine during what historians have called the Song-Yuan-Ming period? The confluence of Confucian and medical learning seemed to be the dominant narrative of the day, so much so that Zhu Zhenheng (1281–1358), a later disciple of the Jin-Yuan masters, claimed that medicine was one and the same with the Confucian pursuit of moral truth through the "investigation of things" (*gezhi*).[29] A unique medical culture developed in South China under the Mongol rulers of the Yuan dynasty, where "medical households" (*yihu*), along with astrologers (known as *yinyang* experts), were recognized by their hereditary status in local administrations. The most successful practitioners attracted literati advocates, established long-standing family reputations, and even occupied key governmental positions by virtue of their art. Even though members of the medical households could not freely mingle and intermarry with literati families—being "not quite gentleman"—their borrowing of Confucian tropes and rituals in their own practices was not necessarily a sign of inferiority.[30]

When Zhu Yuanzhang founded the Ming dynasty after defeating the Mongols in 1368, he staffed the court with a robust presence of technical experts along with scholar-officials and continued the practice of hiring hereditary physicians to staff local medical academies (*yixue*) and philanthropic pharmacies in every county seat. My point here is that, up to the fifteenth century, medical practitioners still possessed solid control over their art, and their status as experts received recognition institutionally by the Yuan and early Ming states. Confucian philosophers looked up to medicine and other technical arts as sources of cosmic reasoning, which in turn left indelible marks on their own thinking.

Wang Lü (1332–?) represents an interesting polymath figure during this period. He composed excellent landscape paintings and reportedly studied medicine with the master physician Zhu Zhenheng. In his literary anthology, Wang made one off-handed remark about the foundational myth of bencao, in which the ancient sage-king Divine Farmer (*Shennong*) allegedly tasted one hundred herbs to tell good medicines from poison. Yet for Wang, it was inconceivable that a sage-king might have to put anything into his mouth in order to know its nature. He argued that the origin of bencao must instead be from divine intuitive knowledge about the workings of the cosmos (for Wang, the Eight Trigrams of the *Book of Changes*), and nothing else.[31] Here we see the compelling power of cosmic medicine that shaped the general epistemic discourses of the day. The rise of intuitive thinking as an essential conduit toward moral knowledge was modeled after the theoretical cosmic medicine of Jin-Yuan times and remained deeply mystical in its outlook. In chapter 3, we will return to see how the hostile attitude toward materiality and sensual knowledge began to give way to one more positive, which in turn impacted literati approaches to the field of bencao.

Decentering Prestige: The Bencao Pharmacopeia and Ming Official Publishing

This brief journey through several centuries now brings us back to the early 1500s, when the Hongzhi emperor took a passionate interest in medicine and commissioned Liu Wentai to revise the pharmacopeia. Since the founding of the dynasty, Ming palace physicians had enjoyed visibility at court, if not always respect. Quite a few of them gained enough prominence in public life that their biographies appeared in the dynastic history.[32] We can now better understand why Liu Wentai, when charged with the task of making a new pharmacopeia, would have wanted to make it concise and simple, for this was how the highest learning in medicine was supposed to be. Going through his medical apprenticeship in the mid-fifteenth century, Liu would have been familiar with the leading Jin-Yuan schools of cosmic pharmacology. In addition, he was also contemporary to an array of "summaries" and "crude commentaries" on the nature of drugs published by commercial printing houses in the southeast, quite independent of literati opinions.[33] These works may have inspired him to condense the pharmacopeia's verbose quotations and reorganize its content, making it more readable in general.

At the same time, however, Liu Wentai's political rivals also started to form their own opinions about bencao. For more than two centuries since the 1249 Pingyang edition, no major new edition of the Song pharmacopeia had been issued. The situation only changed in 1468, when a small number of high-ranking provincial officials of the Shandong Province sponsored a new edition of *Zhenglei bencao* at the Provincial Judge's office in Jinan (map 0.1). In their prefaces, they explained that a lone copy of the 1249 edition had emerged from the collection of a lower-ranking official in Shandong, who said that he had acquired it during a previous post in Pingyang. The printing process, which involved collating and proofreading the existing copy, as well as the carving of a total of 1,340 woodblocks, was completed on schedule under the supervision of several local administrators together with one "sojourning literatus." Graced by an invited preface from the grand secretariat Shang Lu (1414–86), the Shandong edition carries the air of magnanimity that distinguished it from the cheaper commercial imprints. The vivid illustrations and nicely carved blocks faithfully preserved many features of the 1249 edition (figure 1.1).[34]

With the Shandong edition, Tang Shenwei's bencao regained visibility and prestige on the Ming cultural scene, lending fresh luster to the mundane details recorded in the now three-hundred-year-old pharmacopeia. Newcomers to the provincial administration ordered numerous reprints and repair of woodblocks in the years 1523, 1552, 1572, and 1624. A provincial censor noted in his preface to the 1552 edition: "we simply cannot afford to sit here and let the book fall out of use."[35]

Throughout the sixteenth century, official publishing became a fashionable activity among officials who frequently traversed the empire, bringing

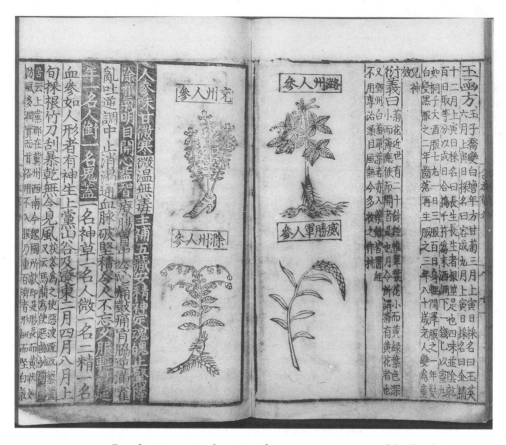

FIGURE 1.1. Page depicting regional varieties of ginseng, in a 1523 reprint of the Shandong edition of *Zhenglei bencao*. Courtesy of the Library of Congress.

newly printed books and handkerchiefs with them as elegant gifts.[36] Unlike the Song and Yuan periods, when local government academies owned land and used the revenue to publish books, Ming law deprived local officials of funding for that specific purpose. Even the publishing of local gazetteers (*difangzhi*) demanded that the magistrate or prefect raise funds on a case-by-case basis.[37] The reemergence of the bencao pharmacopeia in mid-Ming provincial administrations indicated that officials truly saw it as a prestige project that could boost their profile in the world of letters. Similar to the provincial officials, Ming princely households stationed in major provincial locations also actively participated in publishing new editions of different works, including the Song pharmacopeia. In his study of this unique phenomenon of Ming princely court culture, Craig Clunas remarked that each new edition reproduced carried "a local version of a universal virtue."[38] In one extraordinary case, Zhu Su (1361–1425), a Ming prince in central China, conducted pathbreaking work to create a new genre of bencao that focused only on edible plants useful in times of famine. Containing only 414 plants and as short as two *juan* (volumes), Zhu Su's text was remarkably devoid of medical interest. Here, we see an alternative vision for a de-medicalized bencao tailored for governmental purposes, an approach that would win greater sympathy in Qing times (see chapter 4).[39]

Taken together, provincial publishing by Ming officials and princely courts unwittingly moved the prestige of bencao pharmacopeias away from the imperial court down to the localities. The result was a remarkably scattered yet mutually connected landscape of knowledge transmission, in which one famous edition was often taken up and reproduced elsewhere. According to a mid-sixteenth-century survey of regional publishing, various editions of the Song pharmacopeia, in the form of carved woodblocks (over 1,300 blocks in each set), were known to exist in the Beijing and Nanjing Imperial Academies, as well as the provincial and prefectural offices in Nanjing, Shandong, Guangzhou, and as far as Guizhou.[40] Among these, the consecutive reprints of the Shandong edition commanded the most enduring impact. In 1581, *Fuchuntang* (Hall of Wealth and Springtime), a major player in the Nanjing book market, invested in an elaborate edition of the Song pharmacopeia, advertising "original Shandong blocks" (*Shandong yuanban*) with new features.[41] Still later in the seventeenth century, the prolific author Feng Menglong (1574–1646) used the Shandong connection in one of his short stories. The protagonist—an affable old man who obtained a divine panacea by sheer good luck, boasted about his medical learning to curious spectators. "Can't you see that the book of *Daguan bencao* in fact comes from Shandong, my home province?" says the man, in spite of his complete ignorance of medicine.[42]

The localization of bencao pharmacopeia can be seen from two interesting new editions of the Song bencao, both published in 1575. The first came from the Inner Court (*neifu*) in Beijing and was made by order of the twelve-year-old Wanli emperor, who had just ascended the throne three years prior. Solely a palace undertaking, the Wanli edition imitated the popular Shandong bencao, and the emperor's short preface showed no interest in inviting the participation of civil officials, nor did Wanli attempt to commission imperial physicians to improve and revise the book's content.[43] In other words, the imperial center in 1575 was merely reproducing another "local version of a universal virtue," rather than embodying and improving it.

During the same year, another unique edition of the Song pharmacopeia was completed in Nanling, a county located at the southern edge of the southern metropolitan region (*nanzhili*, see map 0.1). The production cost ran as high as three hundred *liang* of silver, a considerable sum at the time, when most local gazetteers—likely the most high-profile cultural projects in an average county office—rarely cost more than 100 liang to produce (figure 1.2).[44] What was remarkable in the Nanling edition was that it was not the local officials who funded the printing of bencao, but a wealthy commoner named Wang Qiu. Growing up a "man of the marketplace" (*fangshiren*), Wang left his name in local histories as a "forthright and wise man." His father had in the past donated grain for poor relief, and Wang Qiu similarly contributed to bridge repair and supported poor students who needed sustenance.[45] Although Wang Qiu himself lacked a good education, two of his sons passed the entry-level examinations and qualified as licentiates at the local academy, and they also participated in the preparation of the new bencao. The sponsoring of a new edition of bencao likely constituted another crucial step for the Wang family to accrue cultural capital with their wealth.

Modern scholars have noted multiple editorial errors in the Nanling edition of the Song pharmacopeia, such as the careless grafting of colophons from one previous edition to the main text of another.[46] Their critique revealed the lingering awareness of the status gap between the old elite and nouveau riche. Yet the Nanling edition clearly became a source of local pride at the time. In their preface, the Wang brothers praised their father's frugality, claiming that they had "no superfluous things at home." The virtue of the self-made "man of the marketplace" enabled him to pursue more edifying exploits, including making a bencao pharmacopeia that "had always been transmitted with official funds."[47] A few decades later, a local magistrate used the carved woodblocks to publish a new reprint, emphasizing that thanks to Wang Qiu's generosity, Nanling "finally has a bencao of our own."[48] Here the boundary between official and private publishing came to be blurred, enhancing the sense that the pharmacopeia could and should be accessible to anyone interested in public welfare.

Portable Treasures: Abridged Bencao and Commercial Publishing

The sheer quantity of new editions of bencao pharmacopeia produced during the sixteenth century offered unprecedented access to the text. As a result, a

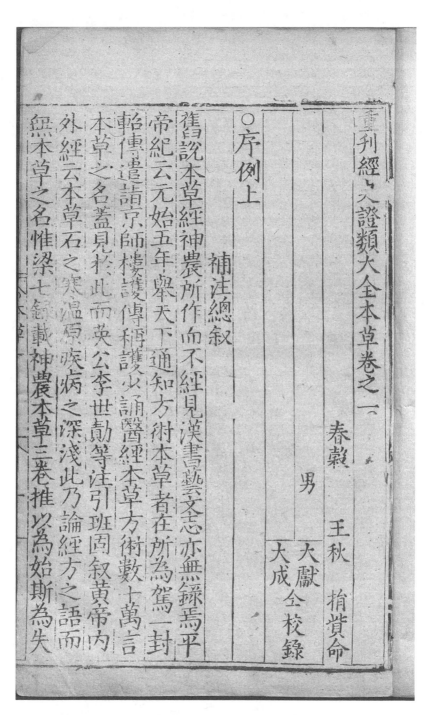

重刊經史證類大全本草卷之一

春穀

男　王秋　梢賞命

　　　大獻　　　　校錄
　　　　大成　仝校錄

○序例上

　　補注總叙

舊說本草經神農所作而不經見漢書藝文志亦無錄焉平
帝紀云元始五年舉天下通知方術本草者在所為駕一封
軺傳遣詣京師樓護傳稱護少誦醫經本草方術數十萬言
本草之名蓋見於此而英公李世勣等注引班固叙黄帝内
外經云本草石之寒温原疾病之深淺此乃論經方之語而
無本草之名惟梁七錄載神農本草三卷推以為始斯為失

FIGURE 1.2. Page with the Wang family's names, in the Nanling edition of
Zhenglei bencao (1577). Courtesy of the Library of Congress.

larger number of middle-range texts emerged that could bridge the gap between a primer text like *Rhymes* and a full-length pharmacopeia. Authors began to compose introductory pharmacy texts that were slightly more sophisticated in format, offering abridged versions of the Song pharmacopeia. Although such attempts had no doubt already started in the Tang and Song times, it was in the sixteenth century that more authors were attracted to publishing their study notes, with a clear goal of achieving personal fame through printed words.[49]

The first major abridged bencao to succeed in print circulation was *Bencao jiyao* (*Summaries of Materia Medica*), compiled by Wang Lun (*jinshi* 1484), a seasoned civil official with a family background in medicine. Picking a total of 545 drugs from the Song pharmacopeia and summarizing the long description into short verse, Wang Lun found a middle ground between the full bencao (~1,700) and popular primers (200–300). In his preface, Wang Lun justified his work by criticizing the "overly complex and repetitive" nature of the pharmacopeia, so much so that the reader could not help but yawn and feel drowsy. Yet he also spoke deferentially about the pharmacopeia's authority, exhorting any serious student who aspired to become a "professional expert" (*zhuanmen zhi shi*) to study "the whole book." Two more editions dated to 1510 and 1529 both enjoyed considerable success.[50]

Wang's work directly influenced at least two others who also composed abridged bencao in the sixteenth century. Both men, Wang Ji (1463–1539) and Chen Jiamo (fl. 1565), were successful physicians from Huizhou Prefecture, where medical practice and publishing flourished.[51] In fact, the lure of celebrity through print may well have given them the idea of expanding their medical practice into something much bigger. Chen Jiamo, in particular, noted how his students begged him to publish his private instructions and explicitly titled his book *Bencao mengquan* (*Instruments for Beginners in Materia Medica*). Chen rearranged the miscellaneous information in the pharmacopeia into pleasant and symmetrical couplets that were conducive to reading out aloud. Despite its considerable length (~20 volumes), the book is a breeze to read.

The abridged bencao quickly found their way into the expanding sector of commercial publishing during the long Wanli reign (1572–1620). Chen Jiamo's bencao, for example, was published by both the long-standing medical publishing houses in Fujian and newer establishments in Nanjing, the southern capital.[52] Also at this time, local gazetteers recorded physicians giving up their practices to focus on the "immortal enterprise" (*buxiu ye*) of authorship.[53] Shorter than the full pharmacopeia yet more elaborate than the Jin-Yuan primers, the abridged bencao offered an ideal genre with which prospective authors could appeal to both publishers and readers. The appeal of publishing success also resulted in plagiarism and, in certain cases, blatant fabrication of authorship in published texts. A short treatise titled *Bencao yueyan* (*Concise Discourse on Materia Medica*) emerged during this period and was attributed to Xue Ji (1487–1559), a highly successful physician who served in the Imperial Academy of Medicine and retired to Suzhou. Scholars now agree that Xue Ji himself could not have composed this abridged bencao.[54] Yet a preface written under Xue's name nevertheless spoke eloquently to the abridgement (*yue*) of bencao as a learned exercise:

> I was born in a later age. Fortunately, all secret texts have been uncovered from their depositories, so I was able to dwell there for many years. I kept compiling indispensable and frequently used drugs from *bencao*, grouped them into two categories [medicinal and dietetic], and classified them by their kinds, so that the account was concise. [In doing so] my book bindings wore out several times; my notes in red ink and corrections in yellow ink covered the whole page to the extent it became illegible.

The preface goes on to promise a pleasant reading experience:

> I thought of the Divine Farmer's profound offerings to the benefit of mankind, which is going to be the model for ten thousand generations. However, the complete book was so vast that one might never reach its end. As for this present volume, the path is short, the effort is easy, and the reader's mind will not be exhausted. At a glance, all the entries and details are presented clearly and in a comprehensive way. This is the kind of book that will enliven your room just by opening it.[55]

"On the desk or in the suitcase, readable and portable," *Concise Discourses* catered to the popular reader by offering an easy path into the "secret deposits of knowledge." The authenticity of authorship mattered less to late Ming readers than the open promise of acquiring useful knowledge without much effort. Perhaps the misfortune of the Hongzhi pharmacopeia lies not in the putative moral failings of its editor, but rather the exclusiveness of its format: as an exquisite manuscript, it could not compete with the impact made by the proliferating number of bencao texts coming in print from multiple loci of the Ming realm.

The rise of abridged bencao as a respectable and practical genre did not escape the attention of leading physicians of the day. In the 1570s, Xu Chunfu (1520–96), a high-ranking member of the Imperial Academy of Medicine and leader of an influential medical association (*yihui*) in Beijing, took to the printed word to spread authentic medical teaching. A long compendium that showcased Xu's erudition, *Complete Collection on Medical Orthodoxy in Ancient and Modern Times* (*Gujin yitong daquan*), received enthusiastic support for publication in Huizhou Prefecture. The subject of bencao, however, only appears quite late in the volume (the seventy-first of a hundred *juan*, or fascicles), and the content simply reproduced Wang Lun's abridged bencao. Elsewhere in the work, Xu indicates that the most important thing for a physician was the capacity to correctly diagnose diseases, and once that is achieved, accurate therapeutics would naturally follow.[56] Here, Xu borrowed Wang's text in a gesture of approval yet also sought to contain the abridged bencao under the structure of a "medical orthodoxy" (*yizong*). In chapter 3, we will see how this tension between amateur literati and orthodox physicians over pharmacological learning later broke into the open in the seventeenth century.

Dietetic Bencao, Master Thunder Texts, and Private Wealth

Another genre of bencao writing that received a great boost from late Ming book culture was dietetic treatises, or texts that focused on the medicinal properties of foods by selectively drawing from the all-encompassing pharmacopeia. Learned readers in Ming China knew that healing through diet had appeared in ancient ritual texts as a separate medical expertise, and that treatises on dietetic advice were incorporated into the Tang and Song pharmacopeias. Later, under Mongol rule, the Yuan court brought forth a fusion of Chinese and Central Asian dietary and medical traditions. Husihui (fl. 1330), a Muslim palace physician, compiled an extensive collection of culinary recipes with rich illustrations of the preparation of food at court. His work was reprinted during the Ming by the eunuch administration and remained popular.[57]

Also toward the end of Mongol rule (the early fourteenth century), Chinese literati in the south started excerpting useful tidbits of dietetic medicine from the Song pharmacopeia. The result (usually short, portable manuals of four to eight volumes) was transmitted under titles such as *Bencao for Everyday Use* (*Riyong bencao*). During the sixteenth century, multiple versions of dietetic bencao appeared in print with varying attributions to different authors (and adaptors), mostly scholar-officials who held office at the district or prefectural level but were not medical practitioners. Their writings catered to the rising demand for self-care techniques among the literati class at large, and urban publishers seized on this demand, producing more easily digestible texts, often with dubious claims to authorship.[58] In comparison to the abridged bencao texts discussed in the previous section, which at least still claimed to facilitate medical training, the "everyday" dietetic bencao more explicitly targeted amateur readers who could afford, or aspired to, a refined lifestyle.

Heightened elite interest in a technical subject, however amateurish it may have appeared at first, helped raise the perceived status of the subject matter. The preparation of foodstuffs is arguably never fully distinguishable from the hands-on preparation of materia medica, a domain controlled by experts well into the sixteenth century (more on this in chapter 4). It is thus quite remarkable that roughly between the 1580s and 1590s, commercial publishers in Fujian, Jiangxi, and Nanjing produced a series of bencao texts with an unprecedented focus on the processing of raw pharmaceutical substances. Distinct from the Jin-Yuan short primers and the midsized, abridged bencao, these texts covered a great number of substances (900–1,200 drugs, almost on the same scale of the full pharmacopeia) but managed to stay much shorter (8 volumes). Like other commercially published texts, these pharmaceutically oriented bencao had long and elaborate titles; here I refer to them as "Master Thunder" texts, after the common titular element that attributed the art of "roasting and preparation" (*paozhi*) to an early medieval tradition with an author surnamed Lei (meaning "thunder").[59]

So what did Master Thunder teach, and how did this tradition find its way into the bencao pharmacopeia? Scholars now agree that a treatise known as *Master Thunder's Discourse on Pharmaceuticals* (*Leigong paozhi lun*) can be dated to a fifth-century author (probably a Daoist adept) named Lei Xiao, whose work was in turn edited and glossed in the tenth century.[60] The main body of *Master Thunder* consisted of instructions on how to deploy (*shi*) about 300 common drugs. It has a preface attributed to Lei Xiao, presenting a dazzling display of sympathetic magic and miraculous cures: touch a tree with dried salmon and it will wither; sprinkling a dog's bile juice on the dying tree would make it bounce back to life. The bone powder of a male rat makes fallen teeth grow again; the juice of the *banxia* plant helps lepers retain their hair and eyebrows. In the late eleventh century, Tang Shenwei decided to incorporate it into his expanded bencao, and it remained there in the subsequent print editions.

It is beyond the scope of this study to inquire into the specific historical circumstances that enabled *Master Thunder*'s remarkable rise in the twelfth century. Yet we can find clues from the ways in which Song polymath scholars such as Shen Gua (1031–95) and later Hong Mai (1123–1202) cited it as credible evidence, which in turn suggests that cosmic resonance, along with its magical manifestations in various esoteric arts, deeply interested the learned literati.[61]

The formative stage of neo-Confucian thought was, in other words, built upon a deep-seated fascination with the occult and an optimism that unexplainable phenomena were fundamentally at one with the coherence (*li*) of the world.[62] Yet no Song authors attempted to elucidate *Master Thunder* on rational terms, content to let the text speak for itself. The late Ming resurgence of interest in *Master Thunder* coincided with unprecedented popularization of bencao texts, giving rise to a new discourse that highlighted the power of pharmacy.

Examined closely, the late Ming *Master Thunder* texts turn out to be an amalgam of excerpts from the Song pharmacopeia. Their scope is definitely wider than the commonly seen primer texts, for they did discuss many esoteric substances not relevant for everyday medical practice. At the same time, each entry is stripped down to the bare essentials, devoid of elaborate quotations or pictures. The most elaborate section in each describes the pharmaceutical processes that turn raw material into a processed form. In addition to copying from the pharmacopeia, these texts include simple, short rhymes that summarize important facts about each drug and were likely to have been newly composed. In some printed editions, the rhymes are featured prominently on the top panels of each page. In short, the authors and publishers of Master Thunder texts, most of whom hailed from humbler backgrounds than dietetic bencao authors, did not thoughtlessly graft material from previous texts, but they also deliberately used the occasion to promote their own teachings in popular pharmacy.

A recent discovery of a manuscript of one late sixteenth-century *Master Thunder* text sheds light on the complex question of readership at the time. The manuscript has a clear date of 1591 and, judging by its appearance and calligraphic style, closely resembles Liu Wentai's ill-fated early sixteenth-century bencao. Scholars have speculated that this manuscript was most likely the work of painters at court, who obtained a printed *Master Thunder* text released in 1587 and produced this richly illustrated copy, probably based on the Wanli emperor's demand.[63] Again, it is notable that no civil officials of the outer court was involved in the production, and the manuscript remained in palace collection till the twentieth century. Aside from the portrayal of over 900 materia medica, the manuscript also featured full-page depictions of the pharmaceutical processes taught by Master Thunder. The opening image depicts a gentleman wearing an elaborate purple and golden robe, who presides over an idealized workspace. Surrounded by nine artisans wielding various tools for cutting, rinsing, and preparing raw medicines, the master looks wise and at ease with himself (see figure 1.3).

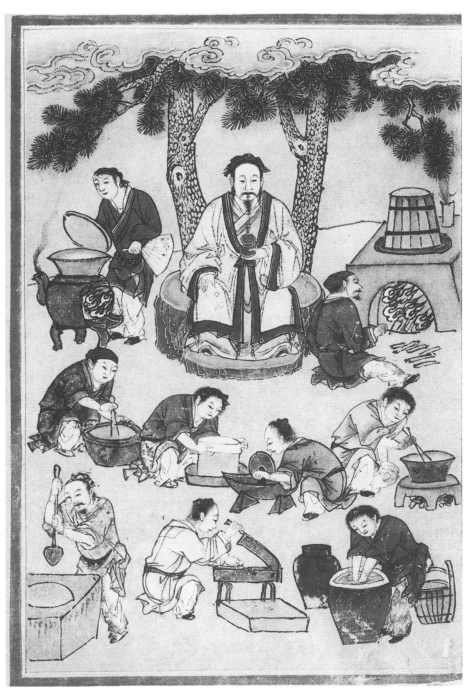

FIGURE 1.3. First page from Anon., *Buyi Leigong paozhi bianlan*.

More research is needed to elucidate the iconographic and narrative approaches employed in these elaborate images. Here again, the boundary between center and local, as well as between public and private, came to be blurred by virtue of a shared fascination with the pharmaceutical processes. Toward the last decades of the sixteenth century, commercially published *Master Thunder* texts almost started to overshadow the scholarly, stern face of the Song pharmacopeia, to the extent of inspiring imperial imitations.

Seen from an even broader perspective, the revival of *Master Thunder* texts in late Ming society was also part of an inclusive "nourishing life" culture, in which the old and new elite—including the Ming imperial family, aristocrats, elite literati, and the nouveau riche—all took an avid interest. By celebrating the transformative power of pharmaceutical processing, this body of texts praised artisanal labor as well as the godly patron of that work. Foregrounding the materiality of pharmaceutical processes, the pictures and texts call attention to the potency of matter and inventiveness of the human mind, with the promise to deliver men from all mundane worries. The archaic prose of the *Master Thunder* tradition intensified this promise by blending in the ecstatic language of Daoist alchemy. In the end, the *Master Thunder* texts deviated from the eclectic approach of the old bencao literature, substituting scholarly deliberation with rapturous promises of efficacy.

This is the lesson that Li Shizhen would learn in the 1580s and 1590s, as he searched repeatedly for patronage for a new pharmacopeia that he had compiled all by himself.

Publishing *Bencao gangmu*: Li Shizhen's Strategies

Li Shizhen (1518–93) was born the son of a physician living in the Qizhou Subprefecture of the Huguang Province, a mountainous town perched on the northern shore of the Yangzi River (map 0.1). Having received a classical education alongside medical training, Li had little luck in the civil examination but started earning his own reputation as a young physician. In his thirties, Li joined the court of Prince Chu and was put in charge of sacrifices at the prince's ancestral shrine. In 1566, Li Shizhen was recommended to serve in the Imperial Academy of Medicine in Beijing, where he stayed for several years before retiring to Qizhou. By that time, Li's own son Jianyuan had achieved more success in the civil examinations and gone off to Sichuan to serve as a county magistrate, raising the social status of his father as well. Back home, Li Shizhen was able to build a new residence with scenic views of a lake, where he socialized with local gentry and conversed about medical and literary matters.[64]

A secure life and local fame, however, did not make Li content. He harbored the greater goal of cementing his—and his father's—medical credentials by writing for a broader audience. In 1578, Li published his first two treatises on the method of pulse diagnosis, featuring a thorough explanation of the so-called irregular conduits (*qijing*) that were notoriously difficult to grasp in needling. One of his literati friends wrote a flattering preface, and the works were printed in his home province.[65] In addition to that, Li announced the completion of a new bencao that would replace the Song pharmacopeia—a grand compendium containing all known information about 1,892 drugs that he had spent twenty-seven years to prepare. In 1580, Li sailed downstream with the manuscript of *Bencao gangmu* and headed for Jiangnan. To publish it, he needed endorsement from someone beyond his provincial circles.

The purpose of Li's visit was to seek a meeting with Wang Shizhen (1526–90), a scholar-official in temporary retirement at his lavish estate in the Suzhou Prefecture. With his towering literary fame and widespread connections, Wang could make or break one's political or literary career, and, as a result, his residence teemed with visitors from near and far. In Wang's own recollection, Li, who was eight years his elder, stood out as slightly awkward and out of place. On the day the two met, Tanyangzi, a female cult-leader whom Wang worshiped as living disciple of the Bodhisattva Guanyin, had just ended her own life in a public spectacle where she "ascended to the heaven" in front of many illustrious witnesses, including Wang Shizhen, who wrote rapturous poems to mark the occasion.[66] His thoughts were still preoccupied when he dashed off another poem to honor Li Shizhen, in which he gently mocked the seriousness of the old man: Li was wrong to have spent such a long time composing the bencao. Had that not been the case, he could have ascended to the realm of immortals long ago.[67]

Li Shizhen's strategy of seeking leading literati endorsement was successful. Ten years after their first meeting, Li finally obtained a short preface from Wang upon a second visit, which may have nudged a minor publisher in Nanjing to invest in this new and expensive text. In 1593, Li Shizhen passed away at the age of seventy-six in Nanjing. His sons and grandsons saw to it that the first print edition of *Bencao gangmu* was completed in 1596. Soon after that, the Li family learned that the Ministry of Rites in the imperial capital was soliciting submissions of recent books that "offered a unique opinion" (*cheng yijia zhi yan*) on any subject matter, in preparation for compiling a general bibliography for the dynastic history. In late 1596, a son of Li Shizhen traveled to Beijing with the book, along with a posthumous memorial to the Ming emperor written in his father's name. The second attempt to acquire imperial patronage ended less well: the court only replied with a short note: "Keep the book for perusal; inform the Board of Rites." Three years later, a fire broke out in the Ming palaces and the historiographical office's book collecting came to a halt.[68] No evidence indicated that Li's bencao received the Wanli emperor's personal attention.

We thus have two very different general accounts of Li Shizhen and his bencao: Wang Shizhen's 1590 preface, as well as the posthumous memorial presented by the Li family to the throne in 1596. In his preface, Wang Shizhen praised Li's bencao in all seriousness, but also sought to downplay the medical relevance of the work. Instead, Wang singled out the erudition displayed in its pages as particularly useful for the Confucian pursuit of the knowledge of things (*wu*), nature (*xing*), and coherence (*li*). In addition, Wang displayed his special knack for words, churning out couplets loaded with marvelous allusions like strings of pearls. While the preface did reveal the existence of some "common intellectual commitment" between lay literati and men of medicine at the time, we must be careful not to overestimate the synergy and rapport between the two very different individuals.[69] It may be more accurate to say that Wang saw a treasure trove in Li's work, which illuminated the former's own fascination with the potency of matter, magic, and immortal transcendence. Posing as the all-powerful arbiter of culture, Wang never truly considered Li his equal, nor took his medical training very seriously.

The posthumous memorial to the throne presents an altogether different narrative of Li Shizhen and his bencao. It is quite likely that Li Shizhen personally drafted the main text of the memorial before he died, or at least played a major role in shaping the final wording of the text. In the memorial, Li presented a long and detailed account of the bencao pharmacopeia, describing it as a genre invested with authority and gravitas, a book that "governed the destiny" (*siming*) of the people. He also confessed that he felt some trepidation over "usurping the power of composition" (*jian zhushu zhi quan*), as he had undertaken the task as only a former minor official in a princely court. It is evident that, in Li's mind, he saw *Bencao gangmu* as a project of public good not necessarily congruent with literati culture. Interestingly, he seems to have misunderstood Tang Shenwei, the Song physician who also participated in pharmacopeia-making five centuries before him. Both were physicians practicing in places relatively remote from major cultural centers; both men achieved the extraordinary task of revising and expanding the official pharmacopeia without a formal role in government. Yet Li insisted that the Northern Song court had commissioned (*ming*) Tang Shenwei to work on the project. In the main text of his bencao, Li again asserted that Tang "presented his book to the court" (*shang zhi chaoting*). Perhaps Li hoped that by framing the history of bencao this way, the Ming court would also grant his pharmacopeia the canonical status that *Zhenglei bencao* had earned from the Song emperor.[70]

The most consistent feature of Li Shizhen as portrayed in the two accounts lies in his deep love of books. Wang Shizhen mocked Li's bookishness, and Li himself confessed to reading books "like craving sugar canes and candies." The two accounts converged on his avid pursuit of "immortality" (*buxiu*) through publishing and authorship. In the end, however, Li Shizhen achieved the fame he hoped for neither from the Wang Shizhen-endorsed Nanjing edition nor from the Ming throne. In 1603, Xia Liangxin (jinshi 1571), grand coordinator (*xunfu*, rank 2a) of the Jiangxi Province, obtained a copy of *Bencao gangmu*. Having served in the Shandong provincial administration, Xia was probably familiar with the official publishing of the Song pharmacopeia there. Citing his own personal health issues, Xia recommended the new bencao with enthusiasm, and soon raised enough funds from colleagues to create a brand-new edition in the provincial capital of Jiangxi. With the supervision of two lower-ranking officials, all carving and printing were completed in only six months (compared to more than three years of preparation for the first edition), and with a higher quality of craftsmanship.[71] The so-called Jiangxi edition was widely distributed, quickly inspiring Huguang, Li Shizhen's home province, to sponsor a similar edition.[72]

It is perhaps paradoxical that imperial China's last great pharmacopeia—a text that heroically aimed at centralizing knowledge—owed its success to the decentralizing cultural trends of the day. Li Shizhen dreamed of an unbroken bencao tradition upheld by imperial authority, under which men of letters collaborated seamlessly with medical experts. Yet this was not to be. Not only was the central government no longer in control of the production, transmission, and assessment of bencao texts, it also faced more vocal challenges over its disposal of material resources. In his preface to the Jiangxi edition of *Bencao gangmu*, the provincial official Xia Liangxin explained that at the heart of all bencao pharmacopeia lies a charitable purpose for the benefit of the people. The populist overtone fits well with Xia's previous record as an outspoken critic of the court's taxation policy and advocate for less centralized control over the local economy.[73] In the next chapter, we will see how pharmaceutical objects were featured in statecraft and scholar-official activism in the sixteenth century. The center will not hold in the control of both texts and material goods.

2

Converting Tribute

Heaven gives life to all kinds of things of uneven quality.
Those that can be used as tribute and tax, clothing and food,
medicinal ingredients, utensils, or toys for play,
such are all of benefit to humankind.
In so far as they are useful, they are knowable.

—*GAZETTEER OF LONGQING SUBPREFECTURE* (1545)[1]

CONSIDER THE ABOVE-QUOTED STATEMENT from a gazetteer of the Longqing Subprefecture, a frontier defense town separated from Beijing to its south by a mountain range, upon which stood the Great Wall. Longqing's jurisdiction consisted of ten administrative communities (*li*), a total of 440 tax-paying households forcibly relocated there in the early fifteenth century to substantiate (*shi*) a frontier defense against the Mongol raids. In 1475, a banished official compiled the first ever local gazetteer for Longqing.[2] Following this, Longqing produced a few successful candidates in the civil service examination who held office in the capital and provinces. One such retired honoree, Su Qian (jinshi 1502), was invited to revise the gazetteer in 1547 to commemorate the town's progress.[3]

Despite Longqing's perceived remote location, a sense of local pride shines through in Su's enumeration of local products (*wuchan*). Starting with grains and legumes (21 kinds), Su moved on to trees (23), garden vegetables (34), melons (6), fruits (15), flowers (20), medicine (44), birds (44), beasts (20), fish (8), and shell-bearing creatures (turtles, clams, and snails). Previously in a dynastic geographical survey, Longqing was only documented as having four local products, all quite homely: sorghum, grapes, hazelnut, and pepper (*di-jiao*).[4] The question is: How did Su Qian come up with the new list that re-flected quite a cornucopia of goods? And what does that tell us about the claim for knowledge in Ming localities?

Su Qian's own answer, of course, was that heaven brought forth all sorts of useful things to benefit humankind, and from that utility sprang the possibility of knowledge. The emphasis on utility, rather than the essence of things seen in isolation from human society, buttresses Chinese scholar-officials' overall approach to technical subjects in Ming China.[5] Yet the idea of utility did not exist in a political vacuum. Are certain things more useful than others? Useful by whose standards? When faced with the problem of scarcity, how does one go about distributing useful things in a just and justifiable manner? Writing as a seasoned bureaucrat in retirement, Su Qian placed the utility of tribute and tax (*gongfu*) on top of the everyday subsistence of the people. Medicine came next, followed by pleasurable things at the very end. In contrast to the bencao pharmacopeia, in which all items on Su's list would have been perceived as pharmaceutical objects, Su defined "medicine" narrowly.

There was a very specific reason for Su Qian's approach to local medicine: the first four kinds of medicine on his list were also designated as Longqing's only local tribute (*tugong*) items to be presented to the imperial court. In the gazetteer's register for taxes, Su listed these "*materia medica* procured annu-ally" (*suiban yaocai*) as follows:

> Licorice (*gancao*): 300 *jin* (approximately 180 kilograms)
> Baical skullcap (*huangqin*): 300 *jin*
> Atractylodes (*cangshu*): 200 *jin*
> Peony (*shaoyao*): 200 *jin*[6]

Locals complained of the hassle (*fanrao*) of procuring such a large quantity of medicinal herbs and dispatching them to the Imperial Academy of Medicine in Beijing. Happily, noted Su, the current magistrate, Liu Yunhong, had since the year Jiajing 27 (1547) come up with an excellent solution to this problem. Gathering the heads of households to deliberate over the matter, Liu proposed to purchase the tribute medicine by introducing a slight surcharge on land tax: distributing the burden evenly across the communities, a half *jin* of medicine, or 0.025 liang of silver, would be added to every fifty *mu* of land. The taxpayers considered it to be a convenient arrangement.[7]

Longqing's self-imposed conversion of 1,000 jin (the equivalent of 605 kilo-grams; see appendix) worth of tribute medicine in Longqing into silver is eminently recognizable as one episode in the broad trend of fiscal reform and social change in mid-Ming China. The so-called Single Whip Law (*yitiaobian fa*) promoted by Grand Secretariat Zhang Juzheng (1525–82) in the early 1570s resulted in the designation of silver as the primary means of fiscal transaction. Ming China's gravitation toward the malleable currency of silver, whose supply became greatly amplified by newly opened mines in the Spanish colonies of America and elsewhere, has been recognized as an event of world historical significance, integrating East Asia into the nascent early modern global trade.[8] Culturally, the infusion of monetized transactions permeated all walks of life and transformed dominant values of the day, inviting much commentary (and lament) from contemporary observers and historians.[9] The ascent of money, in other words, fundamentally shaped the fate of the Ming dynasty and the outlook of Chinese society from then on.

The risk of this familiar narrative lies in our tendency to treat fiscal monetization—and, by corollary, the rise of a proto-capitalist economy—as an inevitable outcome. When money was used to explain historical change on a grand scale, the concrete processes and discourses that justified tax conversion in the first place became emptied of local meaning. The richness of social historical research has provided much insight on the processes of Ming fiscal reform from the local perspective. The offices of the magistrates and prefects were not merely conduits for central commands, but active sites of political negotiation and loci of policy change. The monetization of corvée labor, for instance, reflected the challenge of governance posed by the changing social fabric since the dynasty's foundation in late fourteenth century.[10]

Building on this rich literature, which largely focused on social relations and productivity measured by grain, cloth, and labor, I suggest that it may shed new light on a familiar aspect of Ming history by examining the monetization of tribute medicine. Once we shift our attention to the material specificity of objects, we discover that Ming actors almost always thought through and documented fiscal reform in very concrete terms. Gazetteers of Ming times, such as that of Longqing, were replete with discussions about objects of value: where they were found, how much they were worth, and the specific manners of their deployment in public affairs. Instead of an abstract preference for money, the debates were driven by inherently ethical concerns—and political negotiations—over the distribution of material wealth in official versus non-official domains. The ways in which local administrators came to terms with material resources show more complexity than the straightforward account of fiscal reform offered in dynastic histories. As the case of Longqing indicated, the push for monetization sometimes originated from the bottom up, starting with the county, subprefectural, or prefectural levels before becoming an acceptable practice in provincial and capital offices.

Aside from the concrete processes that led to the ascent of money, a larger question of knowledge is also at stake here: If the Longqing officials, in their strenuous attempts toward better governance, took to buying tribute materia medica and distributing the cost among landowners, to what extent can we still trust Su Qian's claim that these medicines were indeed growing there? The epistemic significance triggered by fiscal reform was not lost on Ming officials, and in fact the politically charged land surveys in Ming gazetteers amounted to nothing short of a reassessment of previous knowledge, including, primary to our interest here, the territorial claims from the Tang-Song pharmacopeias. The proper sourcing of materia medica became one of the favored talking points as Ming actors negotiated between state expenditure and local welfare. We shall see that when deference toward earlier authorities diminished over the course of the sixteenth century, the local elite mobilized other sorts of evidence to buttress their own knowledge claims—and by doing so, they had policy claims in mind. This broadened repertoire of their evidence included references to the mercantile sector and practitioners of folk medicine, amounting essentially to a reconfiguration of local (*tu*) knowledge. In other words, the locals were not only passively impacted by the ascent of money but also played an active role in facilitating it. This process is important to understand before we move on to examine the rapid transformations of pharmacy in the seventeenth century.

Geographies of Materia Medica as Local Tribute in Tang-Song Records

As I have discussed in the introduction, the Tang and Song pharmacopeias internalized the State's administrative geography in their description of drugs as local products. The ability to conduct surveys of the land, in a way, defines the imperial center vis-à-vis the local. The Tang-Song bencao both included a part known as *tujing*, often translated as "map guides" or "illustrated classics," that were essentially compiled reports sent in from local administrations. The rise of tujing as a historiographical genre could be dated to the early medieval period, when regional kingdoms divided their rule over China, and regional regimes maintained a "symbiotic relationship," in Andrew Chittick's words, between asserting local identity and universal literary ideals in their "map guides." Later under the unified Sui (581–618) and Tang (618–907), the imperial court mandated the regular compilation of tujing every three years and archived them as a means of gathering intelligence about its territories.[11] This practice became the immediate context against which courtiers adopted a similar practice to compile the pharmacopeias.

The power of tujing, however, resides beyond the gathering of information; it also concerns the centralized collection of objects unique to the locality. The tradition of geographical writings up to this period attributed their origin to the celebrated deeds of King Yu, the ancient sage-king who, according to records preserved in *Shang Shu* (*Book of Documents*, one of the Confucian classics), "having defined the Nine Lands ... followed the mountains to dredge the rivers, and designated tribute items according to the land."[12] The idea of tribute (*gong*) thus embodied the archetype of knowledge in governance: to know a local product as a ruler is to possess the right to obtain it as tribute. In this book, I refer to this doctrine as the "Principle of Yugong" (tribute of Yu).

The great historian Du You (735–812), in his study of Tang institutions, provided a list of regular tribute items dispatched from "all prefectures under heaven" (*tianxia zhujun*) every year, including more than eighty kinds of materia medica.[13] Three hundred years later, the Northern Song court largely continued the Tang practice of collecting the same items from the same local offices. In both Tang and Song documents, materia medica constituted one of the largest categories of local tribute items collected from prefectures, alongside a variety of specialty textiles, fruits, tea, precious stones, dyes, fur, ivory, mirrors, and so on. If we map the distribution of tribute medicine according to the Song source, however, it becomes apparent that most resources collected by the State came from north of the Yangzi River. The few tribute medicines from the south were aggregated along the axis that extended from the mid-Yangzi region southward to Hainan Island, with the remaining items spread sparsely on the southeastern coast (map 2.1).[14] In sum, the knowledge of local product reflects rather the Tang-Song state's relative extent of control over the territories. Later in this chapter, we will see that the Ming state followed a completely different pattern in procuring its own tribute medicine.

It suffices to say that the Principle of Yugong rarely reflected a perfect match between knowledge and actual fiscal policy. The list of tribute medicine only accounted for up to five to ten percent of the materia medica documented by the Tang bencao. The much richer knowledge about pharmaceuticals likely came from the contributions by master physicians involved in the compilation process. That being said, Sun Simiao (c. 581–682), a master physician whose

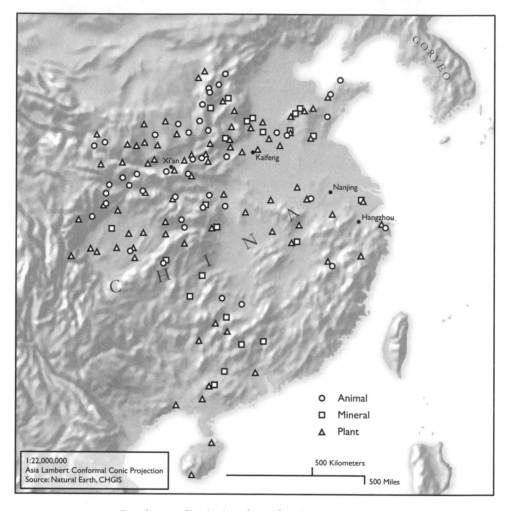

MAP 2.1. Distribution of local tribute (*tugong*) medicine in the eleventh century

skills received the patronage of the Tang rulers, embraced the court's introduction of administrative geography in his own writings about materia medica. In one of his most celebrated medical treatises, Sun discussed the general principle of "materia medica coming out of specific prefectural lands" (*yao chu zhoutu*), providing a detailed list of 519 medicinal substances found in 113 prefectures. Praising the divine (*sheng*) Tang dynasty's unprecedented territorial extent, Sun admonished medical practitioners not to serve incorrectly sourced drugs to patients.[15] The phrase "prefectural land" (*zhoutu*), as a marker of place-based authenticity, kept appearing in Tang-Song medical formulas, indicating that practitioners were, to some extent, educated by the Tang pharmacopeia to trace medicinal ingredients to their designated localities.[16]

Notwithstanding the apparent discrepancies in territorial knowledge, both the Tang-Song pharmacopeia and the designation of tribute remained sources of universal authority. If, in an age of unified imperial rule, the character of a locality became reduced to the content of texts found in the central archive, then the slightest misreading of such a text could have disastrous consequences. A late Tang anecdote made fun of a courtier's misreading of a line in poetry (picking *Pollia* flowers from a "fragrant island" [*fangzhou*]) in enacting tribute policy (let the *Fangzhou* Prefecture present *Pollia* flowers as tribute).[17] A light joke told among courtiers conceals the gravity of the matter for the locality.

We can still see the persistence of such deference to universal authority even after the Song retreated to the south following the mid-thirteenth century. At that time, the writing of "map guides" took on a strong localist turn, giving rise later to the mature genre of local gazetteers in Ming-Qing times. A gazetteer of Lin'an, the capital city of the Southern Song, boasted a long list of local products (*wuchan*), including seventy-three kinds of materia medica. Among them, five kinds were listed first because "the bencao says that they existed in Hangzhou [*Lin'an*]." Three additional drugs not documented by the bencao, however, were acknowledged as regular or previous tribute items. The remaining sixty-five were documented with further details such as the precise sites of production: in neighborhoods of Lin'an, its subordinate counties, or a specific valley.[18] All layers of information are stacked together without apparent conflict: This eclectic approach to different sources preserved what historian Lin Fan has called the "local in the imperial vision."[19] We shall see how this attitude became more antagonistic a few centuries later.

One last observation from the Tang-Song sources is in order here. Du You, reviewing court orders concerning local tribute, pointed out that each year the value of tribute items presented from each prefecture was not to exceed the equivalent of fifty bolts of silk. As a rule, the quantity of tribute was kept meager (*bo*) and the process of procurement carried out with ease. Furthermore, tribute goods now in official (*guan*) possession could be traded on the open marketplace to replenish state revenue.[20] The State's claim to territorial knowledge, and hence materia medica of superior quality, is here entangled with its privileged status in the sphere of commerce. The Song state was especially proactive in utilizing its access to tribute items, such as materia medica, to aid in governmental enterprises, such as charitable pharmacies operated by officially appointed personnel.[21] In chapter 5, we will return to examine how a widening gap began to develop between the geography of administration and the geography of commerce, and the impact of this division on the territorial formation of knowledge.

Medicine as "Material Resource" in Ming Fiscal Records

Before delving into the specific knowledge claims made in Ming local gazetteers, we need to ask how the nature of tribute medicine rapidly changed under the first two centuries of Ming rule. In the sections that follow, I sketch out the changing demand of the Ming state for materia medica and the evolution of tribute medicine as an institution.

The most comprehensive account of tribute medicine can be found in the revised edition of *Collected Statutes of the Ming*, itself the result of intense impetus for policy change in the early Wanli reign (1570–80). Publicly promulgated in 1587, the *Collected Statutes* described the composition and function of governmental offices spanning the inner and outer courts. In so doing, the 1587 *Collected Statues* also offered a historical perspective on policy change by outlining relevant laws and regulations issued since the beginning of the dynasty. The section on materia medica appeared toward the very end, where the office of the Imperial Academy of Medicine (*Taiyiyuan*) was discussed. Early on in the dynasty, a "raw medicine storage" (*shengyaoku*) was built to deposit materia medica "dispatched and submitted (*jiena*) from all under heaven." The storage facility kept an inventory of its holdings, to be updated annually under the joint supervision of the Academy and the Ministry of Rites (*Libu*)—one of the six major ministries that constituted the major organs of the outer court. The Ministry of Rites was also in charge of the Academy's personnel decisions, including running a written examination based on the medical classics. The best personnel could qualify to be on duty at the imperial pharmacy (*Yuyao-fang*), which was, in turn, created in Jiajing 15 (1536) by the eunuch administration for the storage of "tribute medicine from the four directions."[22] The *Collected Statutes* was reticent about how this duplication of storage space may have impacted oversight. In any case, the compilers were likely only to have had access to the inventory of the outer court storage via the Ministry of Rites. The competition between the inner and outer courts to control tribute medicine as material resources mirrored the strife among civil officials and court physicians throughout the sixteenth century.

What follows is a succinct account of how the Ming state procured materia medica from "the places where they were produced" (*chuchan difang*): 55,474 jin (roughly 33,000 kilograms, or over 33 tons) by the end of the Yongle reign (1402–24); 264,227 jin at the beginning of the Jiajing reign (1522–66). By 1587, the total amount of tribute medicine had been slightly reduced to 249,581 jin (see table 2.1). An entry in the *Veritable Records,* which documented major items of the agenda discussed between the emperor and chief officials, confirmed that in the year Zhengtong 1 (1436), the Minister of Rites proposed to cut the amount of materia medica collected by the Imperial Academy of Medicine from 98,100 jin to 55,400 jin, an amount on par with the *Collected Statutes.* Apparently, the palace physicians were not the only ones impacted by the across-the-board cutting of expenses: the Bureau of Astronomy (*Qintianjian*) also received a cut in calendar paper (*liri zhizhang*)—produced locally and dispatched to the Bureau—from 509,700 to 119,500 books.[23] In addition to the staggering demand from the Beijing offices, there were the needs of a second set of offices in Nanjing, the southern capital. Although it did not regularly serve the emperor, the Nanjing Imperial Academy of Medicine operated its own storage for "raw medicines" dispatched to the Nanjing Ministry of Rites, totaling 7,244 jin each year.[24] It appears that despite the rigorous campaigns to save costs, the Ming state demanded and consumed a lot more goods than its Tang-Song predecessors, when the amount of all tribute medicine did not exceed a few thousand jin.

What can we make of the over 250,000 jin (~150 tons) of materia medica that the Ming state claimed to procure each year? First of all, the designated quota was likely to not have been regularly fulfilled, as testified by the court's frequent commutation of overdue shipments. Second, despite an insistence that those materia medica came from "where they were produced," the terminology for procurement shifted from the "meager and easy" local tribute in Tang sources to a more aggressive tone: the State "annually procures" (*suiban*) medicine by "designating" (*pai*) a fixed "quota" (*e*) on local administrations. Last, the distribution of tribute medicine showed a disproportionate reliance on the so-called metropolitan areas (*zhili*), especially in the south.[25] The disproportionate burden on the south was a great departure from Tang-Song precedents, when the north shouldered the lion's share of tribute items (compare with map 2.1).[26]

The diversity of the tax base in early Ming times has been subject to much scholarly discussion. The basic logic of outsourcing a diverse range of productive tasks to the local populace assumes superior knowledge and management

TABLE 2.1. Tribute Medicine in Ming Provinces and Metropolitan Prefectures, 1587

Administration	General materia medica (jin)	Specialty items
Zhejiang	Purple aster (ziyuan) etc., 31,610	Gold foil, 908 sheets Silver foil, 72 sheets
Jiangxi	Aromatic madder (xiangru) etc., 6,142	
Huguang	Fritillary (beimu) etc., 2,738	White flower snake, 9 Black snake, 10 Cinnabar and musk, 104 jin
Fujian	Indigo powder etc., 2,764	Tabasheer (tianzhuhuang), 5 jin
Sichuan	Aconite etc., 14,502	Large aconite, 4 pairs Musk and rhinoceros horn, 9 jin Amber, 20 liang
Guangdong	Patchouli (huoxiang), etc., 5,771	Red lizard, 17 pairs Refined camphor, 30 liang Aloewood etc., 235 jin
Guangxi	Tropical basil (linglingxiang) etc., 3,821	Refined camphor, 30 liang; Bushy sophora root (shandougen) etc., 240 jin
Shanxi		Musk, 10 jin
Shandong	Atractylodes lancea (cangzhu) etc., 8,830	Atractylodes lancea, 22,480 jin
Henan	Gastrodia seed (tianmazi) etc., 8,404	
Shaanxi	Chinese clematis (weilingxian) etc., 8,492	
Liaodong	Bugbane (shengma) etc., 10,312	Realgar etc., 503 jin
	Ginseng etc., 800	
Southern metropolitan area		
Yingtian Prefecture	Raw Corydalis (yanhusuo) etc., 5,859	Atractylodes lancea, 39,690 jin
Zhenjiang Prefecture	Pinellia ternata (banxia), 3,726	Centipede, 45
Suzhou Prefecture	Lygodium (climbing fern) etc., 9,744	Gold foil, 1,000 sheets
Songjiang Prefecture	Shiso, 1,170	

Huizhou Prefecture	Fuling etc., 950	
Ningguo Prefecture	Pinellia ternata (*banxia*) etc., 9,987	Termite-infected wood, 20 pieces
Taiping Prefecture	Elm bark etc., 282	
Chizhou Prefecture	Aralia cordata (*duhuo*) etc., 585	
Fengyang Prefecture	Bupleuri Radix (*chaihu*) etc., 1,777	
Yangzhou Prefecture	Pinellia ternata (*banxia*) etc., 660	
Huai'an Prefecture	Bupleuri Radix (*chaihu*) etc., 3,128	Atractylodes lancea, 24,331 jin
Luzhou Prefecture	Candy drops etc., 86	
Anqing Prefecture	White chalk etc., 459	
Guangde Subprefecture	Fuling, 630	
Chuzhou Subprefecture	Platycodon (*jiegeng*) etc., 1,599	
Xuzhou Subprefecture	Deer velvet etc., 83	
Hezhou Subprefecture	Bupleuri Radix (*chaihu*) etc., 223	
Northern metropolitan area		
Shuntian Prefecture	Dried chrysanthemum etc., 1,946	Atractylodes lancea, 8,594 jin
Daming Prefecture	Honey locust fruit etc., 1,500	
Hejian Prefecture	Hemp seed etc., 2,180	
Baoding Prefecture	Honey locust fruit, 500	
Zhending Prefecture	Honey locust fruit etc., 765	
Yanqing Subprefecture	Skullcap root (*huangqin*) etc., 700	
Bao'an Subprefecture	Skullcap root (*huangqin*) etc., 700	
Total	249,581 (~150,000 kg)	

Source: MHD, 224:2968–71.

Note: Numbers are rounded to the closest integral.

capacity on the part of the government. If, in the ideal scenario, the people in each locality worked industriously to produce a surplus of their renowned local products, the state could rely on their voluntary contribution to get bricks to build city walls and timber to construct palace halls, as well as clothes, shoes, and weaponry to equip its soldiers. Medicine, calendar paper, and wax for candles were requested for the upkeep of the court retinue and governmental offices. The diverse tax base of grains, labor, textile, and material resources enabled the Ming to accomplish extraordinary feats, such as the construction of two capital cities (Nanjing and Beijing) and the building of ships deployed in Zheng He's naval expeditions in the early fifteenth century.[27] The language of "procurement under designated quota" (e'ban) and "ad hoc procurement" (zuoban/paiban) also derived from the first century of Ming rule.

Yet we still need to explain the five-fold increase in procured materia medica between the early 1400s and 1500s, as documented by the *Collected Statutes*. How did the burden become so much heavier? Looking back from the early eighteenth century, the *Ming History* compilers attempted to explain the downfall of the Ming dynasty by dissecting its fiscal woes. Official historians pointed their fingers primarily at the eunuch-run inner court: in the name of bestowing gifts or the maintenance of palace halls, "a piece of paper comes out of the palace in the middle of the night," and no one dared to defy the urgent order.[28] The historians painted an image of the eunuch-run inner court as arbitrary, greedy, and totally out of touch with the welfare of the country. Here again, we hear echoes of the antagonism between civil officials and inner court personnel that I discussed at the beginning of chapter 1.

Is this the only possible cause of the steep rise in the amount of tribute medicine in Ming China? I suggest otherwise. The momentum toward collecting so much medicine as material resources (wuliao) came not directly from emperors or the eunuchs who acted as imperial agents, but rather from the crushing momentum of a bureaucratic government running on paperwork and numbers. Aside from the Ministry of Revenue (hubu)—which oversaw the revenue of grain, textile, and paper money—the Ministries of Works (gongbu), Military (bingbu), and Rites (libu) also jealously guarded their own revenue in all diverse forms, ranging from manufactured goods and weaponry to fattened pigs for ritual sacrifice. The *Veritable Records* recorded numerous occasions when emperors attempted to cut tax and overrule the ministries.[29] Local magistrates could also directly petition the throne for tax relief in defiance of their superiors. The issue of materia medica was highlighted in such a case in 1433, when a local magistrate accused the Ministry of Rites of extorting (zheng-

suo) materia medica from his jurisdiction, where the medicinal plant in question was, according to this magistrate, no longer produced. The magistrate's argument, based on grounds of false information, apparently convinced the Xuande emperor to reallocate the collection of medicine elsewhere.[30] We do not know, of course, whether the medicinal plant in question truly ceased to grow in one locality but not another. The important point is that local officials frequently protested erroneously assigned tribute items and that Ming emperors did sometimes heed their complaints.

One more exigency particular to the late fifteenth century lies in the heightened sense of urgency with regard to border defense. The capture of Zhu Qizhen, the Zhengtong emperor, by Oirat Mongols in 1449, as well as his subsequent release and restoration to the throne, is a familiar episode in Ming history. The gravity of Mongol threat, as a result, inadvertently encouraged ministries to raise their designated quota for material resources in the name of military spending. Aside from items such as horn, fish glue, wood, metal, and string—all essential materials for the making of good bows and arrows—the localities were also asked to supply more overcoats, helmets, and shoes for soldiers. The Ministry of Rites may also have used the opportunity to send for more supply of materia medica under the rubric of "military expense" (*junxu*)—a term that appeared more frequently in late fifteenth-century local gazetteers than the older category of "tribute" (*gong*).[31] The conflation of categories indicated that in practice, bureaucratic actors had little trouble coming up with legitimate excuses for maximizing gains for their agency or themselves.

During the Hongzhi reign (1487–1505), we begin to see more open accusations of the abuse of tribute medicine in official sources. A leading minister of war reported astonishing waste as large quantities of materia medica languished in government storage.[32] Censors accused the director of the Bureau of Astronomy of selling off extra calendar paper for private gains and the chief physician of the Imperial Academy of Medicine of accepting precious medicine as a bribe.[33] In 1488, a censor revealed an astonishing case, in which none other than the long-time Minister of Rites himself permitted family members to embezzle large amounts of tribute medicine for private gains.[34] The surging criticism at the turn of the sixteenth century reflected prevalent discontent in reaction to the steep rises in the amounts of material resources siphoned off from all provinces to the Ming's two capitals. The public outcry resulted in major intellectual reflections on the legitimacy of local tribute itself, giving rise to reformulations of justice in fiscal policy by major Confucian thinkers.

The Wealth of the Nation

The monetization of local tribute items, including miscellaneous materia medica, first appeared as a major national policy proposal in the late Hongzhi reign. In 1503, an outspoken censor named Dai Xian (jinshi 1496) presented a long memorial to the throne with the lofty title *Outline and Details on the Preservation of Good Governance (Baozhi gangmu)*. In it, Dai offered six major governmental reforms and listed eighteen specific measures to be carried out. One item under reform number five argues that making local tribute expedient (*bian*) would be a profitable move. "Today's military expense is an institution coming from local tribute in ancient times," Dai declared. The problem lay in the mismatch between policy and territorial reality: "numerous kinds of dye and *materia medica*" were, in fact, not "local products" (*tuchan*) of places responsible for offering them. Instead of burdening the local people with the thankless task of buying what they did not have, Dai recommended a two-step solution: first, to order a thorough survey of local products throughout the realm; second, to convert the nonlocal products into cash of equivalent value, with which central offices could then purchase the medicine from the capitals. Asked by the emperor to deliberate on Dai's proposal, the Ministry of Revenue replied with approval.[35]

As fate would have it, Dai Xian's proposal for converting tribute medicine took place in the same year when the Hongzhi emperor commissioned a new pharmacopeia from court physician Liu Wentai. Despite their unwillingness to work with Liu, senior officials overseeing the outer court at the time were, in fact, deeply concerned with pharmacy from a completely different perspective. After Hongzhi's sudden passing two years later, his heir, Emperor Zhengde, sided with his eunuch advisor to remove the incumbent grand secretariats from office. Dai Xian and a small clique of die-hard censors protested, and the emperor promptly punished them by public beating in front of their colleagues. Dai died shortly afterward from wounds caused by the beating, and a still greater number of officials were demoted for voicing support of him.[36] One of the sympathizers was a minor official named Wang Shouren (1472–1529), who was dismissed from office and sent into exile in Guizhou. The exile offered Wang, better known as Wang Yangming, a moment of enlightenment through ordeal. Upon his triumphant return to court several years later, Wang's doctrines for achieving good conscience through introspection (*zhi liangzhi*) would inspire countless aspiring "philosophers of the mind." In chapter 3, we will see how this branch of neo-Confucian teachings motivated a major turning point in the study of bencao in the early 1600s. It suffices here to note that during the early decades of the sixteenth century, factional politics at court galvanized more general discussion over controversial policy issues beyond the court, and that tribute medicine became one of the most visible topics of the day.

Reform-minded scholar-officials in Ming times could turn to a rich intellectual tradition that touched precisely on the issue of local tribute. Since the *Yugong* principle of "designating tribute in accordance with the land" was originally derived from the recorded deeds of the ancient sage-king Yu in *Book of Documents* (*Shangshu*), neo-Confucians from the twelfth century onward sought to engage with the ancient classic through new commentaries. Cai Chen (1167–1230), a disciple of Zhu Xi and foremost *Shangshu* scholar of the day, sought to redefine the meaning of tribute (*gong*) as distinct from tax (*fu*): "Tax is what one takes from above; tribute is what one presents from below."[37]

By emphasizing the *voluntary* nature of local tribute, Cai warned that the State should not overlook the will of the people. This reading also implies a categorical divide between agrarian products (grains and cloth) that are uniform in kind and quantifiable, and the diverse, territorially specific tribute items. To define the latter as *presents* from the people to the ruler—and therefore granting the former agency in choosing what, and how much, such *presents* constituted—Cai left open a potential challenge to King Yu's authority to "enact" (*zuo*) tribute based on his privileged knowledge of the land.

Cai Chen's commentary found echoes in the work of another great institutional historian, Ma Duanlin (1245–1322), who dedicated an entire chapter to the issue of local tribute in his comprehensive survey of dynastic institutions from ancient times to the Song. The chapter's main text consisted of a list of historical episodes in which virtuous rulers abstained from taking tribute from their people. Overall, Ma reinforced Du You's claim that the collection of local tribute should remain meager and easy, letting the locals take initiative. Writing in the aftermath of the Song's fall to Mongol rule, Ma imagined an ideal regime in ancient times that satisfied all its needs for material goods (*wuhuo*) through voluntary local tribute. "There was no such thing as the state (*guojia*) engaging in commercial affairs," wrote Ma.[38] One cannot help but wonder whether the diverse tax base designed in the early Ming may have reflected Ma's idea. Yet it was clear that the State's need for material goods quickly transcended what the locals could provide.

Bearing in mind Cai Chen and Ma Duanlin's admonitions, leading Confucian scholar-officials of mid-Ming China sought to create an integrated curriculum that would translate abstract principles into concrete guidance for political action. Qiu Jun (1421–95; jinshi 1454), a child prodigy hailing from Ming China's southernmost territory of Hainan, found a unifying principle that would make this curriculum appeal to all: a completely new commentary on a text that everyone already knew. *Daxue* (*The Great Learning*), one of the so-called *Four Books* that every student taking their civil service examinations would need to learn by heart, exhorted the sequence of moral learning starting from the investigation of things (*gewu*). The Song scholar Zhen Dexiu (1178–1235) expounded on the following steps for the ruler in a popular commentary to the *Daxue*:

> Investigation of Things (*gewu*)
> Extension of Knowledge (*zhizhi*)
> Sincerity of Intention (*chengyi*)
> Rectitude of the Mind (*zhengxin*)
> Cultivation of the Self (*xiushen*)
> Management of the Family (*qijia*)

Going beyond Zhen Dexiu's work, Qiu Jun saw that the final two steps mentioned in *The Great Learning*, "Governance of the Nation" (*zhiguo*) and "Pacification of the World" (*ping tianxia*), could be expounded as a curriculum for the ruler and the official elite. The result of Qiu's lifelong work, *Daxue yanyi bu* (supplement to *Expositions on the Great Learning*, 1487), thus touched on all aspects of government affairs, drawing from his own experience in office.[39]

One can use Qiu Jun's compilation as a reliable guide to respected opinion in late fifteenth-century China. Qiu, too, had much to say on the subject of tribute medicine, under the rubrics of the management of wealth (*licai*) and the proper expenditure of the state (*guoyong*). Qiu concurred with Cai Chen about the voluntary nature of local tribute, a category that encompassed the procurement of cattle, paper, materia medica, foodstuffs, and raw material for making weaponry.[40] Playing with the homonymous terms of "gaining" (*zhi*) and "arriving" (*zhi*), Qiu argued that the state gained (*zhi*) useful goods only by having them arrive by themselves (*zizhi*) and not by demanding them outright.[41] Yet Qiu also acknowledged the difficulty of governing without an adequate supply of those same goods.[42] To reconcile the need of the state and those of the people, noted Qiu, was to make sure the demand for local tribute remained *constant* (*chang*): "To manage the wealth of the state is in fact to manage the wealth *for* the people."[43]

A similarly ambitious attempt at Confucian policy didactics came from Zhan Ruoshui (1466–1560; jinshi 1505). In 1525, the Jiajing emperor (r. 1522–66), who succeeded the childless Zhengde from a side branch of the imperial lineage, issued an edict soliciting straightforward explanations of Confucian classics and history. Zhan, who was then teaching at the Imperial Academy in Nanjing, seized the opportunity to compile a hundred-volume-long guide to sage-learning (*shengxue*), a book that he hoped would rival and supersede Qiu Jun's work that had come out several decades earlier. The title of Zhan's text, *Comprehensive Guide to the Investigation of Things* (*Gewu tong*), captures the essence of his thinking about the fundamental importance of knowledge as the fountainhead of all learning. Writing several decades later than Qiu Jun, Zhan similarly engaged the question of local tribute by seeing products such as materia medica as an endowment from heaven—finite in amount and susceptible to overexploitation. He warned against the tendency to develop a luxurious desire (*chixin*) of the ruler. After all, the wealth (*cai*) that came from the people was not limitless, and rulers must be mindful about the ways in which they obtained (*qu*) and spent (*yong*) this wealth.[44]

The Jiajing reign began with a prolonged fight between the new emperor and many officials, who steadfastly refused to honor the emperor's birth parents with imperial honorifics. Despite the intensity of court strife, Zhan Ruoshui and others still believed that moral suasion could transform sitting emperors into living sages. After presenting the manuscript of *Gewu tong* to the Jiajing emperor, Zhan continued to use it as an outline for his own teaching. Hailing from the far south, Zhan had already developed a solid reputation as "Master South Sea" among younger literati by holding public lectures, often followed by intense debate with the audience. A group of younger disciples built a mobile lodge (*xingwo*) in his honor in the busy city of Yangzhou and used it as a space to teach Zhan's ideas. In 1533, some students raised funds to prepare their own copy of *Gewu tong* for print and obtained crucial help from local officials. Zhan Ruoshui had not foreseen that an instruction manual on sage learning intended for imperial ears would become as a popular guide to self-cultivation and political participation by a much greater number of students, including some zealous commoners aspiring to sagehood. A few decades later, the same social spaces for the spread of popular Confucian teaching would also serve to propagate the science of pharmacy. In the next chapter, we will examine the finer distinctions between competing doctrines on the question of objecthood and selfhood, as well as the centrality of pharmacy in this debate.

By the mid-sixteenth century, the status of tribute loomed large in the ascendant discourse of wealth and profit. A consensus about the wastefulness and injustice of meeting state expenditure through local tribute began to emerge, and would soon gather greater momentum for fiscal reform. We now turn to examine how idiosyncratic solutions proposed by local actors joined the broad intellectual trend and pushed for the monetization of tribute medicine.

The Bureaucratic Logic of Monetization

Converting one kind of tax into another, or between tax and tribute items, did have precedents prior to the sixteenth century. When Ming forces conquered the southwestern province of Yunnan in the late fourteenth century, the region had become known for abundant mineral deposits of silver and copper, but it was relatively weak in agricultural production. In 1384, an edict allowed the province to pay tax with equal value of "gold, silver, shells, textiles, lacquer sap, cinnabar and mercury" instead of grains. A similar decree of tax conversion was extended to the northern part of Vietnam that briefly became a Ming province in 1407.[45] Yet most early precedents applied only to territories distant from the imperial center and converted grains into local products, not vice versa.

As we have seen in the example of Longqing Subprefecture, the shift away from dispatching materia medica as tribute took place at the turn of the sixteenth century, most likely as a local response to drastically increasing quotas for desirable material resources. An early sixteenth century gazetteer of Suzhou, for instance, put it candidly:

> As for tribute items today, they are designated by where they were produced. Sometimes they are also purchased from elsewhere to meet the requirement. Even if demand every year remains constant, the cost of delivering them is several times higher than the price.[46]

The arbitrariness of this kind of local solution was also reflected in the distribution of tribute quota from the level of province to that of prefecture and subprefecture, and then on to counties. Take the southeastern province of Zhejiang as example. Responsible for procuring and shipping 3,000 jin (about 1,800 kilograms) of the porous fungus *fuling* (one of 57 materia medica in Zhejiang's total tribute medicine quota of 31,990 jin), the provincial administration divided it evenly among its eleven subordinate prefectures.[47] Likewise, prefectures in turn designated the task to subordinate counties, sometimes provoking bitter disputes. Since there was no reason to assume the abundance of fuling was evenly distributed across the vast province, local administrations resorted to purchasing the "original kind" (*bense*)—that is to say, medicines such as fuling—from the marketplace as a practical means to make ends (and numbers) meet. Even though the province of Zhejiang, for the time being, still managed to dispatch 3,000 jin of the medicine to Beijing and Nanjing, the tribute items were already dealt with as a "converted kind" (*zhese*) of tax item in prefectures and counties. Fuling became deterritorialized from Zhejiang even though the actual items still shipped from there.

Local gazetteers of the sixteenth century revealed how the impetus for monetization often came from below. In 1550, for instance, the Imperial Academy of Medicine sent to the Yingtian Prefecture (effectively the local administration for Nanjing and adjacent counties) an order of 3,850 jin of *cangzhu*, a fragrant herb that was burned in the summer to dispel evil spirits.[48] While the herb was indeed produced in Jurong County, the prefect assigned the task instead to the neighboring Liuhe County. As a result, the hapless Liuhe community had to buy this large amount of cangzhu from Jurong merchants, who extorted an exorbitant price from their dispatchers. Worse still, the dispatchers from Liuhe were repeatedly mocked and humiliated by Jurong dealers as well as personnel at the Imperial Academy of Medicine. Documenting the whole incident, the Liuhe gazetteer proudly pointed out that in the end, the prefect was persuaded to divert the tribute burden to Jurong.[49] Each similar negotiation further weakened the legitimacy of local tribute by highlighting the inadequate alignment between knowledge and policy.

In fact, incidents of extortion associated with tribute items eventually served to move the loci of monetization up the bureaucratic ladder. Overall, the means of fiscal maneuver was limited at the local level, although magistrates and prefects did manage to invent locally specific solutions to raise the funds, such as the Longqing Subprefecture's proposal to distribute the cost among landowners. A coastal town, for example, exacted an extra fee on households that owned salt yards to mitigate the cost of shipping tribute medicine.[50] Eventually, instead of raising funds and purchasing the medicine locally, as Longqing did in the early sixteenth century, provincial administrations started to allow counties and prefectures to transfer the funds along with other taxes converted to money at the same time, and to purchase the tribute items altogether at the provincial capital, before delivering them to Beijing and Nanjing. Doing so minimized the risk of extortion, for provincial authorities wielded much more bargaining power than county magistrates, who had little choice but to purchase from the few available suppliers in their jurisdiction. For example, Fujian, one of the first provinces to convert material resources into silver, first allowed payment in silver from county to prefecture in 1520, then made it possible to monetize fiscal transactions from prefecture to province in 1548.[51] We can see that by the 1580s, when the so-called Single Whip Law was formally promulgated by the Chief Grand Secretariat Zhang Juzheng to monetize the diverse tax base, many local administrations had been essentially doing so for tribute items for decades.[52]

The overall trend of converting tribute items into a surtax altered the fiscal practice of Ming local administrations. Relieved of the hassle of procuring and dispatching tribute items, prefects and magistrates found themselves engulfed in the minutiae of fiscal bookkeeping. They had to provide the monetary value of various tribute items separately, estimate the summary cost, and calculate the total tax combining all converted items (hence the "single whip" analogy). Sometimes the cost of shipping from the provincial capital to Beijing or Nanjing was in turn distributed among prefectures and counties, adding to the complexity of budgeting. In a popular handbook for beginning officials, the author, Wu Zun (jinshi 1547), advised hiring expert accountants to help in dealing with the calculations involved in tax conversion.[53] A rough survey of Ming gazetteers published during the long reigns of Jiajing (1522–66), Longqing (1567–72), and Wanli (1572–1620) reveals increasingly lengthy documentation of tax items with exact numbers stretching into eight digits after the main unit of liang. In other words, by protesting the injustice and inconvenience of procuring tribute items, Ming officialdom maneuvered itself into relying on monetary transactions that, in however minuscule amounts, still remained a surtax on products that might or might not have been found locally.

A comprehensive study of tribute to tax conversion would necessarily require a more detailed investigation across several hundred Ming local gazetteers, a task that must be left for future research. Having sketched out the impetus and contours of institutional change, I now move to consider the cultural consequences of monetization as a bureaucratic reality. Consider the Longqing Subprefecture again, where a retired official maintained a clear divide that set aside items "fit for tribute and tax" from other useful things.[54] The sense of prioritizing state expenditure was echoed by another prefectural gazetteer in 1530. "While these goods are necessary for the local people," wrote another prefect in 1530, "tributes to the state must take priority." Since everyone was a subject of the emperor, "how can an official forget his lord and listen to his own judgment?"[55]

This earlier sentiment of state-society unison, if not prioritizing the lord over the people, was replaced with an increasingly articulate populism in gazetteers later in the sixteenth century. Similar to the incident recorded in Liuhe County, gazetteer compilers (often members of local gentry allied with the county administration) accused capital clerks and corrupt officials for their mistreatment and extortion of local tribute dispatchers.[56] Many others channeled their criticism through doctrines taught by leading Confucian officials, such as Qiu Jun and Zhan Ruoshui. They drew a clear line between "popular livelihood" (*minsheng*) and necessary supplies for "military and state affairs" (*junguo*), condemning the excessive exploitation of exotic medicines by the court.[57] A medicinal herb growing in the mountains, for instance, could serve either "the everyday use of the people," *or* "the constant demand of (state) procurement."[58] The key to the state's management of wealth (*licai*) lay in restraining expenditure, including the procurement of material resources. "Wherever there are people living, wealth will be generated from them," a prefect commented in the gazetteer he compiled himself. "And this wealth resides either with the state or with the people. Where wealth concentrates, the people disperse."[59] Another prefect elsewhere concurred with this view: "When the state wants of something, it acquires it from the people. But when the people want something, from whom can they get it?"[60] The laborious collection of tribute medicine in particular became a focal point for grievances. "Exhausting the mountain valleys to obtain this drug," noted one magistrate in the 1570s, "is not to cure diseases but to generate more ills."[61] The prevailing sentiment of state-society antagonism in mid-sixteenth-century gazetteers, therefore, was not an inherent feature of Ming political culture, but was encouraged by particular breakthroughs in the process of fiscal reform. In other words, a critical attitude toward tribute medicine only became politically correct after a viable alternative was put in place, namely the move toward monetization.

Redefining Local Knowledge

Historians now generally agree that Ming China's gradual shift from a diverse tax base toward a single fiscal currency of silver constitutes an event of world-historical importance. In this chapter, I have suggested that the significance of this monumental change resides not only in the ripple effects felt elsewhere in the early modern global marketplace of currency and commodities, nor in the short-term stimulations and woes that the newly emerged dependence on silver exerted on Ming domestic economy. Also driving the impetus toward fiscal reform was the question of misalignment between knowledge and policy seen through the Ming actors' own eyes. Materia medica, one of the most richly documented categories of tribute items that were also regionally diverse, came to the forefront of attention in this debate. The questionable existence of certain herbs, animals, and minerals in a particular locality—and the pressing awareness of the limited nature of wealth and material resources— prompted the adoption of money as a compromise between the State and the populace.

In what ways, then, did the cultural battles surrounding Ming fiscal reform alter the landscape of knowledge, in particular the territorialized aspect of pharmaceutical objecthood presented in the Tang-Song bencao pharmacopeias? On the one hand, there was a positive proliferation of local knowledge, once local products no longer risked being wrongfully designated as tribute items. The severance between the singularity of local material resources and state expenditure reoriented the attention of some local elite to the best ways of exploiting this wealth. Going beyond their predecessors in Song and Yuan times, Ming gazetteer authors highlighted the most beautiful (*mei*), numerous (*duo*), and exclusive (*zhuan*) products of their land.[62] "One bird, one beast, one fish, one insect . . . all products of Yingshan are for the profit of the people of Yingshan," declared a gazetteer of the said county.[63] The urge to exhaustively (*jin*) document local flora and fauna in these gazetteers boosted the sense of local pride vis-à-vis the perceived threat of oppression from the center.

Positive affirmation of local knowledge went hand-in-hand with the negative disavowal of previous records. The esteemed stature of earlier bencao as sources of universal authority diminished each time a local actor discovered their shortcomings. "Herbs growing here are mostly used by physicians who treated external wounds (*waike yangyi*)," noted one gazetteer, "and they learned the herbs' names directly from their teachers, making it difficult to check with the *bencao*."[64] "To believe everything in the books is to be obstinate," wrote the magistrate of Dengzhou, Henan. In the local gazetteer, he disputed records of the existence of two rare medicinal minerals—amethyst (*zishiying*) and azurite (*shiqing*)—that had appeared in previous dynastic and prefectural records. Upon his own investigation (*fang*), the magistrate claimed that there was "absolutely no existence" of the precious stones. Worried that an inaccurate record might lead to unwanted tax burdens in the future, he decided to "delete the record according to the facts" (*cong shi shan qu*).[65] His concern was not unfounded: another gazetteer from the Jiajing reign (1522– 66) recorded a dispute that took place in Chunhua County, Shaanxi Province. Rumors went around that *huangqi*, a tonic drug widely used in common prescriptions, grew in Chunhua, and an order for the plant soon arrived from the capital.[66] Unable to find the herb, the Chunhua magistrate sent a similar plant instead. In Beijing, the poor Chunhua physician in charge of dispatching the plant was severely repudiated at the Academy and almost beaten to death. Later, a new magistrate responded to local indignation by deleting the section of materia medica from the gazetteer's list of local products for good.[67] Such cases indicate that the connection between textual knowledge and tribute obligations was still real enough, and locals took to changing the gazetteer records to protest against unjust state demands.

The entangled sentiments of local pride and consternation are best illustrated by a late sixteenth-century gazetteer of Wangjiang County, a river town situated at the border between the Lower Yangzi and Jiangxi (map 0.1). The magistrate, who also initiated the revision of the gazetteers, explained in his preface how he weathered five challenging years of administering Wangjiang. His intimate understanding of the place was, noted this magistrate, enhanced by his personal investigation in the wake of several disastrous floods and droughts. As a result, this magistrate turned vehemently against the preference for "beautiful" and "exotic" products in the previous local gazetteer. In the revised version, he would have none of it: instead, he went to extra lengths in documenting products of actual use to the local people. In practice, however, the magistrate still relied on previous textual sources, including bencao, to supply information on everyday objects such as cotton, vegetables, and domestic animals. His ardent wish to help the local people stemmed from his confidence in the superiority of his education and status.

Yet the most striking move by the Wangjiang magistrate resides in his decision to remove the categories of flowers (*huabu*) and materia medica (*yaobu*) altogether from his revised local gazetteer. He wrote:

Wangjiang had no exotic flowers. For flowers are, after all, flowery; with no use for the people. I will not document them. As for medicine, they are good for conquering diseases, but not good for nurturing life. Medical books document the nature of drugs, and each place has its own products. Wangjiang has several kinds of *materia medica* but they are not documented in the formulaic books and map guides. I will therefore not document them either.[68]

This stance was, even by late Ming standards, quite extreme; later editions of the county gazetteer restored the deleted sections of Flowers and Medicine back to Wangjiang's bounty. Yet the Wangjiang magistrate's categorical denial of medicine's place in local documentation testifies to a widening gap between universal and local discourses. It was not that he denied the textual authority of bencao, for it offered him ample references on plants and animals; he only refused to classify them as medicines. Slowly but surely, local historiography started to overwhelm, and even undermine, the epistemic integrity of the bencao pharmacopeia. We will see the reverberations of this populist sentiment against universal pharmaceutical objecthood after the Ming-Qing conquest.

Here is one final observation on the cultural significance of converting tribute in mid-Ming China. In contrast to the geographical vision of tribute medicine in Tang-Song times (map 2.1), where almost every local administration was associated with one or more tribute items, the sourcing of materia medica in the Ming was pushed farther and farther away from these familiar places. Instead, money flowed from counties and prefectures to provincial capitals, where officials purchased medicines harvested from ever more remote lands through the mediation of commercial actors. Uneven distribution of scarce resources, coupled with the surging demand from state and private elites, stimulated the development of transregional trade that we will discuss in chapter 5. Yet it is important to note that the concept of tribute, once a category applicable to *all* territories under heaven, became marginalized or even eliminated from local administrative vocabulary in central China. The result was an exoticization of tribute, now redefined as the material link between the ruling dynasty and distant peoples residing at its peripheries.

Converting tribute for some, but not all, peoples, in other words, produced a distinction between domestic governance over "our" people and the subjugation of the "other," where the presentation of tribute items persisted. This separation between a human-centered sphere of civilization and its exotic peripheries should be seen as part and parcel of the reformist impetus in mid-Ming times. As a Ming magistrate observed in the mid-sixteenth century:

> Heaven and Earth exist, from which springs forth a myriad of things. Abundance in human talent balances off scarcity of material resources. In the civilization of the Middle Kingdom, we have blessed lands and outstanding

talents. Yet exotic and precious things are often produced from the numerous barbarians overseas. This is fundamentally fair of the Creation.[69]

In chapter 4, we will see how the Qing state continued to apply the trend of exoticizing tribute to its expanding imperial territory and the management of relationships with "numerous barbarians overseas," a relationship that modern historians have labeled the "tributary system," notwithstanding its many inaccuracies.[70] In chapter 6, we will examine how urban consumers in Qing China perpetuated and enriched the imagination of exotica through pharmaceutical commodities.

This chapter has, I hope, revealed the richness and intensity of debates over tribute medicine in Ming dynastic and local sources. It is thus striking to see that neither the Hongzhi pharmacopeia compiled by Liu Wentai in 1505, nor Li Shizhen's *Bencao gangmu* several decades later, took stock of the local knowledge that emerged in this period. Liu Wentai, working in isolation from the outer court, did not possess the political muscle to summon reports and specimens from the provinces. Li Shizhen, on the other hand, consulted 440 nonmedical sources for his great bencao, but no contemporary local gazetteers.[71] It may well have been that the locally published gazetteers were not accessible for Li even if he wished to consult them. Yet in any case, *Bencao gangmu* still presents us with a territorialized geography of materia medica in the Tang-Song tradition, one that sat in awkward contrast to the oft-vociferous denial of tribute designations that swept through the Ming administration. It is perhaps an unintended consequence of mid-Ming activism for fiscal reform that another pharmacopeia built on the legitimacy of local tribute became politically untenable.

Toward the end of the sixteenth century, the composite authority of the bencao pharmacopeia gradually broke down along many axes: a geographically diverse and increasingly competitive publishing sector, momentous tides of Confucian activism that focused on the realignment of knowledge and policy, and a widening gulf between factions of civil officials and technical experts. The next two chapters will take us through the tumultuous events of the seventeenth century by following a new type of pharmaceutical knowledge along scholastic lines: its unexpected rise, flourishing, and demise across dynastic transition.

3

The Nature of Drugs

Student Li is a Confucian scholar.
Why did he write a book on *bencao*?
I taught Student Li Confucian learning.
Why am I writing a preface for his *bencao*?

—LUO WENYING, PREFACE TO
BENCAO YUANSHI (1612)

EVERY THREE YEARS, the Henan provincial civil service examination yielded 80–90 successful candidates (*juren*). Usually at least one candidate hailed from Qi County, a historic town whose name had appeared in ancient historical annals. In good years, it might produce several successful candidates. During Ming times, many Qi County juren did go on to win the high degree of jinshi in the metropolitan examination. Among them, Luo Wenying was particularly fortunate to pass the two consecutive examinations in Wanli 34 (1606) and 35 (1607). Serving in a central governmental office, Luo had his eye on a promotion to a desirable position in the censorate, where he would make his name as an outspoken and upright man. When he learned that a former pupil named Li Zhongli wrote a book on the subject matter of bencao—and requested a preface from him—Luo decided to give Li another lecture on the proper order of things.[1]

Luo Wenying opened his preface with the quote above, pitting the study of bencao against the very concept of Confucian learning. He then deftly came around to find a ground for conciliation:

If one sees Things as Things, how can they have anything to do with myself?
If one sees Things as Images, then a wooden root, a grassy root, a gesture
of flying, wandering, and swimming, the silent coagulations and dim appearances . . . all these are nothing but the awesome manifestations of my
own Nature.[2]

Luo Wenying's tongue-in-cheek approval of his pupil's unusual endeavor can
be read in two ways. It reflected the persistent stigma that distinguished Confucian learning from mere technical pursuits, such as medicine and pharmacy,
but also an increasingly strong movement toward overcoming such barriers.
It was also characteristic of Ming neo-Confucian thought that Luo was able to
make a Confucian study of bencao possible through the concept of nature
(*xing*). This chapter takes this ambivalence toward the nature of things as its
starting point, and argues that the confluence of bencao and neo-Confucian
natural philosophy only took place under specific political and cultural conditions in the first decades of the seventeenth century.

Student Li Zhongli also won the coveted provincial degree in Wanli 40
(1612). No further records existed of him in public life, yet his calligraphy and
drawings are preserved in his *Bencao yuanshi* (*Original Inquiries of Materia
Medica*). Although Li "compiled, wrote, and illustrated" (*zuanji bing shuhua*)
the text all by himself, he did not write his own preface to explain his method
or aspirations.[3] Modern scholars have concluded that Li's bencao relied heav-
ily on *Bencao gangmu* and was likely inspired by the success of this very new
pharmacopeia. The pictorial features of Li's text, however, stood out in their
originality and quality: the several hundred illustrations of materia medica
showed details unseen in previous works. Pictures and texts were interwoven
with each other in a way that later editions failed to preserve (figure 3.1).[4] The
first edition of *Bencao yuanshi* was a product of local prestige in the tightly knit
elite network of Qi County; the freshness and originality were lost in subsequent editions.

This chapter is thus not only about subtle debates within the neo-Confucian
doctrine about the nature of drugs, but also the numerous and diverse attempts to live up to those ideals in late Ming China. Like Li Zhongli, many
Confucian literati who took an interest in the subject of bencao belonged to
the younger generations who came of age during or after the late decades of
the Wanli reign (1572–1620). Not surprisingly, most of them lived and were
primarily active in Jiangnan, the most prosperous and populous region of

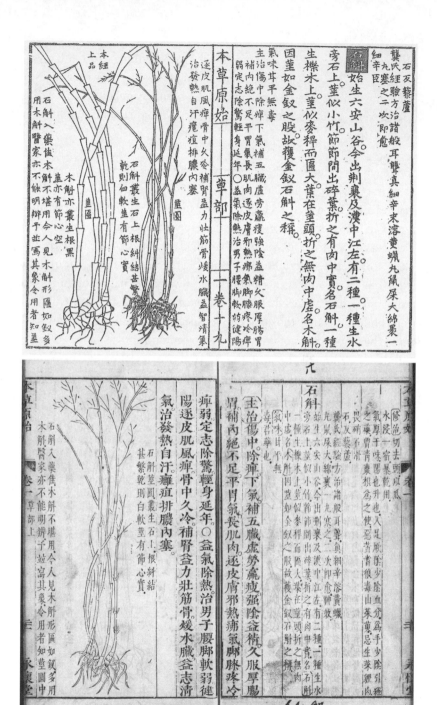

FIGURE 3.1 (top). Page from BCYS depicting Dendrobium (*shihu*).
(bottom) Same page from BCYS-1638. Courtesy of the Harvard-Yenching Library.

Ming China (see map 0.1 inset); but the enthusiasm for bencao did travel outside Jiangnan, as Li Zhongli's case exemplifies. Li was also typical in that he pursued medical learning without practicing medicine for a living. If this description fits quite well what Joseph Levenson and others called "amateurism" in Chinese cultural history then, as I discussed in the introduction, we need to specify the local and personal circumstances that made such intellectual adventures appealing to them.

Let me also say at the outset: it will become apparent that the actors and texts I discuss in this chapter can, and should, also be analyzed through the framework of religion. Syncretism of the "three teachings" (Confucianism, Buddhism, and Daoism) was a dominant cultural trend in late Ming China, and the appeal of bencao was motivated not only by particular doctrines of nature in neo-Confucianism, but also the revival of Chan Buddhism in seventeenth century.[5] I have already suggested in chapter 1 that the reinvention of *Master Thunder* texts on the processing of pharmaceuticals can be seen as part and parcel of the elite nurturing life (*yangsheng*) culture fueled by Daoist ideas. Miao Xiyong, a pivotal figure whose exploits boosted the appeal of bencao learning among literati, followed Chan Buddhist masters and practiced geomancy alongside medicine. The narrative here focuses on the interaction between bencao knowledge and the cultural elite of Ming China, who shared a common educational background and aspired to play a role in public life.

Things and Us

In chapter 1, we saw that the nature of drugs became an issue of common interest for both physicians and neo-Confucian philosophers like Zhu Xi in the twelfth century. While Zhu Xi used the qualities of rhubarb to illustrate the invisible presence of coherence in nature, he was also keen to construct a hierarchy of natures. If all were similarly endowed with a nature (*xing*) through which the coherence of the world (*li*) could manifest itself, why couldn't plants and beasts also become enlightened sages? What made human beings special? Zhu Xi's answer was that not all natures were alike, but each existed with its own particular endowments. In his own metaphor, li, like water and sunlight, was the same everywhere but different in quantity. Different amounts of water or sun, however, would be apparent depending both on the kind of body or vessel and where it was placed; standing underneath a roof that cast a shadow would diminish the intensity of sunlight that could be received.

In the great hierarchy of being in Zhu Xi's metaphysical world, human beings were born with a complete (*quan*) and unobstructed endowment of
li that was conducive to the perfect manifestation of morality, whereas nonhuman things were "partial and obstructed" (*pianse*).[6] Sages, the most enlightened people, possessed a nature that was the purest and most perfect of all;
then came humans with all sorts of imperfections, who could, nonetheless,
aspire to sagehood. The brightest animals sometimes showed humanlike
moral behavior: bees and ants behaved as if they knew the hierarchy between
lords and serfs, while cats took care of their young like human parents. Further
down the hierarchy of moral endowment were other animals, plants, rocks,
and metals—whose bodies, in turn, were made into medicine.

Zhu Xi's formulation of human nature and the nature of things therefore
invited an ethics of nature: that is, one ought to work with what nature had
given, making the most of it—to "let the nature be" (*shuaixing*), or "exhaustively explore one's nature" (*jinxing*), so that the potential to be moral and
good could be realized as fully as possible. An individual was exhorted to follow a path of self-discovery and a life of fulfillment. The negative connotations,
however, were also very clear: there were many perils obstructing the path to
sagehood, all caused by tendencies inherent within one's material existence
that one could not help but live with. Zhu Xi dictated a fixed difference between men and women, whose nature, in his words, was given to "excessive
affection," and hence weakness. Barbarian peoples (*yidi*) fared no better: for
Zhu Xi, they were half-beast beings that resisted the forces of civilization. Nonhuman beings, too, were stuck in their partial, idiosyncratic natures, their bodies resembling a darkened mirror, with "only a few dots of light in the middle."[7]
These arguments reflected the urge to reassure fellow practitioners of neo-
Confucian self-cultivation that they were, after all, already endowed with a
superior nature than that of others.

During the long period encompassing the Song-Yuan-Ming era (the twelfth
through seventeenth centuries), leading scholars of neo-Confucian thought
repeatedly debated the question of nature. The teachings of Zhu Xi, along with
other Song thinkers, offered a range of possible positions on many fronts. One
prominent line of argumentation turned on the question of which was primary: matter (*qi*) or coherence (*li*). The view that held the primacy of "material inventiveness," in Dagmar Schäfer's words, led many to turn their attention to the importance of technology.[8] Others sought to adjust and rejuvenate
the practice of moral cultivation according to their own times: the prominence of Wang Yangming's (1472–1529) teaching in mid-Ming times illus-

trated the vitality of this approach. Exiled because of his support of Dai Xian in 1506 (see chapter 2), Wang found a renewed source of certainty by devoting attention to introspective investigation of one's own moral conscience (*liang-zhi*). Wang's famous dictum, "knowledge and action are one" (*zhi xing he yi*), exhorted his disciples to focus on the intuitive thoughts that sprang forth from "within one's chest."[9] The emphasis placed on introspection by Wang Yangming's teaching should not be interpreted as an argument against materiality: rather, as we will see, it encouraged a more open attitude to reconfiguring Zhu Xi's rigid hierarchy of natures. Most Ming Confucians agreed on the general relevance of nonhuman things (*wu*) to the exploration of human nature. Even Wang Yangming, who famously announced that there was no path toward moral enlightenment through "investigating" a bamboo plant, acknowledged that human existence could not be severed from the knowledge of things.

A range of positions on the commonality and distinction between human nature and the nature of things thus came to be articulated in the sixteenth century by leading Confucian teachers.[10] Zhan Ruoshui, whose comprehensive writings on the investigation of things (*gewu*) enjoyed great popularity (see chapter 2), refrained from embracing a primacy of matter as beyond the mind's grasp. Disagreeing with Wang Yangming's prioritizing of the mind and introspection over knowledge of the material world, however, Zhan exhorted his disciples to "embody and recognize" (*tiren*) the moral principles immanent in things through various encounters in life.[11] Zhan had his own hierarchy of priorities: writing as a prominent statesman, Zhan formulated his concept of *gewu* along the axis of governmental affairs. In chapter 2, we saw that he, like other politically outspoken officials, held rigid opinions on the morality of various policy positions. We could therefore consider his position to be one that emphasized the connection of moral knowledge and action through an insistent institutional realism.

Other prominent teachers of the early sixteenth century, such as Luo Qinshun (1465–1547), emphasized the importance of matter and the nature of things more explicitly. In Luo's own words, "Principle is one; its particularizations are diverse" (*li yi fen shu*).[12] Though Luo seemed to have merely rephrased Zhu Xi's teachings, creatures that inhabited different rungs of Zhu's great hierarchy came to be recast as but different (*shu*) members residing in the great panorama of the world. Each had its virtues and imperfections, which was only natural and appropriate. Some thinkers, such as Wang Tingxiang (1474–1544), even toyed with the idea that the diversity of material existence could function based upon more than one less than completely coherent principle.[13]

In Deng Yuanxi (1529–93), a late disciple of Wang Yangming, we can find an eclectic position that acknowledged the diversity of the material world without compromising the primacy of the human mind. In an encyclopedic text titled *Han shi* (*History in a Casket*), Deng sought to illustrate the omnipresent moral coherence through sampling a wide range of works by both ancient and recent authors. Beginning with Confucian classics, Deng went on to survey governmental institutions and remarkable individuals from dynastic Histories. The eighty-one-volume encyclopedia, constructed with a great sensitivity to cosmology (nine being the greatest yang number, multiplied by nine becoming eighty-one, which represents utmost abundance and efflorescence), ends with a chapter on the "nature of things" (*wuxing*).[14] The fact that nonhuman things came last brought this work in line with Zhu Xi's hierarchy of natures, and yet Deng's account displayed a passionate enthusiasm rarely seen in earlier sources. The main source for Deng was—perhaps unsurprisingly—the Song bencao pharmacopeia, which, as we saw in chapter 1, became widely available through print in the sixteenth century and served for Deng as the standard reference for descriptions of the external world.

Deng accepted the Song bencao's vision for a universal pharmaceutical objecthood and celebrated it. He saw the relationship between human beings and the creatures documented in bencao as one of "mutual nourishment and regeneration" (*xiang yang xiang sheng*). The claim about regeneration (*sheng*) clearly refers to the beneficial action of pharmacy; human life was possible because of the things that nourished and healed us. For Deng, the existence of drugs that could heal offered the most salient proof that the universe revolved around human beings, and understanding that led to discovery of the maximum potential of nature (*jin xing*) for all creatures. Furthermore, this exploration was the proper task for Confucians not only to achieve their own moral perfection through adherence to the heavenly way, but also to apply this understanding to the lordly art of governance (*jundao*). "Behold medicines," he wrote, "are they not the most refined, the most varied, and the most divine of beings?"[15] The overtone of ecstasy is not difficult to detect.

Yet the acknowledgement of matter as a potential source of knowledge did not completely solve the question of epistemology, for, as Deng noted, the interconnected natures of people and things did not reveal its truth so easily. Deng Yuanxi, for one, held that the appearances (*xing*) of things were like handcuffs on the mind, and that true knowledge must be derived from intuition springing forth from its depths.[16] Here, we detect the source of Luo Wen-ying's comment on bencao that I quoted at the beginning of this chapter: the "silent coagulations and dim appearances" of matter were, for Luo, irrelevant noise unless one contemplated them as the "regular images" (*fa xiang*) of one's own (human) nature. The proper way of looking at things was thus to look *through* them without holding on to any sensual distractions. From this detached position, Confucian scholars engaged with the teaching of pharmacy in bencao in an aloof manner. When Dong Qichang (1555–1636), a prominent figure and champion of amateur literati paintings, was invited to write a preface for an early seventeenth-century edition of Li Shizhen's *Bencao gangmu*, he concluded that true knowledge about drugs could not have been obtained through mere senses; the Divine Farmer (*Shennong*) must therefore have *intuited* his knowledge through the eight images (*ba xiang*) of the cosmos, not actual tasting of various substances.[17] We will discover that this mainstream view started to shift at the turn of the seventeenth century.

Donglin Partisans and the Amateurization of Bencao

Doctrinal differences aside, the elite literati of the late Ming found themselves gravitating toward the sensual aspects of pharmaceutical knowledge through making and dispensing compound medicines at home. The elite had, to be sure, always invested in the personal wellbeing of their family members by securing the best ingredients and the means to prepare them. Yet the trend toward setting up private "pharmaceutical chambers" (*yaoshi*, a fancy term with alchemical overtones) at one's own estate became especially pronounced in mid- and late-Ming Jiangnan.[18] The famous painter Qiu Ying (1494–1552), suffering from chronic joint pain, once asked one of his patrons in a letter for an expensive pill "newly-prepared at your household."[19] Gao Lian (fl. late sixteenth century), bestselling author of the celebrated *Eight Discourses on the Art of Living*, gave detailed instructions on how to equip and maintain such a space:

> Choose a quiet room, with no noise from chickens and dogs. Set up one altar for the sage-king of medicine; one large table with a smooth surface fit for compounding medicine; one large iron roller, one stone mill, one small roller, two mortars of different sizes, one pearl grinder, one pounding mortar, three regular sieves, two fine mesh sieves, one broom, one clean cloth, one copper cauldron, one stove fan, one pair of fire-tongs, two

weighing scales of different sizes, one medicine cabinet, one medicine container. As for jars, bottle gourds and bottles, prepare as many as possible. Lock the room when not in use.[20]

Suffice it to say that the elite literati, through their own experience of making and consuming medicine, had every reason to pay heightened attention to the materiality of things. Unlike physicians who had to sustain profitable practices, elite families spared no expense on extravagant and obscure substances. In addition to instructions on how to set up a pharmaceutical chamber at home, Gao Lian's guide to living a good life also offered a large number of recipes that his readers could experiment with. It was this same audience—families of scholar-officials, and the nouveau riche who aspired to imitate them—whose demand would soon motivate the codification of pharmaceutical techniques and an appetite for new inquiries into pharmaceutical objecthood.[21]

The lavish care of the self in late-Ming culture, as summed up by the concern over the "nurturing of life" (*yangsheng*), bears close connections to the Wang Yangming school's emphasis on self-cultivation.[22] Paradoxically, a doctrine invented to encourage the literati's participation in public life was inverted to justify an inward-looking obsession with the self that came close to narcissism. This embrace of ambivalence between public and private engagements found expressions in the amateurization of bencao.

In 1638, Ge Nai (juren 1630), a bibliophile and private publisher who resided in Kunshan (map 0.1 inset), obtained Li Zhongli's bencao and issued a new edition as one of twin volumes, the other being a treatise on military training.[23] In his preface, Ge explained that war and medicine had much in common: they both could "get rid of suffering and save people's lives." Yet fundamentally all goodness emerged from individual moral actions: at root, there was no distinction between selfishness and altruism. In Ge's own words, "to make good use of oneself, one must first pay due respect to the self."[24] Perhaps motivated by this doctrine, Ge Nai altered Li Zhongli's page design to highlight therapeutic instructions, while downplaying the sections on names and morphology (figure 3.1b). He saw no trouble at all in posing himself as an amateur of both medical and military arts, and advertised this twin-volume to his readers as such.

Many would later come to see the self-centered culture of the 1630s and 1640s as a sign of decadence and doom, foreshadowing the dynasty's fall in 1644. Yet it would be wrong to see Ge Nai's defense of selfishness as an aberration from the trajectory of moral pursuits; it was but a logical extension of doctrines taught in *Great Learning* and other neo-Confucian texts. The important point here is that the heightened interest in the care of the self was buttressed by the possession of wealth and status, and was perceived as consistent with the pursuit of the public good. In fact, the same equation between personal wellbeing and public action also figured prominently a few decades earlier in one of the most spectacular displays of personhood in politics—the rise and persecution of the so-called Donglin partisans.

Protracted factional clashes at the Ming court during the sixteenth century led to the consolidation of what historian John Dardess called an "ethical revitalization movement" in the early 1600s.[25] A particular center of gravity formed around the newly renovated Donglin Academy located in Wuxi County (map 0.1). A loosely defined group of like-minded Confucian scholars, banished from office or retired at home, held regular meetings at the academy to discuss doctrinal issues, with an eye toward installing like-minded allies into key official positions and eliminating their enemies. The voluminous literature on this group has, to my knowledge, not yet examined their interest in medicine, in particular the matter of pharmacy. Gao Panlong (1562–1626), one of the founding leaders of the Academy, frequently prepared compound medicines at home and donated them to the poor.[26] Zhao Nanxing (1550–1627), another senior member of the faction, wrote a bencao by taking notes from *Bencao gangmu*, focusing on ingredients commonly used as food and drinks.[27] Ding Yuanjian (1560–1625), a Donglin regular who lived in his hometown in Changxing County (see map 0.1 inset), was particularly interested in medicine and liked to collect efficacious prescriptions from his social circles. In 1613, Ding published a collection of such prescriptions accompanied by short narratives of each case, in the form of a literary miscellany (*biji*). He credited in particular the brilliance of Miao Xiyong (1546–1627), a master physician who treated him and many other Donglin friends, including Gao Panlong and his family members, and generously shared his prescriptions with them.[28]

Who was Miao Xiyong? Anecdotes about him lingered in the Lower Yangzi region well into the eighteenth century. As a "cloth-clad" (*buyi*) commoner without an examination degree, Miao was nonetheless born into of one of the "finest families" (*jiazu*) of Changshu county (map 0.1 inset). Having lost his parents early on, Miao abandoned the pursuit of an official career and dabbled in all sorts of esoteric arts including geomancy and magic, studying for a while under renowned Chan Buddhist masters. Known for his striking appearance ("electrifying eyes and protruding whiskers") befitting an "eccentric gentleman" (*qishi*), Miao traveled constantly through the major towns of Jiangnan on horseback, advising officials informally on governmental affairs. It was through medicine that Miao was able to cement his friendship with prominent Donglin scholars, who "treated him as an elder brother."[29] He collaborated extensively with Ding Yuanjian on the case-prescription collection in which many tales showcased his skills. The success of the case collection further boosted his reputation among elite scholar-officials of Jiangnan; wherever he traveled, he was ceaselessly sought out for prescriptions.

The way Miao Xiyong practiced medicine struck contemporary observers as peculiar. His biography in local gazetteers read that Miao practiced "without bringing a bag of medicine," but "just wrote prescriptions for patients, with incredibly efficacious results."[30] The very act of prescribing became a virtuoso performance that Miao used to impress his audience. Qian Qianyi (1582–1664), a leading figure in Changshu's lettered elite, recalled such a scene many decades later:

> He thinks deeply and observes attentively, as if deep in Chan meditation; now he closes his eyes and falls into hypnosis, and in the next moment he rises with full force, lifting his beard and rolling up sleeves, and proceeds to write a prescription and put together some medicines. He takes command and oversees things, and ideas just spring out from his fingers.[31]

Miao was also known for disregarding the set rules of formula building, and his prescriptions often startled "vulgar physicians" (*suyi*) who could not understand his combination of drugs.[32] These impressions matched Miao's insistence on building a medical practice that was detached from the proprietary concerns of shopkeeping, while claiming superior understanding of the nature of drugs that led to clinical success.

In the early 1620s, an aging Miao Xiyong moved to Jintan County (map 0.1 inset), where he continued to see patients and socialize with the local gentry. At the insistence of a young disciple who also covered his lodging expenses, Miao offered to revise the formerly published case collections with a much more detailed chapter on the methods of "roasting and processing" (*paozhi*) materia medica. The revised case collection was published in 1622 under Miao's authorship, and the chapter on pharmaceutical methods was soon reproduced as a monograph, with the title *Paozhi dafa* (*Great Method of Pharmaceutical Preparation*).[33] The pharmaceutical instructions contained in this text targeted not rank-and-file physicians but elite patients themselves, who preferred to prepare the remedies by instructing their own servants at home. It was no coincidence for historian Paul Unschuld to observe that the literature on pharmaceutical processing reached "the peak of interest" at the turn of the seventeenth century.[34] The textualization of hands-on techniques was motivated by a combination of practical and philosophical interest among elite patients, not professional standardization.

Miao Xiyong was not alone among his contemporaries in promoting amateur interest in pharmacy as a separate branch of knowledge from general medicine. Wang Kentang (jinshi 1589), also a native of Jintan where Miao Xiyong temporarily resided in the early 1620s, became a renowned amateur practitioner after he was demoted from office. Wang frequently conversed with Miao Xiyong on medical matters, the two men sometimes treating the same patient in consultation with each other. Unlike Miao Xiyong's focus on pharmacology, Wang was more concerned with improving the overall outcome of medical treatment through textual teaching. For him, medicine, as a complex art, consisted of five major fields (ke): pulse-taking (mo), etiology (yin), pathology (bing), symptoms (zheng), and treatment (zhi). While the former three fields were difficult for a layperson to grasp, Wang considered it possible to focus on the last two fields alone, for even in the absence of a good physician, the patient could identify a probable treatment based on the symptoms. In 1602, Wang published a general compendium titled *Standard Measure for Symptoms and Treatments* (*Zhengzhi zhunsheng*). In his preface, Wang confessed that the book might be attacked for circumventing the path toward a deep exploration of medicine, yet he argued that the immediate benefits of attaining good treatment would outweigh the potential pitfalls. *Standard Measure* remains in print today as a popular reference for Traditional Chinese Medicine practitioners.[35]

Wang Kentang's willingness to separate pharmacy from general medicine was also reflected in a casual remark recorded in his collection of miscellaneous notes. A friend asked him how to read bencao as an entry point to the study of medicine. "Easy," said Wang, "you just skip all the sections that tell you the main indications of the drug."[36] Here, Wang spoke as a good Confucian philosopher, who insisted that bencao was first and foremost a good source for understanding the nature of things for its own sake; one need not read bencao with the pressing need to put the materia medica into practice. Wang's proposal for keeping bencao and therapeutics separate realms of study resonated with many young scholars who did not see themselves as practitioners of medicine, but nevertheless took a keen interest in the nature of drugs. The appeal of figures such as Wang Kentang and Miao Xiyong lies in the way that they carved out bencao as a field of pure inquiry into the neo-Confucian category of nature (*xing*), distinct from the clinician's pursuit of immediate

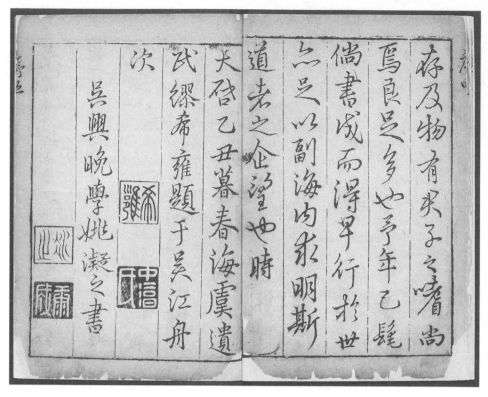

FIGURE 3.2A. Calligraphy by Yao Ningzhi with Miao Xiyong's personal seals, in BCJS-1625. Courtesy of the Harvard-Yenching Library.

results. This vision bears some resemblance to the modern distinction between the basic and applied sciences. Yet this was not how things would turn out later in the seventeenth century.[37]

With the Wanli reign coming to an end in 1620, the young Tianqi emperor delegated governmental affairs to his trusted eunuch advisor Wei Zhongxian (1568–1627). Wei's official allies soon locked horns with the Donglin faction over virtually all policy, from domestic mining taxes to border defense. A fabricated blacklist named 108 Donglin figures, comparing them to the outlaw heroes depicted in the popular vernacular novel *Water Margin*. In at least some versions of the blacklist, Miao Xiyong's name showed up as the "wonderful physician" (*shenyi*).[38] Outspoken officials particularly hated by Wei were arrested and tortured, and many died in prison. Among the martyrs of 1624–25 was Yang Lian (b. 1572), who started off his career as the magistrate of Changshu, and with whom Miao Xiyong had discussed local affairs.[39] Ding Yuanjian, Miao's longtime friend and patron, was also dismissed from his of-

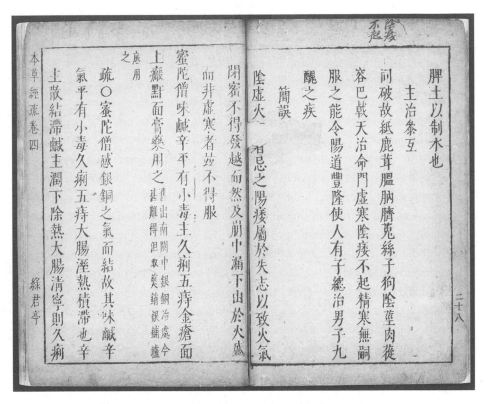

FIGURE 3.2B. Page from BCJS-1625 with Mao Jin's studio name.
Courtesy of the Harvard-Yenching Library.

ficial position and died at home in 1625. Hearing that the secret police had been dispatched to arrest him, the Donglin leader Gao Panlong drowned himself in a lake at home.[40]

In late 1624, as terror reigned supreme among Donglin circles, the old physician Miao Xiyong quietly returned to his hometown of Changshu to attend to some family affairs.[41] While there, he conversed with Mao Fengbao (1599–1659, who later changed his name to Mao Jin), the young heir to a local family related to Miao's lineage. Upon learning that Miao Xiyong had completed a treatise that summed up his understanding of bencao, Mao and a few other young literati offered to help. The resulting text, *Exegesis of the Divine Farmer's Classic of Materia Medica* (*Shennong bencao jing shu*, hereafter *Exegesis*), was released in print in 1625 from Mao's residence in Changshu (figures 3.2a and 3.2b).[42] Just as elite literati prepared their own material remedies at home, private publishing of bencao texts composed by amateur literati would become increasingly common over the seventeenth century.

Miao Xiyong's *Exegesis*: Natural Particulars

Miao Xiyong intended *Exegesis* to be a radical statement on the subject of bencao. The fundamental problem with the official pharmacopeia, in Miao's mind, was that it "talked about how this-is-so without saying why this-should-be-so."[43] Since Tao Hongjing compiled the "collected commentary" (*jizhu*), the corpus of bencao had been constantly expanding as an official pharmacopeia for more than a millennium. Without causal explanations of *why* drugs work the way they do, Miao suggested, the genre of bencao could never go beyond a confusing amalgam of information. Unlike Li Shizhen, Miao had no interest in digging through the several layers of commentary that the corpus of bencao had accrued in the previous centuries, but instead offered a fresh beginning from the ground up. The term *shu* in the title, a word originating from the sense of "dredging a flooded river," connotes an outgoing motion similar to the etymology of "exegesis" (to lead outward). Distinct from the act of adding a commentary (*zhu*) that glosses and ascertains the meaning of a classical text, a shu seeks to bring the hidden meanings of a classical text closer to the reader.[44] The broad coverage of *Bencao gangmu*, Miao reportedly complained to his literati friends, had in fact further "messed up" (*chuanbo*) the subject, rendering it ponderous and lacking in decisive arguments.[45] The *Exegesis*, by contrast, would offer "direct access" (*zhijie*) to the principles with which the Divine Farmer had established the basic rules of pharmacy at the very origin of the genre of bencao.[46]

Published less than three decades after Li Shizhen's *Bencao gangmu*, *Exegesis* discussed only 490 kinds of common drugs in contrast to the 1,892 drugs covered by Li Shizhen and included neither a bibliography nor illustrations. The shortening of bencao also involved departing from the accumulative format of the pharmacopeia. Two densely theoretical chapters preceded the main text, in which Miao laid out his principles of pharmacotherapy. The discussion of each drug had three sections: first, the terse description of the drug in question from the *Divine Farmer's Classic*, followed by a couple of sentences that constituted the "exegesis." Second, Miao included a section called "main indications for mutual reference" (*zhuzhi canhu*), in which each particular substance was applied to the treatment of specific symptoms. A final section called "errors" (*jianwu*) described situations in which the drug should *not* be administered in order to avoid adverse effects. The textual strategies he employed resembled similar exegetical texts to the Confucian classics, and would have been familiar to literati readers of the day.

The agenda of *Exegesis* goes deeper than a simple borrowing of literary styles from neo-Confucian texts. Miao Xiyong's radical reinvention of bencao used the subject of pharmacy to make a statement on the neo-Confucian nature. The importance of the issue is reflected in the first sentence of Miao's preface: "the Way of the nature of drugs is completely recorded in *ben-cao*."[47] Drawing from the cosmic pharmacology of Jin-Yuan physicians (see chapter 1), Miao Xiyong reiterated the metaphysical underpinnings to the nature of things:

> When a Thing is created, Heaven endorses it;
> When a Thing is completed, Earth supports it.
> Heaven gives order, and is in charge of procreation,
> thus Cold, Hot, Warm and Cool, the qi of four seasons circulates there;
> this is Yang.
> Earth condenses matter, and is in charge of substantiation,
> thus Sour, Bitter, Pungent, Salty, Sweet and Balanced, the taste of Five
>   Phases nourishes there;
> this is Yin. . . .
> As a Thing has taste, then it must have qi, and possesses a certain na-
>   ture. This is simply the Way-as-it-is (*ziran zhi dao*).[48]

Here Miao articulates a view of nature (*xing*) that is firmly situated in the neo-Confucian theory of nature, on the one hand, and the basic tenets of correlative cosmology on the other. Unlike Zhu Xi and others who merely alluded to the possibility of knowing the nature of drugs or who used drugs to illustrate their doctrines, Miao Xiyong vowed to investigate the "way-as-it-is" so that the true teachings of bencao could be explained with two primary qualities, qi and taste, that in turn corresponded to the ordering cosmic forces (the dyad yin/yang, and the five phases). All data had to fit into a coherent pattern.

The entry on rhubarb (*dahuang*), for example, exemplifies Miao's procedure of exegesis for individual drugs. First, he quoted the basic qualities of rhubarb from the *Divine Farmer's Classic of Materia Medica*:

> *Rhubarb. Taste: bitter. Qi: Cold. Exceedingly Cold. Not Poisonous.*

He then listed all the "main indications" for rhubarb that Tao Hongjing recorded in his *Collected Commentary*:

> Main indications: Purges congested blood [1].
>   Stops blood flow and fever [2].

Breaks abdominal bumps and stagnated liquid and food in bowels [3].
Raids and cleanses stomach and bowels [4].
Purges the old and to generate the new. Facilitates passage of water
　　and grains [5].
Mediates the inner body, facilitates digestion, harmonizes the Five Or-
　　gans [6].
Pacifies the stomach and brings the qi down [7].
Gets rid of phlegm (tan), congested heat amongst the bowels [8].
Treats swelling and fullness in chest and abdomen [9].
Treats women's obstructed menses, swelling lower abdomen, and
　　misc. stagnation of stale blood [10].[49]

Disregarding the voluminous commentaries made by later bencao authors, Miao decided to work only with the basic qualities, so as to explain why the ten recorded indications should work as claimed in the *Classic*. Miao deduced that its "very cold" qi, "just like" the corresponding motion of descending air in winter, necessarily led its pharmacological action to push downward, achieving metabolic renewal through a forceful purge (*tui chen zhi xin*). Rhubarb's "bitter" taste, in turn, matches it to the heavy yin endowment, which creates a higher affinity toward the visible, material flow of blood vessels. In this way, he was able to link rhubarb's nature to the main claims 1–3 recorded in the bencao. The rest, he argued, belonged to secondary symptoms that could also be treated with rhubarb, but one had to be careful about the physiological context of the condition. For instance, although claim 6 indicated that rhubarb could be used to "moderate the bowels and facilitate digestion," Miao warned readers that the benefit was only secondary, depending on the primary action of purging. Thus, it should only be administered in situations when the cause behind indigestion was real blockage, not depletion of vital forces.[50]

　　Being no philologist, Miao treated the text of bencao as largely transparent in meaning. When his deductions reached a dead end, he would not hesitate to cast doubt over the authenticity of a sentence. Dried ginger, for instance, was recorded as being able to resolve the vomiting of blood, but Miao decided that since ginger's nature is pungent in taste and warm or hot in its qi formation, the pharmacological action of ginger should always be dissipating (for pharmacological action of the pungent taste, see table 1.1) and warming. There was simply no way for a warm drug like ginger to cure blood vomiting, a sure sign of excessive heat in the body.[51] His approach to bencao strove for a coherence and certainty that sometimes overrode textual evidence.

Miao Xiyong's approach to pharmaceutical objecthood also departed from Jin-Yuan pharmacology (see chapter 1) in his approach to *differences* (*chabie*) and material diversity. No longer content with setting up the basic principles of cosmic correspondence, Miao sought to ascertain their veracity by working through the nature of individual substances. He wondered whether the simple system might, after all, fail to explain everything: Why did some drugs that were bitter and cold have the effect of drying up bodily liquids, while others replenished them? Why could some drugs with a sour taste be cold and others hot in nature?[52] Even more perplexing was the ever-present danger of poisoning, as seemingly benevolent cures like ginseng could do harm when used improperly. As Miao stated in the introductory chapter:

> Medicines are endowed with the idiosyncratic (*pian*) and extreme *qi* of Heaven and Earth. Even the effects of mellow and virtuous supreme drugs, since they still possess idiosyncratic qualities (*pian*), must nevertheless be dangerous. If one uses them in ways inappropriate for their nature, they will inevitably wreak havoc by their idiosyncratic forces.[53]

It was therefore not only necessary to explicitly explain the "virtues" of drugs, but also to warn people of their potential harm. There was no inherent distinction between medicine and poison, or good and bad natures, but all things were idiosyncratic and could exert opposite effects depending on the context.

Miao Xiyong's usage of the term *pian* (unbalanced) warrants close attention here. In classical medicine, the issue of pian was most commonly evoked in a pathological context, indicating a loss of balance among the vital forces residing in various organs.[54] In the *Inner Canon*, for instance, it was written that the consumption of each of the five flavors would feed into one of five main organs to which it corresponded (see table 1.1). When the intake became imbalanced (eating too much of one flavor over others), one organic system would prevail over others and become pathological over time.[55] Wang Bing (fl. 762–63), an important early medieval commentator on the *Inner Canon*, glossed the paragraph as follows:

> If the *qi* [derived from ingested food or medicine] accumulates incessantly, the *qi* of certain organs will overwhelm others (*piansheng*) and result in extreme imbalance (*pianjue*). Once an organ falls into an abrupt imbalance, it will result in sudden death.[56]

Overall, the medical discourse of pian denoted a deep anxiety about the stagnation and congestion of vital breath that could result from excessive intake of potent substances. The focus of the gaze fell on the internal balance of the body, not on the substances themselves.[57]

Miao Xiyong's explanation of the pathologies of imbalance, however, turns the focus of discussion outward to the metaphysical makeup of drugs. The term *pianxing* (imbalanced nature) clearly derived from the neo-Confucian context as we have seen earlier this chapter. According to Zhu Xi's hierarchical notion of nature, humans were ranked on top of all other creatures as possessing the most complete (*quan*) nature. Yet the nature of things was not categorically different, but merely less complete (hence pian) along a spectrum. Humans and nonhuman creatures thus saw in each other partial familiarity instead of absolute otherness.

Building upon the schools of thought that emphasized the interconnected nature of people and the world, Miao Xiyong used his *Exegesis* to document the *differences* in the nature of drugs that, he argued, offered the key insight to achieve excellence in medicine. By blurring the boundary between benign and poisonous pharmacological actions, Miao pointed out that the pian nature of each medicine should be grasped in the specific circumstances of the creature's life history. It is in this sense that I translated pianxing in Miao's bencao as "idiosyncratic" instead of "unbalanced nature."[58] An endlessly diverse mixture of creative forces gave rise to the diversity of things, which then lent themselves to be used as medicines. They were, in other words, natural particulars.[59]

According to one sympathetic recollection, Miao Xiyong in his prime years often dined with luminaries of the Donglin Academy. As the party went on into the late night and everyone became a little drunk, Miao would stand up and give passionate speeches about the lost teachings of the Divine Farmer and the moral degeneration of the present age. If anything, argued Miao, the medical classics and bencao might be the most certain textual remnants from which to retrieve the lost teachings of antiquity. He would then admonish the illustrious guests for failing to change the status quo, and, upon hearing this reproach, the guests would all shed tears of remorse and weep loudly.[60]

The intersection between a master physician's career and a political movement's most spectacular moments of triumph and defeat in the person of Miao Xiyong is no coincidence. Miao articulated the agenda for a new type of bencao that was tailored to scholarly interests at a time of deep conviction in, and public display of, moral certainty. Despite their militant commitments to reform court politics, the Donglin partisans failed to prevail over their opponents. At heart still an esoteric magician, Miao Xiyong impressed them not only with his display of medical virtuosity, but with his promised mastery over the nature of drugs. *Exegesis* summed up this message in its explication of particular natures: the capacity for pharmacological action became a microcosmic reenactment of the capacity for moral action; the diversity of matter a direct metaphor for the diversity of humanity. Despite the immediate defeat and persecution of Donglin partisans, this sentiment would last well into the final years of Ming rule.

Discourses and Lectures: The Social Milieu of Late Ming Literati Science

The exegetical analysis presented in Miao Xiyong's reinvention of bencao was not, to be sure, a solitary endeavor. According to one anecdote, Miao worked through the most difficult passages of *Exegesis* while traveling on a boat, accompanied by his closest disciples.[61] Mao Fengbao, the young literatus in Changshu who published *Exegesis*, saw the book as imparting the greatest benefit to people with "middling talent and above" (*zhongren yi shang zhi zi*), just like himself.[62] Mao's comment suggested a moment of generational shift: If the senior, founding members of the Donglin partisans found direct inspiration from Miao Xiyong's inquiry into the nature of drugs, what options did the younger and "middling" members of their lineages have, in the wake of the turbulent partisan politics of the 1620s?

One answer was that the surviving followers of Donglin did not have to wait very long for their revenge. In 1627, a new emperor, Chongzhen, was sympathetic to the Donglin cause and reinstated many Donglin partisans to office, after ordering Wei Zhongxian to commit suicide. The conflict between Wei's former allies and the Donglin lingered through the 1630s and 1640s, and proactive literati in Jiangnan organized new associations (*she*) to rally support and voice their political agenda.[63] It may seem, then, as if the political participation and activism of the late sixteenth century persisted unabated as the younger generation came of age.

A closer look at post-Donglin cultural life suggests that there was more to the story. While the traumatic experience of the 1620s may have further galvanized some to fight back, it also encouraged others to seek fulfillment and purpose elsewhere, away from factional struggles at court. This resulted in the growth of private scholarship and cultural reproduction, a trend that would survive the dynastic transition after 1644. One example we have already encountered is Mao Fengbao (later known by the name Mao Jin). Having tried his hand at private publishing with Miao Xiyong's *Exegesis* and a couple of literary anthologies, Mao refashioned himself with a new studio name, *Jigu ge* (Pavilion of Inspiration from Antiquity), and vowed to propagate Confucian erudition by publishing a wide range of texts. Over the next twenty years, Mao published complete sets of the *Thirteen Confucian Classics* and *Twenty-One Dynastic Histories*, as well as reprints of several hundred rare Song-Yuan philosophical and literary texts, all the while without seeking public office.[64] This severance between the pursuit of learning and participation in governance would have been severely admonished a century ago by neo-Confucian statesmen like Qiu Jun. The sacred, integral curriculum taught by *Daxue*, one that began with the cultivation of the self and eventually led up to the pacification of the world, fractured along an emerging fault line that demarcated the private and the public lives of literati elite. This process of fissure had already become quite pronounced before the Qing conquest in the mid-1640s.

The privatization of learning, increasingly estranged from the official sphere, also sustained amateur interest in the field of bencao. Many bencao authors of the 1620s and 1630s were not political activists. Instead, we detect in their works a willingness to build social circles around the common love of "natural" studies in the neo-Confucian sense. Within these circles, the articulation of personal experience came to be validated as a reliable source of good knowledge.

In 1624, a young scholar named Ni Zhumo completed a treatise titled *Collected Discourse of Bencao* (*Bencao huiyan*). Ni was descended from a prominent Jiangnan literati clan; a grand uncle of his, Ni Yuanlu (1593–1644, jinshi 1622), wrote a preface for his nephew's bencao. Describing Zhumo as a "quiet man who loves antiquity," Ni Yuanlu expressed none of the skepticism in Luo Wenying's preface quoted at the beginning of this chapter. Ni Yuanlu would go on to hold high office in the Chongzhen reign, lobbying hard for revenge on the former enemies of Donglin, and die at the eve of the fall of Beijing in 1644.[65] Once a diligent student who "buried his head in preparing for the civil service examination" (*mai shou changwu*), Ni Zhumo lived the rest of his life degreeless. He was remembered, along with other medical physicians in the local gazetteer, as someone "quiet in nature" (*xing chenmo*) with a "love for antiquity" (*haogu*).[66] His bencao was published posthumously in 1645 by his son.

Lacking a track record in an official career, the text of his bencao therefore remains the only source through which we can recover any information about Ni Zhumo's life. In it, Ni agreed with Miao Xiyong in criticizing Li Shizhen's systematic reorganization of the pharmacopeia as lacking in scholarly rigor. He also believed in the possibility of understanding the nature of drugs through rigorous reasoning.[67] Yet the most remarkable feature of this text is the social character of the "collected discourse." To compose this book, Ni Zhumo traveled "through cities and markets, and over the quiet and hidden mountain valleys," seeking out experts and texts on the subject of bencao. Altogether, he consulted more than a hundred interlocutors (including scholars, physicians, and learned monks) and compiled these exchanges into written form. Of the people he interviewed, he acknowledged twelve as mentors (*shizi*), among whom Miao Xiyong ranked in third place. He also listed 136 fellow scholars (*tongshe*), whose names and hometowns he carefully recorded. Ni considered them all "remarkable Confucian scholars active during the Wanli reign, also deeply learned in medicine."[68] The majority of these people were from the Lower Yangzi area, although some did hail from the north and west. The book shows that in late Ming times, a common interest in the nature of drugs, rather than familial or political agendas, became a social glue among like-minded literati.

Another hub of scholarly association was Hangzhou, the picturesque provincial capital located on the southern side of the Lower Yangzi Delta (map 0.1 inset). Famous literati and officials, including "many gentlemen of Wulin [Hangzhou]" (*Wulin zhu junzi*) frequented the house of Lu Fu, a man who held no degrees and never pursued an official career. The Lu family apparently enjoyed enough respect and prosperity that Lu Fu became known for his generosity toward students of medicine and the advancement of this art. His son Lu Zhiyi inherited a love for medicine and Buddhism. In his own recollection, Lu Zhiyi described how he used to sit quietly at the lectures hosted by his father, listening to scholars debating difficult issues in classical medicine and Mahayana Buddhism. One day, the usually reticent Lu Zhiyi stood up and, to everyone's surprise, posed a string of sharp and challenging questions to a senior guest, challenging the latter to yield the lectern to him. After that, Lu Zhiyi's fame as a real prodigy soon exceeded that of his father's, and they started to collaborate on a new treatise of bencao.[69]

Lu Fu and Lu Zhiyi both had high praise for Li Shizhen's *Bencao gangmu*, which they used as a systematic collection of relevant sources. They were also familiar with Miao Xiyong's *Exegesis* and frequently referred to it. Unlike Miao, who led a peripatetic life in the Lower Yangzi region, the Lu family used their Hangzhou home as a stable venue to develop a wide-ranging network of bencao scholars. After Lu Fu passed away, Lu Zhiyi continued to work on their bencao and tested his ideas through public debate, all the while treating patients who were attracted by his growing fame.[70] His bencao manuscript, a philosophical treatise infused with Chan Buddhist terms, was near completion in the early 1640s, and the carving of woodblocks for publishing started in earnest at his home studio in Hangzhou.

If we were to eavesdrop on one of the lectures held at the Lu house in the 1630s, we might overhear a conversation like this:

> GUEST: As far as I can see, bamboo grows leaves in Year One, becomes lush in Year Two, dense in Year Three, emaciates in Year Four, then becomes further sparse in Year Five before it dies in Year Six. How can there be such thing as flowering every sixty years?
>
> YI [LU ZHIYI]: The ancient author meant that the bamboo root could live for a Sexagenary Cycle, not just referring to the growth and death of one stalk.
>
> GUEST: Bamboo has knots as soon as it is born. How is it that its growth fits the seasonal cycle?
>
> YI: Bamboo prepares its bud in mid-winter, grows out in mid-spring, changes its leaves in mid-summer, and elongates its root in mid-autumn—how clear is its seasonal punctuation! "Growth" should not be understood merely as penetration of the earth.[71]

In his manuscript, Lu recorded this conversation in the entry for the bamboo plant, under the section he called "Meditation" (can). Here, the "guest" questioned Lu about the literal meanings of the *Divine Farmer's Classic*, and Lu managed to find a plausible explanation in this case.

Compared to Miao Xiyong's concise prose in *Exegesis,* Lu Fu and Lu Zhiyi showed a stronger interest in incorporating an additional body of literary and nonmedical sources in their metaphysical speculations. The Tang-Song bencao pharmacopeia juxtaposed literary sources with medical instructions but never rigorously cross-examined them. Lu Zhiyi, however, considered the philological study of names (ming) as containing the key to elucidating the nature of drugs.[72] On the question of bamboo leaves, for instance, he speculates that:

> Bamboo is a thing that has sinews and knots. That is why the characters for "sinew" (jin) and "knot" (jie) both have a bamboo radical.

Lu Zhiyi rejoiced in the abundance of signs in the world. In one move, he conflated the actual bamboo plant with the character for "bamboo," which in turn appeared as a signifying part in composite characters that meant "sinew" and "knot":

> Bamboo has knots on the stalk, and its branches grow out from the knots. The knot repeats itself after three branching points, just like three five-day periods makes up of a solar period (*jie*). Therefore, bamboo cures the overflow of *qi* caused by loss of punctual rhythm, or anxiety brought by overly rigid sinews.

There are still more ways in which the characteristics of the bamboo plant can be deciphered and associated with its medicinal properties:

> Its fruit is conducive to divinity, and lightens the body, because bamboo blooms into flowers every sixty years, that is a full cycle of stem-branch combinations.

Here the number sixty, significant due to the sexagenary cycle that contained a complete run of combinations between the ten heavenly stems and the twelve earthly branches of the Chinese calendar, assumed the added meaning of divine perfection. By eating the rare fruit of bamboo, Lu imagined that it would return a body's tired and turgid constitution to tranquility.

Aside from abundant nonmedical textual references, Lu also drew much from his own observation. In the section called "Verification" (*he*), Lu went beyond descriptions of morphology in bencao pharmacopeias and emphasized the importance of looking (*kan*), for important signs that suggested the nature of drugs might be hidden in plain sight. In the entry for the calamus plant (*changpu*), Lu observed that:

> Its leaves begin to grow from within the stalk, and therefore one can discern its opening effect on the heart vessels. The twisted shape of its stalk and branches is a perfect match for the shape of the conduits that wrap around the heart. All such various methods of discerning a drug's indications must be understood through morphology (*shengcheng*). This is not only to elucidate the supreme principle, but also to articulate the method of looking (*kan fa*).[73]

Lu's hermeneutics of bencao thus oscillated between texts and senses, resorting to correlative thinking and numerology as he saw fit. The free-flowing associations he made in conversations were designed to impress his interlocutors. In response to a visitor's accusation that he was "deliberately seeking strange explanations," Lu Zhiyi replied that the "embodied nature and preferences of things" (*wu ti xing qing*) must be grasped through unexpected means of *reading*, lest one be trapped (*fu*) by the most banal meanings of words.[74] The audacity of Lu Zhiyi's bencao allowed him to include direct observation as valid data for the understanding of nature in all its idiosyncratic manifestations. The nature of drugs was not only coherent but also ecstatic.

Li Zhongzi's Integrated Curriculum:
Amateurism and its Discontents

In literati associations, open lectures, and elegant conversations, bencao became a fashionable topic for educated men, especially the generation who came of age in the 1620s and 1630s. The reading and writing of bencao became a respectable pastime, and even occupation. In rhetoric, studying the nature of drugs was considered congruent with the neo-Confucian pursuit of moral truth. Yet in practice, younger literati championed techniques that could safeguard and maintain their own lives, but would not necessarily go on to offer that life for a higher purpose.

The publishing market for bencao texts flourished in the 1620s to 1640s as a result of rising popularity of the subject matter. The original woodblocks of *Bencao gangmu*'s first edition in 1596, which sold poorly at first, were recycled by at least two publishing houses in 1640 to issue new editions with new prefaces.[75] The mid-sixteenth-century bencao primer by Chen Jiamo, originally a plain text with no illustrations, was further expanded with added illustrations in the 1620s. Still fancier editions of dietetic bencao emerged from Suzhou in 1621, cobbled together by Qian Yunzhi, a cultural entrepreneur who declared himself as "having learned no medicine, but good at editorial matters."[76] The rebranding of previous editions, plain plagiarism, and false attribution of authorship abounded in the late Ming decades, as exemplified by Barbara Volkmar's study of physician Wan Quan's bestselling pediatric medical texts.[77] In 1634, a different Suzhou publisher promoted its own dietetic bencao under the fake authorship of Li Shizhen, even fabricating a preface in Li's name, complete with personal seals. The pseudo-Li Shizhen claimed that following on *Bencao gangmu*'s success, he was happy to bring a second volume on dietetics to the reading world. He reassured potential buyers that this volume would help them live well "under all climates, in Chinese or foreign lands . . . roaming about free of worry, with a full belly!"[78]

The alliance between amateur literati and commercial publishing thus created a nexus of wealth and fame unimaginable to authors several decades earlier. The care of the self, nominally the fountainhead of moral behavior, now became an opportunity for achieving celebrity status as a professional author, aesthete, or cultural critic. One of the most successful figures in this age, Chen Jiru (1558–1639), offered another preface for the 1634 edition of the dietetic bencao. In his signature witty prose, Chen declared himself an "old gourmet" (*laotao*), and cajoled the reader to appreciate the importance of bencao:

> Physicians (*yi*) are those who control people's lives. Rather than entrusting my life to their whims, why not take my fate into my own hands? Everyday needs and dietetics are indeed a realm where I am in charge. If you know the true flavors, you will know temperance; knowing temperance, your body and mind will be both fine.[79]

Two seemingly contradictory rationales are at work in marketing this new dietetic bencao: on the one hand, the fake authorship of Li Shizhen invoked medical authority; on the other hand, however, the more immediate appeal of the book resided in the promise of a worry-free, well-fed life, where one would "take one's fate in his own hands." The appreciation of beauty extended to bencao as well; in 1640, Qian Weiqi, one of the most resourceful publishers in Hangzhou, reprinted the Jiangxi edition (1603) of *Bencao gangmu* with newly carved illustrations.[80] In his preface, Qian praised their artisans' dexterity and masterful depiction of plants and animals, so much so that this new edition would "revitalize" Li's work.[81] Talking candidly about the capital he invested in bencao, Qian sought to inject pleasure and beauty into the scholarly inquiry of the nature of things.

The flourishing market of medical texts benefited more than amateur literati authors. In 1618, another medical treatise enjoyed quick success, possibly owing to its elegant title, *Subtle Discourses on the Preservation of Life* (*Yisheng weilun*). The author, Li Zhongzi (1588–1655), however, did not wax lyrical on the pleasures of life. Li had grown up in a military garrison located at the tip of the Yangzi Delta, near modern-day Shanghai. His ancestors had been re-located there as soldiers when Zhu Yuanzhang founded the Ming dynasty. His grandfather and uncles were officers killed in pirate battles in the mid-1550s; his father, orphaned at a young age, studied hard for both civil and military examinations and aspired to greatness, only to take ill and die shortly after winning the coveted jinshi degree in 1589.[82] Still a boy, Li Zhongzi took the loss to heart and became determined to study medicine well.

Despite its reference to the cultivation of the self, *Subtle Discourses on the Preservation of Life* posited the centrality of a "medical orthodoxy" (*yizong*) that set forth a standard reading list for students of medicine. His list of "medical lineages" only endorsed the Divine Farmer as the first author of bencao, while leaving out the numerous commentators on later pharmacopeias. In a short chapter devoted to the subject of pharmacy, Li selected only 140 drugs, insisting that "abundance begets confusion" (*fan ze huo*).[83] In other words, Li attempted to dissociate the orthodoxy of medicine from the all-encompassing corpus of bencao and to exert some control over which parts of the pharmacopeia were deemed relevant for a practicing physician.

Shortly after the success of *Subtle Discourses*, Li produced a second popular text, this time dedicated to the subject of pharmacy. In 1622, *Explanation of the Nature of Drugs* (*Yaoxing jie*) was published by Qian Yunzhi, the same man who aggressively marketed dietetic bencao. Picking up on the long-lasting popularity of Jin-Yuan pharmacology primers, Qian packaged Li's text as a modern gloss on the well-known *Rhymes on the Nature of Drugs* (see chapter 1) and an accompaniment to the *Master Thunder* manuals on pharmaceutical processing. Li's new commentary, wrote Qian, was superior to the "abundant imprints on pharmacology" in that it was thorough in its explanation and yet short and comprehensive.[84] In his own preface, Li lamented the degree to which medicine had degenerated since ancient times. "Confucians like to self-aggrandize" (*ru zhe hao zi zhangda*), he wrote, "and put physicians into the Nine Currents [of minor professions]."[85] How can one expect effective cures if physicians were so dismissed and disrespected?

The difference between Li Zhongzi and Miao Xiyong belied an important issue in the diversification of bencao works in early seventeenth century. Both men claimed no direct lineage from a medical master, dabbled in Buddhism and esoteric arts, and established their reputations as effective physicians by treating patients in literati families. Miao Xiyong in the 1620s had already enjoyed a highly prominent career among the Donglin partisans and targeted his *Exegesis* at young literati readers, such as Mao Fengbao, who took delight in complexity and subtle discussions about the nature of things. In contrast, Li Zhongzi was an up-and-coming young author who hailed from a military lineage and never fully identified with the values of scholar-officials. He took the thwarted political career of his father as evidence of the perils of officialdom and quickly identified himself as the new champion of medical orthodoxy. His prolific writings appealed to a wider audience with simple, transparent prose, always limiting the scope of his pharmacy treatises to a small number of 200–

300 drugs. Later in 1637, Li repeated the message more explicitly with another treatise titled *Must Reads for the Medical Orthodoxy* (*Yizong bidu*).[86] In this way, he was able to bring the haughty literati to his heels, their "boats and carriages ceaselessly docked at his door."[87]

As I have discussed in the introduction, the possibility of Confucian amateurism depended on the depoliticization of other professions (according to Yang Xiong, "artisans do not comprehend human affairs"). Late Ming times witnessed a further assertion by Confucian literati to prove that they were, in fact, better than technical experts in their professional domains. The aggressive refashioning of bencao according to neo-Confucian theories of nature allowed amateurs to claim authority over the science of pharmacy. Li Zhongzi's message posed a critical stance toward the free-wheeling demonstration of virtuosity by Miao Xiyong and other amateur authors. If, based on a deep understanding of the nature of drugs, anyone could invent and propose new treatments and interpretations that had never existed before, what, then, would be the difference between an expert healer and an amateur philosopher?

In the end, however, the reality of the 1630s and 1640s was that neither amateur literati nor technical experts could derive much effective power in public affairs from their knowledge. We hear angry protests from others at this time—for example, the Jiangxi local educator Song Yingxing's frustration over the unfulfilled transformative potential of technology.[88] For all his success in becoming a bestselling author, Li Zhongzi also complained that while he saw himself as more than someone with "expert skills" (*zhuanmen xue*), his own success had confined him in the narrow image of a master physician. Like his father, he sometimes dreamed of using his knowledge to "investigate Heaven and Humanity, meditate on the hidden secrets of Zen, and consult in affairs of state," and yet people "held my arms and forced me" in exchange for "a small dose of drugs."[89] We might well see the downfall of the Ming in 1644 as a result of the prolonged impasse over the legitimate ownership of technical knowledge.

PART II

4

Virtuosity and Orthodoxy

What Heaven has conferred is called Nature;
an accordance with this nature is called The Path of Duty;
the regulation of this path is called Instruction.[1]

—ZHONGYONG (*DOCTRINE OF THE MEAN*)

FANG YIZHI (1611–71) was from a prestigious lineage of scholar-officials in Tongcheng County. Growing up in 1630s Jiangnan, Fang was closely involved in political activism through literati associations. In 1640, he obtained the highest degree in the civil examinations and earned a coveted official position in the Hanlin Academy. While in Beijing, Fang was nevertheless haunted by the dynasty's uncertain political prospects and his own intellectual perplexities.[2] He pursued two paths simultaneously, leading to the completion of two written works: a long, annotated dictionary titled *Comprehensive Refinement* (*Tongya*), and a shorter treatise, *Notes on the Principle of Things* (*Wuli xiaoshi*).

Medicine, and pharmacy in particular, occupied Fang's attention in both works, and he engaged with the tradition of bencao according to two distinct methodologies. First, in *Comprehensive Refinement*, Fang collected thousands of names and dissected the origin, variations, and classical references of each term, drawing from bencao as only one of many textual sources. To do so, he paid particular attention to the phonology and orthography of ancient times and showcased the power of philological research. In *Notes on the Principle of Things*, however, Fang started from the neo-Confucian premise of cosmic unity and worked his way through the affairs of Heaven, Earth, humanity, and (nonhuman) things. Three out of twelve chapters dealt with subjects pertaining to medicine, including human anatomy, general medicine, and pharmacy.

Fang discussed the nature of drugs in particular in one essay he included in the "General Discourses" (*zonglun*) for *Notes on the Principle of Things*. Reviewing the bencao literature's historical origin as product of "imperial power" and collaboration between "famous physicians and official historians," Fang marveled at the recent developments in the genre, praising in particular Li Shizhen's erudition, Miao Xiyong's concision (*jian*), and Li Zhongzi's judiciousness (*zhe*).[3] By declaring that "everything is a medicine" at the outset (see the quote at the beginning of the introduction to this book), Fang aligned himself with the surging interest in using bencao to study "natural particulars"—to comprehend the nature of individual drugs as a source of knowledge and action.

Fang Yizhi's two-pronged approach to the understanding of things revealed a moment of uncertainty and tentativeness, as if he were experimenting with these methods to determine which one was better. The belief in the unity of man and the world, of knowledge and action presented in sixteenth-century neo-Confucian works such as those of Qiu Jun and Deng Yuanxi, had met grave challenges in the downward trajectory of the dynasty. The rise and persistence of Donglin-style political activism, as mirrored in the exegetical maneuvers of Miao Xiyong, claimed to have found lost truth in antiquity. It is no coincidence that many bencao authors in the 1620s and 1630s (such as Ni Zhumo and Lu Zhiyi) were remembered for their "love of antiquity" (*haogu*). For these people, as well as the new generation of cultural entrepreneurs such as Mao Jin, the love of antiquity was still inseparable from the epistemic optimism that one could indeed fathom a cosmic unity behind the myriad effects of pharmaceutical substances and derive meaningful action from them. Writing around the year 1640, Fang Yizhi still insisted on fathoming the "supreme principle" (*zhili*) from "the norms of things" (*wuze*). Yet he also harbored no illusions about the challenges of explaining the differences (*chabie*) among things: the known data of bencao was replete with errors and might not be a reliable guide after all.[4] A more systematic reconfiguration of knowledge was inevitable.

The Ming dynasty was under siege on all fronts as soldiers turned into murderous rebels, invading one province after another. On the northeastern front, the threat from the Manchu Qing regime mounted as Ming forces could not hold on to territories beyond the Shanhai Pass. Fang Yizhi's tenure at the peak of Ming civil officialdom did not last very long: in 1644, Beijing fell to the rebel leader Li Zicheng, who would, in turn, be defeated by Qing forces the following year. When the young Manchu ruler ascended the throne as the Shunzhi emperor of the Qing dynasty, Fang Yizhi headed south to serve in multiple regional courts of Ming princes, only to lose hope for restoration and go into hiding as a tonsured Buddhist monk. He roamed the coastal region and the deep mountains of the war-torn far south, bringing manuscripts of *Comprehensive Erudition* and *Notes on the Principle of Things* with him and making notes for revisions.

In the published version of *Notes on the Principle of Things*, we can see many of Fang's post-1644 notes that reveal the transformative effect of exile. Stripped of his book collection and thousands of miles away from the imperial library, Fang saw and touched many novelties he had not even heard of before. In the far south, he saw tropical plants that grew in winter and matured in spring. He smelled tiger fat preserved by hunters. He investigated the peanut plant, which he called "foreign bean flower" (*fan dou hua*), and wondered how it could have seeds grown under the soil.[5] He learned to identify regional varieties of herbs that came from the southwestern provinces Yunnan and Guizhou and briefly engaged in the pharmaceutical trade himself. The metaphor of pharmacy permeated other philosophical works he composed in his late years.[6] Overall, Fang seemed concerned less with finding out how the nature of drugs exercised its power in general, and more with the experience of discovering exotic cures and applying them.

Hailing from an elite gentry family in Jiangnan, which set him up for success in the civil service examination and an official career, Fang Yizhi ended his life in an exile that also brought him into contact with the frontier and the market town. The trajectory of Fang's life prompts us to consider the complex impetus for intellectual change as an immediate consequence of dynastic transition. In his influential study of Fang's later life, Yu Ying-shih characterized his pre-Conquest works as exemplifying the tendency of late Ming Confucian learning to "move from the abstract to the concrete" (*she xu jiu shi*), and his post-Conquest philosophical writings as "tracing the abstract without abandoning the concrete."[7] The case of Fang's interest in pharmacy in both his pre- and post-1644 works, however, suggests a consistent interest in the concrete materiality of things marked by a shift in epistemic strategy: before the conquest, Fang joined others in believing in the validity of systematic deductions based on correlative cosmology. During exile, he took an "empiricist" approach to sensory data and personal experience, to use Ya Zuo's characterization of the Song polymath Shen Gua's intellectual dissention back in the eleventh century.[8] The political activism that Fang espoused in his youth had come to naught; his written works would continue to be read for centuries. We will encounter him again in the next two chapters.

War-induced trauma and displacement during the Ming-Qing transition not only shaped Fang Yizhi's late works but also the lives of countless less-privileged individuals. With the Qing reforms in government and culture came a parallel, albeit less pronounced, reconfiguration of natural studies within Confucian learning. The centrality of pharmacy and the nature of drugs in the pre-Conquest years also came under intense questioning in postwar decades. In a move that was hardly premeditated, the Qing rulers found themselves in the company of new allies from the elite strata of literati and physicians who were championing a new approach to the field of bencao.

Continuities and Change in Early Qing Bencao

When news of the Ming house's dramatic fall reached the south, Ni Zhumo, the introvert scholar who visited many provinces to compile his bencao, had long died and left his young widow to raise their son through famine and war. Remarkably, Ni's bencao got published in the midst of political chaos in 1645.[9] In Hangzhou, one of the regional courts set up by Ming princes, the recluse Lu Zhiyi seized the opportunity to offer himself in the service of Prince Lu and obtained a minor official title. Yet when the Qing forces approached Hangzhou after capturing Nanjing in 1645, Lu Zhiyi went into hiding, and when he returned, it was to find his home and estate in ruins, and the carved woodblocks of his bencao destroyed. Lu was able to quickly recover half the manuscript and put the incomplete manuscript to print in 1647. The once boisterous lectures and intense debates on the nature of drugs were over for good; Lu spent the rest of his life at home, blind and bedridden, tended to by his filial daughter-in-law.[10]

Across the Hangzhou Bay in Changshu, Mao Jin, who commanded great respect as a scholarly publisher, managed to protect his estate and negotiate a peaceful handover of the county to Qing forces. Toward the end of his life, Mao wrote a poem to commemorate the first book he ever published—Miao Xiyong's *Exegesis*—praising the electrifying moments of Miao's bencao lectures.[11] After Mao's death in 1659, his immense collection of books and carved woodblocks was dispersed by auction and theft among various Jiangnan collectors.

New provincial administrators appointed by Qing authorities continued, for a brief period of time, the practice of issuing new reprints of bencao pharmacopeias. Zhang Chaolin, a veteran commander of Qing forces back in the 1630s, commissioned a new edition of *Bencao gangmu* after assuming the governor-generalship of Jiangxi, where the carved woodblocks of the 1603 edition were stored. Also in the 1650s, Jiangnan commercial publishers recovered from wartime disruption and issued new illustrated editions of *Bencao gangmu*, ensuring the text's continued availability in print throughout the next centuries.[12] Dietetic bencao remained popular, inviting literati readers to savor the goodness of life and overcome traumatic memories of the dynastic transition.

Away from the main battlegrounds, Liu Ruojin (jinshi 1625), a retired official living in his hometown Qianjiang County in central Huguang, spent the rest of his life composing a thirty-two-volume treatise titled *Bencao shu* (*Narrating Materia Medica*). The densely written ontological speculations and correlative inferences echoed Miao Xiyong, Lu Zhiyi, and other late Ming authors. Liu's son, who served under the Qing as a magistrate, published the text to little fanfare, suggesting that this mode of inquiry had gone out of fashion by the 1690s.[13]

During the war, the physician Li Zhongzi lodged with his patrons and continued to teach medicine. His fame soared in the postwar decades, and Li continued to publish medical treatises written in his signature concise and accessible style. One last set of three treatises was published in 1667, combining instructions on diagnostics, etiology, and pharmacy, testifying to the success of Li's insistence on an integrated curriculum of medicine, with pharmacy prominently featured but never separated from discussions of disease. With his explicit consent, some of Li's disciples imitated his style and openly attacked the legacy of Miao Xiyong.[14] Li's late works were so popular that, in 1678, a new edition was funded by the grandson of Wu Sangui, a former Ming general who had surrendered to the Manchus and was now leading an open rebellion against the Qing. In a roundabout fashion, Li Zhongzi found the subtle balance between asserting his own virtuosity and teaching a standard curriculum.[15]

The scattered evidence presented above suggests that the appeal of bencao persisted in the peculiar intellectual climate of post-Conquest Jiangnan. At the same time, a critical reassessment of pre-Conquest bencao, in particular Miao Xiyong's expansive approach toward a deep understanding of the nature of drugs, started to emerge among Li Zhongzi's circles and beyond. One of the most outspoken critics of Miao Xiyong's bencao was a physician named Yu Chang (1585–1664). Hailing from a humble background in Jiangxi, Yu Chang was known for his eccentric manners early on. Yu took the civil examinations repeatedly without success, yet when he was finally recommended for office, he relinquished the opportunity in a cynical gesture. He also dabbled in monastery life as a Buddhist monk but then abruptly quit.[16] While his behavior resembled that of Miao Xiyong in many ways, Yu was unable to achieve the same prestige and respect as the latter until the postwar years, when he traveled to Changshu—Miao's hometown—to seek the patronage of the remaining luminaries there, many of whom were Donglin sympathizers and knew Miao Xiyong's work very well.

Even before the conquest, Yu Chang had been attacking amateurism in medicine in his writings. The only way to achieve excellence, wrote Yu, was to engage in deep thinking and intuitive understanding based on personal experience. Yu abhorred the notion that one could ever grasp the principles of medicine by merely reading. Many such self-styled "Confucian physicians" (ruyi), observed Yu, were in fact just mediocre scholars who had no other career option but to seek profit in medical practice.[17] Rather, the physician should practice inward meditation (neizhao), which would allow the physician to think, feel, and empathize with the patient to the extent of "transforming one's own body into theirs."[18] Virtuosity was not meant to be easy.

Yu Chang's medical works spanned a wide range of topics, but the critical focus on pharmacy remained a consistent theme. Texts, especially those that advocated for the expedient use of drugs, were not to be trusted too quickly. With an acerbic tone he pointed out how "everybody rushed to get a copy" of Miao Xiyong's Exegesis, without realizing that all it offered was grandiose talk on the nature of drugs that served only to impress the readers. It was lamentable that people only read books in search of ready-made recipes (fang), wrote Yu, and that "books without recipes" such as the Inner Canon received scant attention. Difficult books were shunned in favor of explicit instructions for how to use drugs. All the abridged bencao, rhymed primers, and promises of causal explanation in books like Exegesis, argued Yu, made the art of medicine look cheap. Worse, the proliferation of pharmacy texts resulted in a decisive shift of discourse in clinical encounters: Should we not blame them that doctors and patients nowadays "only discuss drugs but not diseases" (yi yao bu yi bing)?[19]

Yu Chang remained active as a physician after the Qing conquest of South China, residing in Changshu until his death in the 1670s.[20] Despite his open attack on Miao Xiyong's bencao, Yu in fact concurred with the latter's claim about the sanctity of an ancient tradition of pharmacy. His objection targeted Miao's discursive strategy of making the nature of drugs accessible and easy to comprehend. For Yu, the proliferation of medical discourses "adulterated sagely knowledge with vulgar knowledge, like sewing beautiful silk with broken wadding."[21] His late work, titled *Rules and Commandments for the School of Medicine* (*Yimen falü*), set up a rigorous regimen that sought to train a physician's body and mind. Borrowing the strict commandments (*lü*) practiced by Buddhist clergy in monasteries, Yu Chang envisioned a medical profession with similar aspirations for discipline and compliance with a moral code. The lack of focus and permissive speculation that characterized the late Ming bencao had put it at odds with his vision. It is telling that throughout this treatise, which was organized according to different etiological conditions, Yu Chang made no reference to the bencao pharmacopeia. For him, the hierarchy between a well-trained physician and patient ought to be absolute, and there should be no more grounds for dispute over the prescription of drugs. Virtuosity was to be tamed under orthodoxy.

Regularity Prevailed

Yu Chang's austere call to reestablish medical authority should be understood against the background of a dramatically enlarged pool of practitioners in postwar Jiangnan. An "enlightened physician" named Zhang Lu, who resided in Suzhou, described the breakdown of preexisting boundaries during wartime.[22] In the midst of displacement and misery, wrote Zhang, patients "did not get to pick their physicians," and practitioners practiced at will, defying previous divisions between specialties such as internal and external medicine, or pediatrics and gynecology. As a result, all sorts of illnesses came to be treated by the same practitioners. The implication, then, was a rising demand for integrated medical training and a unified ethics for all who practiced this art. Second, Zhang also noticed, not without a dose of sarcasm, how "Confucian gentlemen of elevated status" (*rulin shangda*) quit official careers and "deigned to set their mind" (*jiangzhi*) on medicine. Zhang, who started practicing in the 1630s when he was just teenager, observed the swelling ranks of medical practice with disapproval. Yet he too felt compelled to solidify his legacy by way of written words as a response to the Confucianization of medicine in post-Conquest Jiangnan.[23]

At the age of seventy-nine, Zhang Lu prepared to publish his collected treatises, titled *Comprehensive Medicine* (*Yitong*), with the help of his descendants. Covering a wide range of topics from comments on the *Inner Canon* to specialized treatments in ophthalmology and smallpox, Zhang was determined to emerge as an all-around virtuoso who also rigorously adhered to orthodoxy. In the volume, Zhang chose an appealing title for the chapters on general pharmacy: *Encountering the Origin with the Bencao Classic* (*Benjing fengyuan*).[24]

Toeing the line of the rhetoric of antiquity championed by earlier authors such as Miao Xiyong and Lu Zhiyi, Zhang Lu's bencao nevertheless offered much fresh insight into his contemporary practice in the busy commercial hub of Suzhou. His prescriptive style was remembered as eclectic and flexible. He was enthusiastic about novel cures and modern-day drugs that never appeared in ancient texts, including the so-called swallow's nest (*yanwo*), an exotic tonic drug newly available during Zhang's lifetime (see chapter 6).[25] While Zhang duly quoted the Divine Farmer's original text before offering his own "interpretation" (*faming*), he never explicitly disavowed the contributions of previous commentators but enthusiastically engaged with their opinions. Overall, Zhang's text gives one the feeling that he was constantly distracted by more interesting things beyond his touting of a return to classical antiquity. Zhang Lu explained his view of the relationship between classical studies and medical practice as follows:

> The fact that medicine has *The Divine Farmer's Classic of Materia Medica*, is just like artisans having their own standard measuring tools. Once there is measure, then there are rules; with rules then comes the room for flexibility and innovation. Flexibility and innovation derive from intelligence and dexterity, yet are still grounded in the basic measures.[26]

Here and elsewhere, Zhang Lu stressed that all innovations in medicine derived from a classical core of bencao: the regular use of a small number of materia medica (~300–400), whose truths had already been spelled out in the earliest textual records dating back a millennium. The understanding of the nature of drugs could thus only be achieved through the careful parsing and study of the classics, instead of a comprehensive intuition of the unity of all things. The locus of knowledge was no longer found within the self of the aspiring student, but externalized in the words of the ancient sages.

After all, Zhang Lu wrote what his audience was ready to hear. His argument for a classically rooted medicine ran parallel to a similar turn to classical textual criticism in Confucian learning. The fact that an experienced (and established) physician who was not particularly scholastic in training could affirm this neoclassicist position belies the overwhelming power of orthodoxy in the 1690s. In so doing, Zhang Lu claimed the truth of bencao for a comprehensive curriculum of medicine, and medicine alone.

The most successful work of pharmacy emerged toward the end of the seventeenth century, promoting an eclectic combination of regularity and individual insight. In 1694, *Complete Essentials of Materia Medica* (*Bencao beiyao*) was published as the work of Wang Ang, a native of Huizhou Prefecture who did not practice medicine. Wang Ang's career as a medical author took off in his sixties, when he realized the demand for books that not only shared medical recipes but also *explained* them. Wang gradually built his publishing studio, Huanduzhai, into a successful enterprise that had outlets in multiple cities across the Lower Yangzi region.[27] In the 1690s, Wang set his mind to creating the most definitive book on bencao. With the astute eye of a cultural entrepreneur, Wang reminded the reader that the pharmacopeia-style books like *Bencao gangmu* were too long to master: "reading it always makes me want to lie down and fall asleep."[28] To remedy this situation, Wang borrowed passages from Miao Xiyong's *Exegesis*, especially the best explanatory parts that provided the reader "something meaningful to chew on."[29] *Complete Essentials* was thus designed to be a readable combination of Li Shizhen's erudition and Miao Xiyong's discerning insight, a portable volume that discussed a modest number of 240 common drugs. The first edition of *Complete Essentials* proved so successful that Wang produced a second edition in a mere five years with some expansion, now covering 400 drugs.[30]

If the nature of drugs could be taught as a matter of skillful manipulation of previous accounts, then pharmaceutical processes too witnessed a new round of textualization. In 1704, Zhang Rui, a Confucian physician (*ruyi*) serving in the Imperial Academy of Medicine, compiled a short guide to the handling of materia medica titled *Xiushi zhinan* (*Definitive Guide to the Art of Pharmaceutical Processing*). The text itself was an amalgam of quotes from previous authors, ranging from Master Thunder to Li Shizhen and Chen Jiamo in the sixteenth century, focusing on only about two hundred kinds of materia medica with no illustrations. This short text leaves many puzzles for modern-day historians: Why did Zhang, an experienced medical expert in his own right, not offer any new opinions in this short text with a grand title?[31]

One hint of the text's intentions can be gleaned from Zhang's elaborate discussion of the range of methods employed in the processing of drugs:

> Sometimes one uses (non-medical) ingredients to process drugs;
> Sometimes one uses drugs to process drugs.
> Sometimes hot-natured drugs process cold-natured ones;
> Sometimes moist-natured drugs process dry-natured ones;
> Sometimes slow-acting drugs process fast-acting ones;
> Sometimes benign-natured drugs process poisonous ones;
> Sometimes purgatives process tonics[32]

The list went on for pages. While earlier authors such as Chen Jiamo and Miao Xiyong also liked to display their mastery over a wide range of methods, their terminology had a clear focus on the material processes (roasting, frying, baking, soaking, washing, steaming, etc.) and the specific ingredients (honey, licorice, lard, vinegar, boy's urine). Zhang's account further abstracted these techniques into a language game of warring natures: the process of cultivation (*xiu*) and production (*zhi*) was, in essence, the technique of pitting things of idiosyncratic natures against one another. The moral overtones of pharmaceutical teaching in Zhang's account are hard to miss.

In 1714, another northern physician published a sequel to the *Master Thunder* texts. The preface also aligned pharmaceutical processing (*xiuzhi*) unequivocally with moral instruction (*jiao*) as articulated in the first sentence of *Zhongyong* (*Doctrine of the Mean*), another one of the four books in Zhu Xi's neo-Confucian curriculum:

> Master Zisi said: "What Heaven has conferred is called the Nature (*xing*); an accordance with this nature is called the Path (*dao*) of duty; the regulation of this path is called Instruction (*jiao*)." I say that all pharmacy books are rooted in this principle. How so? The various natures of drugs—Yin and Yang, soft and hard—are conferred by Heaven. If we use their kingly natures, then they can save people; if we unleash their idiosyncratic natures, then they can also kill people. So to adjudicate and supervise them, we need sages who cultivate the Path. . . . The *bencao* books speak to heavenly-conferred nature, whereas the teaching of *Master Thunder* focuses on instruction, that is to say education.[33]

Here we see a fundamental shift in the discussion over the "idiosyncratic nature" (*pianxing*) of pharmaceutical objecthood: the late Ming authors, including Miao Xiyong and Lu Zhiyi, celebrated the potency and diversity of pharmacological action springing from their natures. Here, evoking *Zhongyong*, the early eighteenth-century compilers of pharmaceutical techniques emphasized the need for corrective processing, issued by higher beings who "cultivate the Path." Pharmaceutical expertise therefore became a metaphor for taming the unruly nature of drugs *before* they had a chance to wreak havoc, just like a good Confucian scholar and teacher should concern themselves with the education and disciplining of human nature. Here we see the beginnings of what Andrew Schonebaum has called the "pharmaceutical dramas" of Qing vernacular literature.[34] In these novels and popular plays, idiosyncratic drugs became human characters whose natures were fixed from the beginning; good was meant to prevail over evil, and the hierarchy of moral perfection was transparent for all to see. The nature of drugs, in other words, was transformed into a theater of morals.[35] And in almost every Qing pharmaceutical drama, there presided an emperor of drugs (frequently ginseng) who was always right.

Taming Pharmaceutical Objecthood in the Kangxi Reign

In 1699, the Kangxi emperor embarked on an imperial tour of the southeast for a third time. The rule of the Qing dynasty had never been more secure: in the three decades since Kangxi assumed personal rule at the young age of fourteen, he had held the reins of the empire so successfully that no one seemed capable of posing a credible challenge. He defeated powerful regents at court and rebellious Ming generals in the provinces; he deterred Russian forays into Manchuria through the negotiation of a treaty and vanquished the formidable navy of the Zheng family who occupied Taiwan until 1683. The Manchu emperor proved himself worthy of the Mandate of Heaven through the demonstration of his mastery of all knowledge, from Confucian classics to astronomy and mathematics taught by the Jesuits at court. During his stop at Suzhou, he granted an audience with Zhang Lu's descendants, who presented their father's medical works to the emperor.[36] What would Kangxi do in the realm of medicine?

The early 1700s would prove to be a watershed moment that fundamentally shaped Qing cultural policy during the entire eighteenth century. Having secured their control over not only former Ming territories but also lands beyond, the Manchu elite turned their attention to forging a firm ideological foundation that would justify, once and for all, the legitimacy of their rule over China. Unruly elements among the literati class received stern warnings through high-profile cases of literary inquisition that often resulted in long exiles or the death penalty. At the same time, competition intensified over the recruitment of talent in the highest echelons of power, starting from the imperial court and encompassing the personal entourage of princes, aristocrats, and high officials. Particularly appealing to elite literati was the opportunity to participate in the compilation of the official history of the fallen Ming dynasty. The *Ming History* office opened in 1679, and the complex work of drafting, editing, and printing took sixty years, involving hundreds of scholars with or without formal official titles. In a clear break from Ming times, Kangxi and his successors sought to restore the imperial state's firm command of elite culture.

The imperially sanctioned version of *Ming History* offers a comprehensive review of the accomplishments and shortcomings of the previous dynasty on all fronts. Following previous conventions, the official historians conveyed their verdict through a carefully selected set of individual biographies. The arrangement of these biographies reflected the perceived importance and moral stature of the lives included. The subject matter of medicine fell under the category of formulaic arts (*fangji*), which appeared very late in the whole work, just ahead of illustrious women, eunuchs, evil officials, bandits, native rulers in the southwest, and foreign countries. In a short summary, the historians dismissed the importance of mere "artisans and technicians" (*yiren shushi*) as being incapable of pursuing the "Path of Virtue" (*daode zhi tu*). In their mind, the most extraordinary practitioners were those who could "achieve utmost erudition" from classical books of their trade and "comprehend the principles." Given this rationale, it is no wonder that Li Shizhen earned a place in dynastic history with his *Bencao gangmu* that surpassed previous pharmacopeias in its coverage. Miao Xiyong also received a brief nod for his "deep thinking and analysis" of pharmacy. Overall, however, the biographies were brief and contained obvious errors. The official biography conflated Miao Xiyong's *Exegesis* with another work of his, apparently not bothering to find out the exact title. They also claimed that the Wanli emperor had ordered Li Shizhen's bencao to be transmitted "all around the realm," an act that Li himself had hoped for but never took place.[37] The erroneous assumption rather reflected the new reality under Qing rule, when emperors became much more proactive patrons of elite culture, including scholarly projects that illuminated the fundamental patterns of the universe.

For all his eagerness to embrace science, the Kangxi emperor did not commission a new bencao pharmacopeia, though he came rather close to doing so in 1702. At some point during his reign, the 150-year-old manuscript of the unpublished Ming pharmacopeia, *Bencao pinhui jingyao*, was discovered in the palace collections. Upon examining the richly illustrated work, Kangxi ordered Hesihen, a trusted Manchu bondservant, to take it to the Imperial Academy of Medicine and have a duplicate copy made there. Further, Kangxi also specified that the gaps of knowledge between Liu Wentai's pharmacopeia and Li Shizhen's *Bencao gangmu* should be compiled in an addendum. Two palace physicians started the work immediately, and within a few months a print edition of the ill-fated Ming pharmacopeia was published by the newly established printing house at the Wuying palace, supervised also by Hesihen.[38]

It would be a mistake to see the mere existence of this new edition as the rebirth of pharmacopeia-making at the Qing court. Only two palace physicians—not even the highest-ranking members of the Imperial Academy—participated in the editorial process. There was neither any collaboration with civil officials nor a systematic survey conducted in the provinces.[39] No new imperial endorsement graced its pages, nor did Kangxi follow up with a formal promulgation. In other words, there was to be no new bencao pharmacopeia under the aegis of Qing rule.

The inaction of Kangxi toward bencao could not be explained away by resource constraints or lack of political will to resurrect a cultural tradition. Neither is it satisfactory to blame the Manchu emperor for cutting off a venerable precedent in the Chinese tradition. Rather, we might see Kangxi's decision *not* to pursue another pharmacopeia as nothing more extraordinary than following the consensus of his time: that medicine should be kept separate from Confucian learning. As a result, pharmaceutical objecthood was narrowed down to a small number of materia medica instead of a universal lens through which to explore the larger issues of nature (*xing*) and coherence (*li*). In lieu of bencao, the Kangxi emperor, together with the elite scholars that flocked to the court, chose to follow the other path laid out by Fang Yizhi in *Comprehensive Refinement*: to study the myriad things through historical and philological inquiries. In other words, the separation between natural history and pharmacy—and hence the demise of bencao pharmacopeias—was well under way before the midcentury dynastic transition. The Qing court did not initiate the division of different fields of inquiry, but its actions consolidated their boundaries.

The separation between Confucian natural history and orthodox medicine is clearly seen in two cultural projects sponsored by the Qing court and completed in the 1720s and 1730s. The first one is an encyclopedia (*leishu*) that encompassed, as its title suggests, "pictures and books of ancient and modern times" (*Gujin tushu jicheng*). Chen Menglei (1650–1741) started compiling this ambitious encyclopedia under the patronage of a prince (the third son of Kangxi), before the emperor granted Chen access to the imperial book collection, including several hundred titles of recent local gazetteers. Following Kangxi's death, Chen became estranged from the newly enthroned Yongzheng emperor and went into exile. Yongzheng then appointed a different group of officials to edit and publish the encyclopedia. The initial print run (1726–28) yielded sixty-four copies, each totaling more than 750,000 pages, using copper-cast moveable type manufactured at the Wuying palace.[40]

The classification of knowledge in *Gujin tushu jicheng* (see table 4.1) represents a consensus between elite Confucian scholars and the Qing court that would go on to influence scholarship in Qing China for a long time.[41] Without dwelling on the details of this encyclopedia's indebtedness to previous works,

TABLE 4.1. Classification of Knowledge in *Gujin tushu jicheng*

Category (*huibian*, "collection")	Section (*dian*, "tomes")	Subheads (*bu*, "parts")	Chapters (*juan*, "fascicles")	Citation of *Bencao gangmu*
Celestial Matters (*Lixiang*, "calendrical phenomenon")	**The Heavens** (*Qianxiang*)	21	100	8
	The Year (*Suigong*, "year-long accomplishments")	43	116	43
	Astronomy and Mathematics (*Lifa*, "calendrical methods")	6	140	
Geography (*Fangyu*, "localities and territories")	**Strange Phenomena** (*Shuzheng*, "omens")	50	188	3
	The Earth (*Kunyu*, "earthly territories")	21	140	15
	Political Divisions of China (*Zhifang*, "local administrations")	223	1544	3
	Mountains and Rivers of China (*Shanchuan*)	401	320	1
	Foreign Countries ("frontier peoples")	542	140	
Human Relationships (*Minglun*, "illuminated relationships")	**The Emperor** (*Huangji*)	31	300	
	The Imperial Household (*Gongwei*)	15	140	
	The Government Service (*Guanchang*, "official routines")	65	800	
	Family Relationships (*Jiafan*, "familial norms")	31	116	
	Social Intercourse (*Jiaoyi*)	37	120	
	Clan and Family Names (*shizu*)	2694	640	1
	Man and his Attributes (*Renshi*, "worldly pursuits")	97	112	12
	Womankind (*Guiyuan*, "fine women of the inner chambers")	17	376	1

Category	Subcategory			
Science (*Bowu*, "erudition of things")	**Arts, Occupations and Professions** (*Yishu*, "arts and techniques")	43	824	30
	Religion (*Shenyi*, "divine and extraordinary")	70	320	
	The Animal Kingdom (*Qinchong*, "birds and beasts")	317	192	113
	The Vegetable Kingdom (*Caomu*, "herbs and trees")	700	320	210
Literature (*Lixue*, "Learning of Principle")	**Canonical and other Literature** (*Jingji*, "classical texts")	66	500	1
	The Conduct of Life (*Xuexing*, "conduct of students")	96	300	
	Branches of Literature (*Wenxue*)	49	260	
	Characters and Writing (*Zixue*, "etymology")	24	160	2
Polity (*Jingji*, "statecraft and governance")	**The Examination System** (*Xuanju*, "Selection and promotion [of talents]")	29	136	
	The Official Career (*Quanheng*, "evaluation of officials")	12	120	
	Foods and other Articles of Commerce (*Shihuo*, "sustenance and commerce")	83	360	37
	Ceremonies (*Liyi*, "ritual ceremonies")	70	348	
	Music (*Yuelü*)	46	136	
	Military Administration (*Rongzheng*)	30	300	
	Law and Punishment (*Xiangxing*)	26	180	
	Industries and Manufactured Articles (*Kaogong*)	154	252	27
Totals		6100	10000	514

Source: Adapted from Giles, *An Alphabetical Index*, appendix II. Giles's translation is presented here in bold, with a literal translation following the Chinese term when necessary.

we need to recognize that its classification scheme resonated with Zhu Xi's hierarchical nature that I discussed in chapter 3. Following heaven and Earth came the affairs of humanity and the "Erudition of Things" (*bowu*) that led the way to the "Investigation of Patterns" (*lixue*) and its practical applications for statecraft (*jingji*). Importantly, the sections on animals (*chongshou*, "insects and beasts") and plants (*caomu*, "grass and trees") were further divided into hundreds of subheads (*bu*), of which the category pharmaceuticals (*yao*) only applied to a small portion of plants (but not animals). Also absent was the premise of unity among all natures: instead of seeing the cosmos as a giant pharmacy, *Gujin tushu jicheng* divided nature into various realms of existence that in turn called for specialized ways of knowing them.

By contrast, the only state-sanctioned medical encyclopedia in Qing times presented a circumscribed vision for the field of medicine. Titled *Golden Mirror of the Medical Orthodoxy* (*Yizong jinjian*), the ninety-volume compendium was commissioned by the young Qianlong emperor in 1739. Wu Qian, one of the chief palace physicians at the time, assembled a large team consisting of several dozen imperial physicians, with editorial support provided by court scholars and scribes. Historian Marta Hanson's study of the *Golden Mirror* suggests that the imperial encyclopedia became a venue of legitimization for preexisting regional trends of medical practice. More importantly, the text was designed to "reach as broad an audience as possible" and was replete with "mnemonics, diagrams, and illustrations."[42] Throughout the book, any discussion of the scholarly tradition of bencao was conspicuously absent. Wu Qian and his colleagues fostered a vision of a medical orthodoxy (*yizong*) that resonated with the earlier claims of Yu Chang and Li Zhongzi against the amateurization of pharmacy. To empower physicians in their professional practices, they should be taught a standardized curriculum and prescribe medications accordingly.

In sum, the first decades of the eighteenth century saw the hardening of disciplinary boundaries between Confucian scholarship and medical learning. As a result, the dominant notions of objecthood for each field also diverged, with a unified pharmaceutical objecthood replaced by philologically informed natural history on the one hand and standardized pharmacy instructions on the other. The contracting universes of Confucian scholarship and medical learning still resembled each other in the shared notion that a small number of ancient classics constituted the fountainhead of truth. Specialists in each field pursued their own sort of truths and were not encouraged to cross-examine their knowledge across disciplinary boundaries. Ultimately, the final arbiter of their learning remained the one whose nature reached closest to that of a living sage—the emperor, whose sagacity required no further proof other than his power to govern all under heaven.

In Search of Bencao in the Emperor's Complete Library

Their differences notwithstanding, the sheer scale of erudition achieved by the *Gujin tushu jicheng* and the *Yizong jinjian* is indicative of the zeitgeist of the so-called High Qing era. In chapter 1, I discussed how the Song pharmacopeia only became widely available in print toward the end of the sixteenth century. The palpable excitement of "portable treasures" had, two centuries later, yielded to an increasing pressure to compete for attention in the publishing world. The monumental texts of the sixteenth century—the Song pharmacopeia and Li Shizhen's new bencao—became commonplace to the point of banality. The most celebrated medical authors of the eighteenth century consistently championed a reduced scope of inquiry for the subject of pharmacy: encyclopedic bencao appeared too cumbersome for their needs. Overall, bencao lost its potential as a field of liaison between Confucian learning and medical expertise.

Anxieties over abundance brought about new initiatives to selectively curate knowledge, resulting in the rise of collectanea (*congshu*) within official and scholarly circles especially from the midcentury onward. In contrast to encyclopedias (*leishu*) that dissected earlier texts into bits of digestible information grouped under universal categories, collectanea featured past titles stitched together from fragmentary quotations. Such a move was logical in an age when the sources of knowledge were considered to reside in uncontaminated antiquity. In the early 1770s, the Qianlong emperor joined the fray to announce the compilation of an imperial collectanea that would present the best selection of learning on all topics. Whereas rare, ancient texts were to be reconstructed by a team of scholars from past encyclopedias, the edict also called for recent works to be systematically culled from private collections and reviewed by an imperially appointed editorial team. The review naturally led to methodical censorship of "inappropriate and jarring" (*wei'ai*) content in the name of preservation. In the end, the *Complete Library of Four Sections* (*Siku quanshu*) preserved a total of about 3,500 titles in full length, reviewed twice as many, and banned the circulation of over 2,800 titles.[43]

For our purposes here, the Siku's selection offers a sampling of learned opinion about the field of bencao, as well as the proper relationship between

Confucian and medical learning in the late eighteenth century. In the so-called "Four Sections" of the collectanea, medicine (*yijia*) joined a host of miscellaneous subjects constituting the "*zi* section," following the Confucian classics (*jing*) and histories and proceeding anthologies of belles lettres (*ji*). Customarily translated as "masters" of "philosophers" of all kinds, the amalgam of subjects under the zi category shared a subsidiary status below the scriptural teachings of Confucianism proper.[44] Altogether, only ninety-six medical titles were selected for inclusion in the imperial collectanea, with another ninety-four titles reviewed but not included. The Siku editors lumped bencao together with other medical works and arranged them chronologically. In so doing, they affirmed the medical orthodoxy's claim that the subject of pharmacy should be classified as a subfield of medicine, instead of a form of general inquiry into the nature of all things.

Out of the hundreds of bencao texts that had been compiled and circulated in print, the Siku editors picked only a handful to preserve in full. Beginning with Tang Shenwei's Song pharmacopeia, they also included a representative work of the Jin-Yuan era cosmic pharmacy, together with Li Shizhen's *Bencao gangmu*. In a nod toward the seventeenth-century literati amateurs, they also included Miao Xiyong's *Exegesis* and Lu Zhiyi's *Shengya*, seeing them as two colorful figures representing intellectual trends in late Ming Jiangnan. These five titles together made a statement about the historical origin of bencao learning, with an eye toward its more recent variations.[45] The Siku editors' opinions have deeply shaped our notion of what constitutes the "core" literature of China's medical tradition and what falls outside of it.

The reviewed titles (*cunmu*) present a more complicated picture. The editors had few good things to say about popular primers such as *Pearl Pouch and Rhymes on the Nature of Drugs,* dubbing them the "most ugly" work done by "unenlightened physicians."[46] Their reviews also touched on a number of maverick authors who sought to overturn received wisdom via their radical writings. In the 1750s, for example, a physician named Huang Yuanyu made his name known in Beijing with his bold assertion that all previous writings on pharmacy, except for the classical formulary of one ancient author, should be completely discarded. Huang wrote numerous treatises to promote this view, which impressed many if failing to convince all. Probably lobbied by one major editor who patronized Huang's works, the Siku editors reviewed all of them, while politely pointing out that the author was rather "good at badmouthing others" (*shan ma*).[47] The arbitrary inclusion of one author at the expense of others belied the lack of consensus at the time. The competition over medical orthodoxy created its own spectrum of positions that escaped the attention of mainstream scholars, who found themselves unable to adjudicate their doctrinal disputes.

One conspicuous omission from the Siku library concerned the revived following of an early Qing author, Zhang Zhicong (d. 1674). Zhang's name was quite obscure at first, until his writings on medicine, and especially the subject of pharmacy, were propagated by his disciples in many popular editions during the mid-eighteenth century. Based in the city of Hangzhou, Zhang lived out the post-Conquest decades as a recluse and developed his unconventional doctrines on medicine with a small number of disciples. The social makeup of Zhang's circles was quite distinct from the Lu family's open lectures only a few decades earlier. One eccentric feature of their doctrine lay in the claim that the main purpose of pharmaceutical processing was *enhancement*, rather than subduing and controlling the nature of drugs. Whereas it was common practice to soak aconite for an extended time in water to reduce its toxicity, Zhang Zhicong proposed heating it over fire, so as to enhance the hot nature of aconite with yet more heat. For a cold-natured drug such as Golden Thread (*huanglian*), Zhang recommended soaking its bitter roots in water to enhance its coldness. He fiercely opposed the idea of preparing drugs with the opposite quality to "curb in" an unruly nature, and argued that doing so would be equivalent to letting a soldier fight with his hands and feet bound up.[48] Similar to his contemporaries Yu Chang and Zhang Lu, Zhang Zhicong also promoted the return to the classical teachings of medicine, and his monograph on pharmacy was aptly titled *Venerating the Origins of Materia Medica* (*Bencao chongyuan*). Considered too difficult at the time, Zhang's teachings were revived after his medical works were published in a successful medical collectanea in 1767.[49] Later on, other authors used Zhang's works to advance still more controversial claims, such as banning the excessive use of ginseng as a panacea. They concurred with Zhang that the classic account had ginseng's nature as "cold," which rendered it unsuitable in curing cold-natured pathologies. Zhang's posthumous fame was such that he earned a place in the dynastic history compiled after the Qing's fall in the twentieth century.[50] While Zhang's doctrines hardly had any real impact on the practice of pharmacists (see chapter 5), the popularity of his polemical written works indicated a new anxiety over the soundness of medical orthodoxy as taught in common textbooks.

The Siku editors' silence about Zhang's polemic against pharmaceutical processing may have been more than accidental. To reject the "curbing-in" of pharmaceutical natures could be read metaphorically as a parallel argument against the corrective education of human nature. Launching his arguments from a literal reading of ancient classics, Zhang set himself up as the lone harbinger of truth while the world was cloaked in mediocrity and deception. The medical orthodoxy that was constructed and espoused by many during the first hundred years of Qing rule now faced new challenges from revived performances of virtuosity, a phenomenon that resonated with newly insurgent classical criticism in Confucian learning toward the end of the long Qianlong reign (1736–96).[51]

By all accounts, Xu Dachun (1693–1771) was the unsurpassed favorite of the Siku editors. Of all the medical authors we have encountered in this book, he alone had four treatises preserved in full, with additional titles reviewed favorably by the editorial office.[52] Back in the late seventeenth century, Xu's grandfather Xu Qiu qualified during one of the special examinations opened by Kangxi and was recruited to work in the Ming History office as a Hanlin academician. Unable to keep his court position, Xu Qiu was forced to retire early, and his son (Dachun's father) also did not pursue an official career, but was known instead for his deep knowledge of hydraulic engineering. Xu Dachun inherited a wariness of politics from his father and was a self-taught polymath. According to his biography in the local gazetteer, he was good at astronomy, music, martial arts, and medicine. He frequently impressed local magistrates with his insight on engineering projects. Eventually, Xu's name reached the ears of the Qianlong emperor, who twice summoned him to Beijing to treat high officials. The posthumous fame of Xu Dachun and his high-profile encounter with the emperor may have contributed to the eminence of his work in the Siku collection.[53]

Xu Dachun's mastery of the medical orthodoxy is on full display in a short treatise on bencao, where he selected only one hundred kinds of materia medica from the *Divine Farmer's Classic* and wrote lucid commentaries on them.[54] In this regard, he followed the classically oriented paradigm of late seventeenth-century authors such as Zhang Lu but did so with more literary refinement. Elsewhere in his writing, Xu gave a full-throated criticism of previous authors on doctrinal differences. He portrayed himself as someone who possessed amazing talent in hydraulics and medicine but could not rise up to greater positions due to his unwillingness to pursue office at all personal costs. He was, in other words, a reluctant amateur who was precluded from the main aspirations of his upbringing.

We shall end this chapter with a unique insight from Xu's works that directly concerned the nature of pharmacy. Among the many problems Xu saw in contemporary medical practice, he paid close attention to the fact that physicians ceased to stock and prepare their own remedies (*yi bu bei yao*). Just as in late Ming times, some elite patients still prepared compound medicines at home, but Xu noted extravagant waste in their practice. Drawing from ancient sources where, as we will see in chapter 5, physicians always prepared their own remedies, Xu saw the practice of leaving all pharmaceutical production to commercial pharmacists, who were driven entirely by the pursuit of profit, as indicative of medicine's degeneration.[55] How did this situation come about?

In another essay, Xu hinted that the root cause of the separation between general medicine and pharmacy was money. The prohibitive cost of setting up a pharmacy and preparing compound medicines in one's own shop deterred most physicians of his day. In addition to the lack of capital (*ziben*), there was the laziness of practitioners. When all the patient wanted was a written prescription, the average physician would do nothing more than provide that prescription, and eventually he would end up forgetting all the methods taught in medical classics, such as needling, moxibustion, and even the hands-on preparation of pharmaceuticals. Pharmacies became the requisite intermediaries of healing, whereas elite medicine could not exert any oversight over the shopkeepers.[56]

For all his brilliance, Xu Dachun came across as an embittered man. He lived at odds with the all-too-human weaknesses on full display in the medical marketplace: the shirking of risk, the pursuit of wealth and fame, and the warring rhetoric of orthodoxy without any substance. He portrayed the medicine of ancient times as a pragmatic, flexible, and respectable art and lamented the loss of this art in his own lifetime. It is ironic, however, that High Qing elite culture in fact appreciated Xu's cynical criticism of the degeneration of medicine and ensured that his works occupied a prominent place in the historiography of medicine ever since. In the next chapter, we turn away from those learned complaints and try to hear from those who actually ran the marketplaces and shops that supplied the bulk of material remedies in late imperial China.

5

The Marketplace and the Shop

IN 1636, THE PORTUGUESE JESUIT Alvaro Semedo (c. 1585–1658) set sail back for Europe after serving as part of a mission to China for more than two decades. To the home audience, Semedo described the abundant supply of medicinal "herbs, roots, fruits, seeds, etc." in distant Ming China:

> [B]ut of all others the Physicians are well provided; because they never write any receipt, but give the medicine themselves to the patient whom they visit, And all is done at the same visit, therefore the Physician hath alwayes following him a boy, carrying a Cabinet with five drawers, each of them being divided into more than fourty little squares; and all of them furnished with medicines ready ground and prepared.[1]

In unequivocal terms, Semedo affirmed the Chinese physician's intimate command over the therapeutic arsenal. The wonderful medicine cabinet—portable, capacious, and compartmentalized into numerous small drawers—epitomized its owner's claim to expertise in the business of healing.

One and a half centuries after Semedo's comments, Nakagawa Tadahide, a Japanese official overseeing foreign trade in Nagasaki, interviewed Chinese merchants there and compiled an illustrated description of everyday life in Qing China. According to Nakagawa's informants:

> There is absolutely no such thing as medicines dispensed from the physician. No matter how grave and acute the illness is, physicians do not bring their own medicines. They only take their medicine cabinet when invitations [from the patient] come from rural and remote places. This is because there is no pharmacy in rural areas, and the distance is too far from a mar-

ketplace, so that it becomes the case that physicians would bring their medicine cabinet with them.[2]

The merchants' answers described a world in which the division of labor between physicians, who prescribed without dispensing medicine, and pharmacists, who filled the formers' prescriptions and dispensed compound drugs,
was normalized in urban communities with good access to a marketplace. The
places where physicians had to bring their own medicines then came to be
defined as "remote" and "rural." It was the intensity of commercial exchange,
not the official ranking of the local administrator, that defined a place's centrality or marginality in Qing culture. Access to pharmaceuticals became synonymous with access to capital.

A well-established literature has examined the history of pharmaceutical
enterprises in premodern China. Most scholars agree that between the sixteenth and eighteenth centuries, two major developments shaped the ways in
which patients in Ming-Qing China acquired their remedies. First, what Richard von Glahn has called the "maturation of the market economy" during this
period gave rise to an extensive network of wholesale trade that supplied materia medica in bulk to retailers.[3] This pharmaceutical trade was interregional
by nature, for medicinal ingredients harvested from very different geographical
regions must be combined to furnish a complete pharmacy. As a result, market
towns (*shizhen*) specializing in pharmaceutical trade became important nodes
of exchange, setting the price for key commodities on a national scale.[4] Second, historians of the nineteenth century frequently noted the rising prominence of urban dispensaries of compound medicine. The most successful
entrepreneurs of these shops were able to market their brand-name products
nationwide, accumulating staggering wealth that translated well into local influence and beyond.[5]

To what extent did the growth of the pharmaceutical trade, both wholesale
and retail, shape claims to knowledge vis-à-vis the orthodox medicine we have
examined in chapter 4? To what extent was Xu Dachun's aversion to pharmacists justified? By and large, men and women of the marketplace did not find
their voices recorded in past bencao pharmacopeias. If anything, compilers of
bencao, ranging from Tao Hongjing of the fifth century to Su Song in the
eleventh century, warned readers against the deception and fraud of the trade,
and sought to impose clarity and order with the pharmacopeia. The uniform
presentation of thousands of drugs made it difficult to see that, after all, the

production and dispensing of medicine relied on the labor and entrepreneurship of those whose foremost concern had always been the wellness of their own businesses. We can gain no insight, for instance, about the prices of particular drugs from Li Shizhen's *Bencao gangmu*, although, as a practicing physician still invested in compounding his own cures, he no doubt had intimate knowledge about these kinds of things. We hear hardly any testimony from the numerous middlemen who took part in buying and selling thousands of ingredients, sourced from different regions of China and distant foreign lands. One could argue that the claim to universality of the bencao pharmacopeias hinged precisely on the deliberate omission of fluctuating cost, price, human labor, and the pursuit of profit.

Yet it would be wrong to assume that the world of commerce made no difference to the world of elite medicine. In chapter 2, we saw that the commodification of materia medica responded to fiscal policy in sixteenth century and shaped the documentation of local products. The Qing conquest and prolonged warfare facilitated the disruption and mingling of formerly separate lives, thereby generating a new sense of value that also shaped the self-image of traders and pharmacists. This chapter examines the *cultural* significance of the medicinal marketplace through two interconnected case studies. First, I examine the rise of a sub-county-level market town named Zhangshu, located in the Jiangxi Province (see map 0.1), where wholesale traders of materia medica gathered and traded, and supplies from all over the country were pulled together for redistribution. Second, I revisit the well-documented history of the pharmacy Tongrentang (Hall of Common Humanity), which opened for business in Beijing circa 1702 (Kangxi 41). My argument is that metropolitan pharmacies like Tongrentang could only exist and function after an integrated wholesale market came into existence in the late Ming. The shops not only took over the State's role of collecting and redistributing materia medica, but also out-competed the businesses run by individual physicians in dispensing compound medicines. Both the marketplace and the pharmacy shop were highly successful in articulating and injecting their values to mainstream Qing culture.

Division of Labor in the Song-Ming Medical Marketplace

In Tang-Song times, physicians were essentially shop owners who compounded their own remedies. The Tang pharmacopeia preserved in full Tao Hongjing's earlier instructions on pharmaceutical processing and instructed physicians on how to prepare an existing formula into dosage forms, such as pills, powders, ointments, and tinctures. Languishing in the Tang capital city Chang'an, the poet Zhang Ji (c. 766–830) complained about being overcharged by "physicians of the pharmacies" (*yaopu yiren*).[6] In the designated neighborhoods of Chang'an where markets were held, physicians were perceived as liable to the greed and deception that killed virtue. In his exile, the banished official Liu Zongyuan (773–819) wrote an essay commemorating an extraordinary man named Song Qing, who traded in the west market of Chang'an and supplied raw medicine to artisanal physicians (*yigong*). Unlike other merchants, Song never pursued his debtors who were poor; in the end, he was repaid handsomely with their gratitude. At the end of this celebrated essay, Liu lamented the rarity of Song Qing's virtue in an age where the "Way of the Marketplace" (*shi dao*) reigned supreme, even in officialdom.[7]

The medicinal marketplace in the Northern Song further diversified at a time when cities were no longer bound by strict rules separating residential and commercial quarters.[8] At the height of its prosperity, the Northern Song capital Kaifeng boasted over a dozen medical shops (*yipu*) in various neighborhoods of the city. The Song government's active promotion of medical learning gave official ranks to many elite physicians who opened shops proudly displaying their titles and specialties ranging from pediatrics to obstetrics. One such shop, "medical officer Zhao's home" (*Zhao taicheng jia*) was depicted in *Qingming shanghe tu* (*Along the River during the Qingming Festival*), arguably the most celebrated scroll painting of urban life created at the Song court. The artist depicted the physician Zhao treating a young patient in his shop opening onto the busy street, with multiple signs on display advertising his compound medicines (see figure 5.1). Others devised eye-catching trademarks such as "Silver Baby," "Dr. Du the Golden Hook," "Dr. Ren the Big Shoe," or "Ugly Granny's Medical Shop."[9] The commercial nature of medicine was likewise proudly celebrated in documentations of the urban scene in the Southern Song capital Lin'an (later Hangzhou), where medical shops continued to boast official prestige ("Home of Defense General Ban").[10] One could imagine the bustling street scenes, in which practicing physicians' shops were an commanding presence.

Historians usually cite an anecdote dated to the thirteenth century as the earliest evidence for the emergence of general pharmacies in China, where the manufacturing space of a workshop (*zuofang*) was melded with the retail shop. Upon closer scrutiny, however, the author, Zhou Mi (1232–98), was in fact describing peddlers selling "raw medicine cut in pieces for decoction"

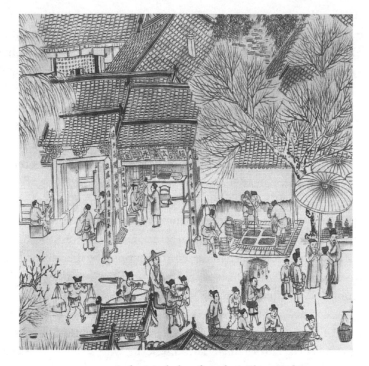

FIGURE 5.1. A physician's shop front from Zhang Zeduan,
Qingming shanghe tu. Wikimedia Commons.

(*shengyao yinpian*) and "cooked medicine in pills and powders" (*shuyao wansan*), along with steamed buns, roasted meats, preserved candy jujubes, and kumquat tangerines. Zhou noted that businesses of Lin'an became so "proud and idle" that they would not make everything from scratch but would purchase these half-processed products from "workshops" instead.[11] The anecdote reflected the sophistication of manufacturing processes in Song urban culture, and yet the assumption remained that medical shop owners should prepare their own remedies.

While managing and running their shops, Song physicians recognized the fact that most of their common ingredients had origins in distant regions. Beneath the uniform designation of tribute medicine in official geographical sources, a consensus emerged that the most precious medicinal ingredients came from the western and southern frontiers of the dynasty. Overall, the Song state's access to certain local products through tribute was probably hampered by its reduced territorial extent and, as a result, the State actively took part in the pharmaceutical trade. In essence, the pharmacies of central China drew a disproportionate share of their major ingredients from the regions of Sichuan (bordering the Tibetan Plateau) and the subtropical habitat of Guang (a short form for Guangnan, later split into the provinces of Guangxi and Guangdong). The source of medicines and the center for elite medical practice did not overlap: a late tenth-century author recorded a proverb that delegated Sichuan as the home for the best medicines, whereas only in the capital city of Chang'an could one find the best physicians.[12] A shorthand term, Chuan-Guang, consisting of (Si)chuan and Guang(nan), was used by commentators in praise of a government-sponsored charitable pharmacy assembling every imaginable product of the world.[13] Travelers recorded their observations of "medicinal market fairs" (*yaoshi*) regularly held in Chengdu, the major administrative center of Sichuan.[14] Further north from Chengdu, the district of Zhangming became known for large-scale production of the hot-natured aconite root (*fuzi*) in Song times (map 0.2). At its height, Zhangming sent over 160,000 pounds of aconite roots eastward every year, and the best batch always went to "noble people" (*guiren*).[15] In urban centers such as Lin'an, regular medicinal fairs were held as a part of the famed Cocoon Bridge (*Jianqiao*) fair, where cultivators of the city's well-known variety of white chrysanthemum traded during its harvest season.[16] Specific solutions for sourcing the best pharmaceutical ingredients shaped the local culture of each urban community.

Commercial culture in Song China thus extended the pharmaceutical repertoire of practicing physicians. Depending on one's location of practice, a physician might choose to rely on a combination of suppliers: market fairs (if possible); local collectors who picked herbs from mountains and forests; and one's own medicinal garden, for a limited number of domesticated medicinal plants.[17] The centrality of pharmacy in medical practice was highlighted by the rise of the so-called pharmaceutical chambers (*yaoshi*), a term derived from Daoist alchemical treatises that came to be used as a common appellation for the space of proprietary medical practices. From the thirteenth to fifteenth centuries, many physicians solicited commemorative essays from famous literati and used the opportunity to get a good brand name for their shop, often along the Confucian lines of benevolence and altruism.[18] The maintenance of a pharmaceutical chamber became essentially a family business as recognized by the Yuan and early Ming state in the status of hereditary "medical households" (*yihu*). The hereditary branding of pharmaceutical chambers would provide an important precedent for Qing metropolitan pharmacies, although as we shall see the centrality of the owner's medical expertise would drift out of focus in later times.

An unusual account in an early fifteenth-century source gives us a rare peek into the day-to-day management of a physician-run pharmaceutical chamber. The professional life depicted in this text was far from glamorous and had everything to do with the mundane concern of managing propriety, courtesy, and cost incurred by material expenses:

> Rise early and retire late, do not leave your shop even for a moment. When a patient comes, make a careful diagnosis, and dispense the drugs. Never ever entrust it to your assistant.
>
>   . . .
>
> Price [your remedies] according to local custom; this is good for you and also will not annoy your fellow practitioners. You might want to occasionally give away drugs for free, but do not lower the price.
>
>   . . .
>
> When dispensing a remedy for the first time, write out the prescription according to the Classical formula. Do not invent fake drug names or write nonsense secret recipes, for people will later scold you on that.
>
> As for assistants and compounding laborers, only hire a couple of them, depending on your income. Don't say that it makes your shop look good with more helping hands. Although the labor is cheap, lodging and food are very expensive.
>
> If you receive gifts from solicitous courtesans or theatre troupes, such as tea, fans and handkerchiefs . . . never accept them. Return them with a couple packs of medicine for decoction.[19]

The text indicates the extent to which a physician's professional authority and social standing depended, in many ways, on the effective management of a shop and the dispensing of actual remedies. The scientific and entrepreneurial qualities of a medical practitioner, so to speak, were not seen as being in conflict with each other. We shall see how such assumptions faltered toward the end of the Ming dynasty.

Reconfiguring Authenticity in the Late Ming

Ever-extending supply chains of pharmacy made many wary of the capriciousness of the marketplace. We saw in chapter 2 how editors of local gazetteers went so far as to delete records of local products so as to avoid unwanted attention. An early sixteenth-century gazetteer complained that wealth was being extracted from poorer places in favor of the rich: "Abundance comes from the assembly of things; profit stays meager where they are produced."[20] The weavers could not get adequate clothing; those who picked medicinal herbs did not use them to cure their diseases. It was thus not without irony that many activists for fiscal reform in late Ming found themselves advocating for more, not less, dependency on mercantile interests. In late Ming times, the latter's terminology and values did eventually seep through the general culture of the day.

One of the most salient discursive shifts lies in the specific connection be- tween the pharmaceutical trade and a new notion of place-based authenticity, articulated by the term *daodi*. Literally meaning "routes and places," the term acquired the meaning of place-based specificity—and hence authenticity to one's origins—no later than the thirteenth century.[21] Following the conver- sion of tribute medicine into silver, merchants made good fortunes from wide- spread governmental purchases all over the country, supplying materia medica to the places where the greatest profit could be made. If the monetization of tribute medicine delocalized a medicinal herb from its traditional origins, commercial exchange relocalized them to new places, thereby creating at the same time new discourses of sameness and difference. "Medicines gain their value from authentic sources (*daodi*)," noted a gazetteer in the 1640s, "or else they are mere weeds."[22] The language of authenticity now came not from gov- ernmental stipulations but from the world of traders.

The rise of integrated long-distance trade in materia medica quietly altered the attitudes and assumptions held by consumers of medicine. The playwright Tang Xianzu (1550–1616), also a native of Jiangxi, used the term "daodi materia medica" in his famous play *Peony Pavillon*. In a personal letter, Tang explained how he could not possibly relocate to Beijing, for "authentic and refined medi- cines mostly do not reach the North."[23] Similarly, writing in the 1630s, the Hangzhou-based bencao scholar Lu Zhiyi casually commented on the supply of materia medica:

> The production of medicine is different in ancient and modern times. . . . Ancient people harvested from the Central Plains and got more than what they needed. Nowadays, most medicines are obtained from distant lands and faraway peoples (*xiafang yuanyi*), for products from nearby sources are by no means adequate.[24]

To sophisticated urbanites like Lu Zhiyi, it was a banal fact that the *general* supply of medicines, not just precious or expensive ingredients, now depended on long-distance trade from faraway places.

Rising expectations on the part of elite customers posed new questions for the physicians' ability to maintain good quality for the material remedies they dispensed. In his bencao primer published in 1565, the Huizhou physician Chen Jiamo quoted a folk idiom to express this power imbalance between pharmacists and physicians: "The drug-seller has two eyes; the physician has only one eye; the patient has no eye at all."[25] It was physicians, not pharmacists, who frequently became popular targets of ridicule in late Ming literature. A late Ming short story describes how a self-made physician received help from a generous trader for the start-up funds and supplies of his business. The trader describes that business as follows:

> I only accept cash when other people buy medicine from me, except for physicians who practice in shops, who are my long-term customers. If they need anything, they just take it from me and leave a note on the account book. I collect money from them every season [three months] or every month according to the sums, and this is called half-loan-half-cash.[26]

In very clear terms, the trader laid bare the fact that physicians relied on him for supply of their pharmaceutical chambers, and that he alone had claim on the latter's debt. We might recall, as I discussed in chapter 3, that the Wanli reign (1573–1620) was also when virtuoso physicians such as Miao Xiyong started to practice by prescription alone, "without carrying a bag of medicine." We could start seeing the migration of traders and suppliers—perhaps comparable to the trade of "apothecaries" in early modern Europe—into the realm of healing, making it possible to see them as pharmacists.

Urban landscape paintings of the late Ming, such as the many versions of the so-called Suzhou Scrolls (*Suzhou pian*), also suggested the indeterminate tension between medicine and the marketplace.[27] One of the most finely executed scrolls, in imitation of the style of the famous artist Qiu Ying (c. 1494–1552), adopted many motifs from the twelfth-century Qingming Scrolls, including the physician's prominently featured shop, in which he could be seen treating a child and writing prescriptions. In contrast to the dignified shop front of the physician, a pharmacy shop supplying "authentic materia medica" (*daodi yaocai*) was depicted in a different quarter of the city. Densely packed with waiting customers, the pharmacy clerks busily chopped herbs and filled the prescriptions. Strings of fresh and dried plants and calabash gourd containers hung on the wall, and shelves and cabinets overflowed with various materials. A reptilian animal with an intact tail and four limbs was fixed to the ceiling of the shop. The animal was probably a *tuo* specimen, a small, freshwater alligator native to the middle and lower Yangzi waterways. In *Bencao gangmu*, Li Shizhen noted that the skin of the tuo was useful in pharmacies, for it was believed that the animal could "dispel moths and worms and prevent the *materia medica* from decay."[28] By depicting two very different spaces of healing, scrolls such as this one offered prototypes of urban spaces that met the needs of different consumers.[29]

The long-distance trade of daodi medicine formed the background against which the late Ming vernacular novel *Jin ping mei* (*Plum in the Golden Vase*) set up its narrative. Ximen Qing, the main protagonist, is the wealthy owner of a pharmacy (*yaopu*), which he inherits from his deceased father, Ximen Da. The senior Ximen had made a solid fortune by "traveling to *Chuan-Guang* and trading *materia medica*" before settling down in Linqing, a key stop on the Grand Canal (see map 0.1).[30] Upon taking over the shop, however, the young Ximen Qing does not travel to Chuan-Guang like his father but instead stays in Qinghe as a "settled merchant" (*zuogu*), waiting for itinerant dealers of materia medica to come to his door. In chapter sixteen of the novel, Ximen Qing's secret rendezvous with the beautiful widow Li Ping'er is interrupted by the arrival of several "guests (*keren*) from Chuan-Guang." Waiting in the shop, they offer Ximen a deal for a batch of "fine stock" (*xihuo*), demanding a down payment of 100 liang of silver, with the remainder to be paid off in several months. His romantic evening spoiled, Ximen Qing curses the uninvited guests:

> Bloody bastards! They never come knocking at your door, trying to unload their goods, unless the market is slow and they've got nowhere else to dispose of them. . . . I've got the largest store in the whole Qinghe district. It wouldn't matter how long I kept them waiting, they'd still have to come looking for me in the end.[31]

Owning a big shop—and thus being in possession of capital—allowed Ximen to beat the market by buying cheaply when trade was moving slowly, and selling high when prices picked up. To do business with him, traveling traders were willing to sell off their merchandise quickly, even if it meant getting the payment in delayed installments.

The anonymous author of the novel demonstrated an intimate understanding of long-distance trade in the late Ming.[32] In chapter 67 of *Jin ping mei*, Meng Rui, a young man in his mid-twenties and brother of Ximen Qing's third concubine, pays an amiable visit to his sister before setting off for a business trip. He described his itinerary as follows:

I'm scheduled to set out on the second day of next month, but how long I'll be gone is impossible to say. I'm going to buy paper in Jingzhou, and sell fragrant wax in *Chuan-Guang*. It will probably take a couple of years. I will come home when I'm done selling off my goods. On this expedition I will take the overland route by way of Henan-Shanxi-Hanzhou on the way out, and return on the water route by way of Xiajiang and Jingzhou. The round-trip will amount to seven or eight thousand *li*.[33]

Individual dealers such as Ximen Da and Meng Rui crisscrossed Ming territory along the water and land routes that were documented in the thriving genre of travel guides and route books. Meng Rui's itinerary may well have been typical for an average "Chuan-Guang" guest merchant in late Ming times (see map 5.1 below). By taking the onerous westbound route overland, Meng would have bought manufactured goods such as paper and wax in east and central China, and then sold them in Chuan-Guang. For the westbound return trip, he would have bought daodi products from Chuan-Guang, possibly including materia medica, and brought them to sell as consumer products back home. High in value and likely perishable, the fresh products of Chuan-Guang traveled best on boats first downstream on the mid- and lower Yangzi River, and then back north along the Grand Canal.[34] The toil of traveling merchants was motivated by the prospect that, with enough accumulated capital, they could one day settle down in a good location and establish their own shops. The story of *Jin ping mei* suggests that it was not uncommon for successful dealers to pass on their wealth to the next generation.

The inversion of the roles of physician and pharmacist was also seen clearly in the plot of *Jin ping mei*. On more than one occasion, physicians become the targets of bullying and mockery by Ximen Qing, who is himself ignorant of medical theory. In chapter 17, Li Ping'er becomes estranged from Ximen and instead marries an ordinary physician named Jiang Zhushan. Whereas Jiang only earns about five cents of silver for each medication he prescribes to a patient, he receives three hundred liang of silver from Li to open a large shop front with an abundant supply of Chuan-Guang medicine. Two chapters later, a vengeful Ximen Qing sends his men to harass Jiang. They beat him, demolish his shop, and force him to leave Li Ping'er, who eventually becomes Ximen's sixth concubine. Losing all the capital he had gained haphazardly, Jiang Zhushan moves out with only the "medicines, grinders, sieves, and medicine cabinets" to his name.[35]

In chapter 54, Li Ping'er's health has deteriorated due to the premature death of her son with Ximen Qing. A lineage physician (*shiyi*) surnamed Ren is summoned to treat her. Although Ren acts with the air of a learned physician, Ximen Qing makes him hasten his service with the additional tip of one ounce of silver. The 1613 edition of the novel highlights the moment when Ximen opens the medication package delivered from Ren's "pharmaceutical chamber" and comments that Ren is courteous enough to send along not only the ingredients to make a decoction, but also compound pills he prepared in advance.[36] In a later edition of the same novel that appeared in the 1640s, however, the portrayal of Ren's encounter with Ximen Qing was revised significantly. Gone was the detailed description of a delivery from Ren's pharmaceutical chamber, and the satire focuses instead on the Confucian doctor's (*ruyi*) obsequious conversations with Ximen Qing.[37] It may very well be that by the 1630s, the detail of getting compound medicine delivered from a physician's medicine chamber already appeared out of fashion to elite readers. The trace of respect for physician Ren's medical skill recedes into the background, and all that remains is the ugly face of wealth and power.

The Making of a "Medicinal Wharf"

Let us now turn to another story told about late Ming medicinal traders. It is included in a collection of cautionary tales titled *Dupian xinshu* (*The Book of Swindles*), first published in 1617. The main protagonist, a trader named Yu Dingzhi, hails from the southwestern province of Yunnan. Yu's business trip starts with the sale of a batch of dried gardenia fruit (*zhizi*) for eighty liang of silver in Sichuan. He then uses the cash to buy several loads of angelica (*danggui*) and Sichuanese lovage (*chuanxiong*), both native plants of Sichuan frequently used in medical formulas. Yu hires a few laborers to carry the loads and rents a boat to sail downstream along the Yangzi River. Their destination, however, was not the densely settled area of Lower Yangzi, but a small market town called Zhangshu, located in the province of Jiangxi along the Gan River (see map 5.1). The shipping costs amount to two liang and six *qian* per load.

In Zhangshu, Yu checks in to a lodge run by a local broker (*yaren*), who proposes to buy his angelica at ten liang per load, and lovage for six liang per load. Yu decides to wait for a better deal and declines the offer. Day after day, more guest merchants (*keshang*) arrive in Zhangshu with even more abundant supplies of Sichuanese drugs, and the buying-in price drops lower and lower.

In the end, Yu is forced to leave the town with his herbs and head further east, eventually selling off his wares in the Jianning Prefecture, Fujian, at the dismal rate of three liang and seven qian per load.[38]

The moral of the story is that a wise merchant should be wary of excessive greed, and that the blind pursuit of the highest profit only results in financial ruin.[39] Although the characters and their adventures were fictional, the story nevertheless gives us a very real sense of the geographical logic and seasonal rhythms that dominated the wholesale trade of materia medica in late Ming China. Individual dealers such as Yu competed with one another to transport local Sichuan products downstream, and their demand nurtured a supply chain of laborers and shipping services along the waterways. The frequency and intensity of business transactions were enough to generate a centralized marketplace in the town of Zhangshu. Unlike the story of *Jin ping mei*, the dealers did not travel into cities to bargain with potential buyers, but instead assembled in one town, where brokers (legally licensed by the government) hosted all business partners to make deals. The marketplace was also sensitive enough to fluctuating supply and demand that a short moment of delay could result in major losses. The seasonal rhythms of harvest in Sichuan promptly resulted in the plunging prices at Zhangshu, thousands of miles away down the river. When someone like Yu saw no room for profit in Zhangshu, they would have to make the extra effort to travel to places further away from the main trade routes (for example, hinterland Fujian) and sell off their goods with the local prices there.

Where is Zhangshu? In the administrative hierarchy of Ming China, Zhangshu was a town (*zhen*) that fell under the jurisdiction of the magistrate residing in Qingjiang (clear water) County. The walled city of Qingjiang, which also served as the administrative seat of the Linjiang Prefecture, and the unfortified town of Zhangshu were located respectively on the west and east bank of the Gan River, facing each other and connected by ferries. The town's name, meaning "camphor trees," may have been related to the abundance of such trees in the region, whereas a legend attributed it to an ancient warrior who once chased a deer and shot an arrow into an old camphor tree. The mighty Gan River originates from the northern ridge of the Nanling Mountains and flows north from there, cutting through the Jiangxi Province before finally joining the Yangzi River. Along the way, minor waterways connect the Gan route to Fujian in the east and Huguang in the west. At Qingjiang-Zhangshu, the Gan is joined by the Yuan River, a navigable waterway that leads to the hinterland of Hunan. Since the thirteenth century

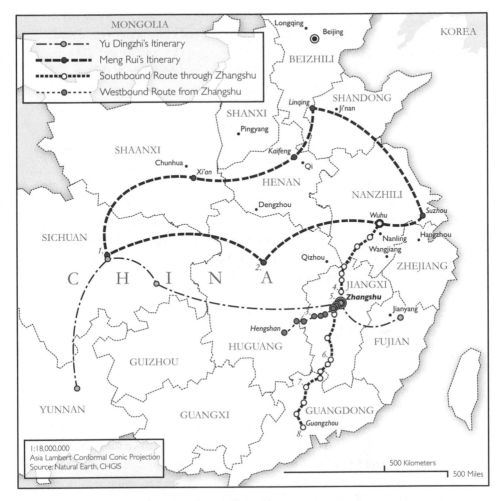

MAP 5.1. Ming travel itineraries through Zhangshu, based on literary sources
and route books in Yang Shitai, *Mingdai yizhan kao*, appendix 3, 325–27.

the region of Qingjiang and Zhangshu had been associated with the medicinal trade, owing in part to the fame of the nearby Gezao Mountain as a Daoist site.[40] Hou Fengbing, a literatus who moved to Zhangshu after the Mongol conquest, was known for his charitable pharmacy that distributed effective cures for free. Yet there is no evidence indicating that interregional trading of materia medica concentrated in Zhangshu prior to the fifteenth century.[41]

Locals suggested two narratives that explained Zhangshu's rise into a central marketplace for interregional trade. One story, favored by local literati, had to do with the ill-fated rebellion of Zhu Chenhao (d. 1521), a Ming prince whose fiefdom was located at the provincial capital of Jiangxi. Legend had it that merchants relocated across the river from Qingjiang to Zhangshu in order to get away from the heavy tax imposed on them by the tyranny of the prince.[42] A second story attributed the cause to the Gan's sudden change in course during the Jiajing reign (1522–66). Instead of meeting the Yuan right at the foot of the walled city of Qingjiang, the Gan now cut directly north and met the Yuan at the doorstep of Zhangshu. River traffic to and from Guangdong therefore increasingly docked at the town of Zhangshu, bypassing the county seat.[43] During the mid-sixteenth century, locals rebuilt temples and constructed impressive dykes that lined the town's waterfront.[44] By the late sixteenth century, Zhangshu's fame as a "medicinal wharf" (*yao matou*) had been firmly established.[45] Merchant handbooks referred to the town as the "meeting place of medicines from all country," where "merchants from north and south" came together.[46] Wang Shixing (1547–98), a well-traveled author, estimated a total of over ten thousand households "thriving" in the "imposing town" (*xiongzhen*).[47] Locals noted that not only materia medica but also timber, utensils, and clothing were traded in Zhangshu and then sold "to the southeastern prefectures."[48] In sum, a formerly obscure sub-county-level market town started to attract national attention.

Local administrators in the late Ming reacted to Zhangshu's newfound fortune with mixed feelings. Similar to the widespread activism that had surrounded the reform of local tribute, the Qingjiang elite detested eunuch envoys sent from Beijing to purchase goods from the market town for the throne, seeing it as disruptive of local order.[49] The gazetteer also documented, with certain wariness, the increasing tax burden on the town beginning in the early seventeenth century, first from the prefecture, then directly from authorities in Beijing.[50] By the 1630s and 1640s, the Ming state's desperate attempt to fund border defense and antirebellion campaigns resulted in even more punishing surtaxes on the south. The local magistrate thought that the good fortune of Zhangshu was over.[51]

Further complicating local politics was the influx of traders who lived in Zhangshu but acted to maximize their own transregional interests. In one magistrate's words, the "guests were overwhelming the natives" (*ke sheng zhu*).[52] Other river towns along the Gan waterway posed a constant threat to Zhangshu as trade moved up and down the river depending on local circumstances. In the 1630s, a group of salt merchants from the Huai region (north of the Yangzi River) floated the proposal of raising funds to build a bridge over the Gan at

Zhangshu, so that an additional station could be built there to collect extra levies from passing ships. A local literatus named Guan Daxun argued strongly against the proposal, pointing out that the Huai merchants only suggested this so that their competitors from Guangdong would be rendered unable to out-sell them with cheaper salt. Yet according to Guan Daxun, one more round of levies on shipping traffic would be enough to convince merchants traveling along the Gan to choose another spot to dock their boats and trade, ruining Zhangshu's good fortune.[53] This episode indicated that the local community understood the logic of commerce very well, and that it took constant vigilance to keep the center of trade in their town.

Trade stalled and rebounded in the immediate aftermath of the Qing conquest wars. In the early 1660s, Fang Yizhi (whose writings and post-Conquest exploits I discussed at the beginning of chapter 4), now an ordained Buddhist monk, traveled to Qingjiang and lodged in a local temple.[54] While there, he visited the town of Zhangshu and wrote one last addition to the chapter on pharmacy in *Notes on the Principle of Things*. The title of that entry was "Different Forms at the Medicine Market" (*yaoshi yixing*):

> In Zhangshu, it has been said that:
> *Mutong* from the Huai region can facilitate the flow of *qi*. Its color resembles frankincense, and has a radiating texture like spokes of a wheel. *Mutong* from Sichuan is white in color, and can only be used as a diuretic. The false kinds are in fact grapevines.
> Also, *Xuanshen* from the Huai region is black, whereas *Xuanshen* from Sichuan is white;
> *Niuxi* from Huai is slim and long, yellowish white in color, for use by women; *Niuxi* from Sichuan is bulky and blackish, for use by men.
> All such information has not been previously recorded in *bencao*.[55]

The marketplace of Zhangshu offered Fang Yizhi an abundance of differences coded in regional origins (Huai versus Sichuan) and measured by sensual data (color, texture, shape). Here, Fang Yizhi simply recorded what he had learned without attempting to explain the varieties in terms of their cosmic natures. Fang was reticent about how this kind of knowledge could pave the way to a clearer understanding of the principle of things (*wuli*); yet he was also open to its influence. The epistemic skepticism of earlier sources on the trustworthiness of commerce was gone. Instead, Fang pointed out the inadequacy of bencao pharmacopeias to document such an abundance of "different forms." In chapter 6, we shall see how those who held a similar attitude of curiosity and openness toward the marketplace would give new meanings to the learning of bencao in the eighteenth century.

Qing Mercantilist Policy toward Pharmaceutical Trade

Uncertainty loomed large in the initial decades following the Qing conquest, as the Manchu rulers of the new dynasty reckoned with the institutions and customs of the vast land they now governed. Would they continue the late Ming push toward monetizing a diverse tax base or revert back to earlier principles of collecting local tribute in kind? To what extent would local officials be allowed to negotiate tax relief for their jurisdictions? Would they encourage transregional and overseas trade? If so, where would such transactions be permitted to operate, and how much would the State extract from the profit? Just as in the cultural realm, it took some time for Qing fiscal policy to reconfigure the relationship of the State vis-à-vis its tax base. The issue of pharmaceutical objecthood is again indicative of the Qing approach to governance, as an abundant supply of materia medica remained essential for the sustenance of the State. The ways in which different branches of the Qing government acquired their remedies thus formed an important context for the continued development of the pharmaceutical trade and other business enterprises in the eighteenth century.

In 1648, four years after the Qing seized Beijing and claimed the Mandate of Heaven, an imperial decree arrived in the Ningguo Prefecture (see map 0.2) demanding the tribute medicine Golden Thread (*huanglian*), a bitter, knotty root known to grow in Ningguo's famous mountains. Following a systematic review of the backlog in tax payment accumulated during the last decades of Ming rule, it was determined that a total of 1,700 jin (over 1,000 kilograms) of the precious medicine was to be dispatched immediately.

The decree stirred a small crisis in the local community, still reeling from the traumas of war. The prefectural gazetteer recorded that back in the eleventh century, the Song state collected twenty jin of Golden Thread as tribute from Ningguo each year. The Ming quota, although much higher in quantity, had long been converted to payment in silver. The local gentry reasoned that the sudden request from the Qing administration was probably triggered by the diminished market supply of Golden Thread from Sichuan as a result of the recent rebellions and warfare, which had caused the price to soar. As a result, someone in the Beijing ministries had turned to Ningguo as an alternative source for the essential medicine.

In search of a solution, the Ningguo prefect teamed up with local gentry and sent crews to search for the valuable plant in the mountains. The provincial governor shortly received word that native Golden Thread had been "completely dug out" and there was none to be had as tribute. The prefect offered further details by saying that all previous shipments of Golden Thread had in fact been purchased from Wuhu, a commercial hub on the Yangzi River.[56] The prefect offered to pay for the 1,700 jin of Golden Thread in silver cash as a surtax and gathered additional support from Ningguo natives among the capital civil officials. Authorities in Beijing eventually settled for a combination of silver and the medicine itself to be fully monetized in eight years' time.[57]

This case shows how the familiar pattern of bargaining between central and local administrations continued across dynastic transition. The elite of Ningguo mobilized local knowledge (the nonexistence of Golden Thread) to resist centralized demand for tribute items, a trope that we have seen in chapter 2. In so doing, they offered oblique insight into the interregional pharmaceutical trade, for Wuhu was situated at the northern tip of Jiangxi, and much of the materia medica on sale there would have been supplied from market towns upstream of the Gan River such as Zhangshu (map 0.2). The regional varieties that Fang Yizhi saw in Zhangshu in the 1660s were corroborated by the Ningguo prefect's argument about the differences between the Sichuan and the Huai (of which Ningguo was considered a part) varieties of the same herb. In the end, both the Beijing ministries and the local players looked to the marketplace as the final arbiter of value.

Historians have pointed out that the so-called Single Whip Law reforms of the late Ming, intended to convert diverse forms of taxation into silver, only came to be fully implemented in all provinces under Qing rule.[58] Money became the central instrument and chief unit of accounting for the Qing state to use to extract and allocate surplus wealth. In the process, the nature of governance came to be disassociated from the state's direct claim to the specific products of the land, hinging instead on the commodification of labor and natural resources. If the marketplace was able to supply Golden Thread from Sichuan, the State was willing to buy it with revenue gathered from Ningguo.

In 1663, the Qing court ordered that all agricultural taxes, labor levees, and local tributes be paid directly to the Ministry of Revenue in Beijing. Medicines, livestock, and calendar papers would no longer be shipped in bulk from local administrations to the Ministry of Rites. Instead, the Imperial Academy of Medicine directly purchased ingredients for their pharmacy and got reimbursement from the Ministry of Revenue.[59] In this way, transactions between the inner and outer court came under the closer scrutiny of book-keeping and periodic reviews, and the various offices of the Qing government became direct customers of mercantile suppliers. Occasionally, provincial administrators still procured tribute items in kind and sent them to the emperor. Yet remarkably materia medica were largely taken out from regular tribute lists, giving way instead to regional varieties of fine tea, porcelain, and other manufactured goods. Conversely, Qing emperors in the eighteenth century frequently ordered the manufacturing of "ingot medicine" (*dingzi yao*) to be given out as gifts to officials.[60] The directionality of medical gift-giving had been reversed from bottom-up to top-down.

Later in the eighteenth century, the familiar tension between the emperor's inner court personnel and the outer court ministries was epitomized again in the allocation of medicine. The Imperial Household Department (*Neiwufu*), a sprawling organization run by the Manchu rulers' trusted bondservants (Ma. *booi*), was in charge of all inner court affairs and ran a separate Imperial Pharmacy (*yuyaofang*) that came to eclipse the authority of the Imperial Academy of Medicine.[61] The Imperial Household Department's exclusive source of income included rent collected from its vast tracts of land and transit tax extracted by domestic and maritime customs houses.[62] Early eighteenth-century records indicate that the Qing state regularly monitored the trade of 200–300 common kinds of materia medica near major urban markets and maritime trade hubs such as the port city of Ningbo, where ships to and from Japan's Nagasaki carried large quantities of medicine native to China or brokered by Chinese merchants (these sojourning merchants were the ones interviewed by Nakagawa in Japan about everyday life in Qing China). The most valuable daodi medicine from Sichuan was subject to a higher duty on par with other luxury items.[63] Medicine continued to be a significant component of regional and global trade well into the nineteenth century, as China remained a major exporter of pharmaceutical ingredients and also imported new varieties from Japan, Korea, Southeast Asia, and, famously, ginseng from America. We will examine the impact this trade had on pharmaceutical knowledge in chapter 6.

Unlike the outer court ministries, the Imperial Household Department was not merely content with making ends meet but aggressively invested in trade and commerce to maximize profit. Throughout the eighteenth century, the Department made high-interest loans to private businesses, calling it "silver that grows and proliferates" (*shengxi yinliang*). Another profitable activity was licensing the dealership of ginseng harvested from the Manchu homeland, now strictly prohibited by state power from outside exploitations. According to historian Chiang Chu-shan's study, the Department's relentless pursuit of additional income did much to cause the market price for Manchurian ginseng to rise to exorbitant levels in the late years of the Qianlong reign.[64] Starting with the continued monetization of the tax base, the Qing regime pursued a mercantilist policy to encourage trade in commoditized local products, reaping extraordinary profits from selected venues to which it laid exclusive claim. In so doing, the emperor's personal agents worked with designated business partners and nurtured their privilege in society. Since the ventures of the Imperial Household Department took place almost entirely outside of regular civil bureaucracy, there was little room for criticism or external review. At this time, not many of the civil officials would have dared to raise objection to the emperor's private wealth.

In a way, the partitioning of regular state fiscal practices from the unregulated investments of the inner court mirrored the reclassification of knowledge in public culture: that the orthodoxy of medicine resembled in rhetoric, but did not need to be entirely commensurable with, the orthodoxy of Confucian learning. If the ultimate ground for unity and authority over moral truth resided in the hands of the monarch alone, then his personal actions, including indulgence in the pursuit of wealth and power, would also remain immune to regular bureaucratic oversight. The late Ming officials' critique of the ruler's abuse of his power became muted in an age of mercantilist logic, symbiotic to autocratic rule.

Among the mercantile actors who benefited from business liaisons with the State, the exclusive purveyors of materia medica for the Qing court eventually became highly successful entrepreneurs who boasted their imperial connections to earn a competitive edge in the marketplace.[65] Such was the case of the Beijing pharmacy Tongrentang that we will examine next.

The Pharmacist's Progress

In 1736, five artists at the Qing court collaborated to create a new scroll painting after the style of *Along the River during the Qingming Festival*. The urban landscape depicted resembled the twelfth-century original and late Ming Suzhou Scrolls in its organization: a meandering river, a boat passing beneath a bridge, a magnificent city wall and bustling street scenes. Yet many details were quite different.[66] For example, in the 11.5-meters-long scroll, the Qing palace painters depicted urban pharmacies at much more prominent locations than the shops of physicians, which became almost inconspicuous. A pediatrician stands on a side street, bowing to his visiting patients, his shop only featuring one sign, "the poor are treated without concern for profit" (*pin bu ji li*). Another quiet building was the residence of an "incantation exorcism specialist" (*zhuyou ke*). Two pharmacy shops, by contrast, appear much more dynamic and appealing: apprentices are busy cutting herbs, carrying trays of materia medica up to the roof for drying, and weighing packages delivered to the shop's front door (figure 5.2). Both shops feature multiple signs, advertising "authentic (*daodi*) medicine from Chuan-Guang." The colorful depiction of materia medica is coupled with packaged shipments that indicate the business connections of the shop owners. Later in the eighteenth century, *Prosperous Suzhou*, another scroll painting of urban landscape commissioned for the occasion of the Qianlong emperor's southern tour in 1759, also depicted various pharmacies featuring merchandise from "Chuan-Guang-Yun(nan)-Gui(zhou)" but not a single physician's office.[67] Overall, High Qing urban landscape paintings indicated that pharmacists were expected to play a much more active role in city life than individual physicians.

The paintings confirm Xu Dachun's complaint about the inability of physicians to exert any real control over pharmaceutical processes. The separation between prescribing physicians and dispensing pharmacists replaced the earlier composite image of the medical expert as master of the pharmaceutical chamber. Just when bencao was rendered into its most accessible textual form, physicians lost control over the artisanal techniques that had once been the pride of their trade.

The popular image of the pharmacist was derived from that of the physician but also explicitly distinguished from it. The pharmacy shop Tongrentang (Hall of Common Humanity) opened for business in 1702 (Kangxi 41), at a prime location in the Dashilan commercial district of Beijing. At first, the owner, Yue Fengming, referred to the business as a pharmaceutical chamber (*yaoshi*) after the Ming fashion. In Yue's account, the shop's unique products came from the medical training of his late father, Yue Zunyu, who had served as a clerk (*limu*) in the Imperial Academy of Medicine. Having descended from a lineage of itinerant healers, the senior Yue was well known for his ability to "tell the subtle features of authentic [*didao*] materia medica," and the compound medicines he made were popular and efficacious. Despite its alleged origin in the skill of an individual physician, Tongrentang came to be consistently referred to as a pharmacy shop (*yaopu*). Descendants of Yue Fengming no longer practiced medicine but saw themselves as "knowing the remedies

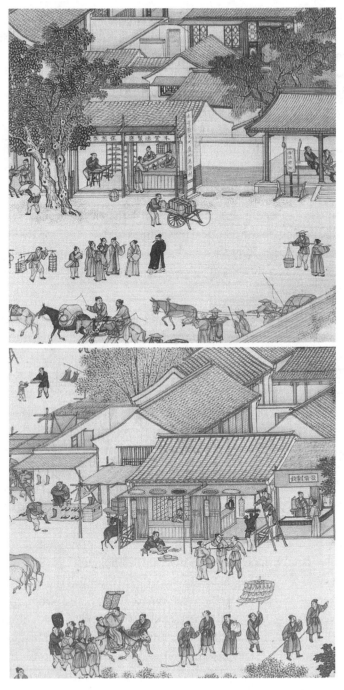

FIGURE 5.2. Two urban pharmacies depicted in Chen Mei et al.,
Qingming shanghe tu. Wikimedia Commons.

but not [the art of] medicine" (*zhi yao bu zhi yi*). In the mid-1700s, the Yue family sold Tongrentang to another owner who also did not practice medicine.[68]

If the pharmacist was not necessarily a healer, then how could he vouch for the efficacy of what he sold to the customers? Tongrentang's owners started off by asserting the timeless efficacy of ancient recipes (*gufang*). In his 1706 preface to Tongrentang's first catalog, Yue Fengming insisted that if a drug failed to cure, the problem must have been either the quality of ingredients or the process of compounding. Hence Yue laid out the pharmacy's promise that would become the shop's guiding mantra:

> Follow the *Recipes at Hand*, and distinguish the products' places of origin; Complex as the pharmaceutical procedures are, we never spare our labor. Costly as the ingredients are, we never compromise on the material expenses. Gods and ghosts will judge us, and our products will respond to all sorts of illnesses.[69]

The dual emphasis on material and technical authenticity dovetailed nicely with the dependence on well-known, "ancient" recipes. Although the pharmacist did not profess to know medicine, he vowed to render recipes into potent cures. The smooth translation from text to commodity was in turn guaranteed by access to daodi authentic ingredients on the one hand, and fastidious execution of pharmaceutical processes on the other. In doing both, pharmacies held a competitive edge over individual practitioners who, on average, possessed less capital to purchase ingredients from the wholesale marketplace or to hire labor.

In addition to that, the pharmacist also asked for customers' trust by pledging undisputable piety. As another business slogan of Tongrentang asserted, "no one sees how we compound / yet Heaven alone knows our mind." Urban pharmacists competed to appear as the best exemplar of moral piety. Taking up a similar logic to the Qing state's mercantilist policies, elite pharmacists of the eighteenth century sought to convince their customers that the efficacy of medical remedies was congruent to their market value. The wellbeing of individual lives, just like that of the polity, could be rejuvenated with money.

Grandiose rhetoric aside, the few extant catalogs published by Qing pharmacists hinted at their struggles amid fierce competition. The transition from individual, physician-owned pharmaceutical chambers to pharmacy shops that employed up to 15–20 hired hands was not easy.[70] Heniantang (Hall of Crane-like Longevity), another established pharmacy in mid-eighteenth-century Beijing, only issued a printed catalog in 1758, after "a few decades of careful practice." Located only two kilometers from Tongrentang and adjacent to the busy vegetable market intersection (*Caishikou*), Heniantang also claimed access to the Qing imperial court as a purveyor of materia medica and nurtured close ties with capital officials, as seen from the multiple prefaces written by five mid- to high-level bureaucrats in the catalog.[71] The owner also confessed that he "had not mastered my family's art of medicine" but pledged to "insure the authenticity of our *materia medica*, and the appropriateness of pharmaceutical procedures." Perhaps in response to Heniantang's challenge, Tongrentang also reissued a new edition of its own catalog in 1764.[72] Both pharmacies offered a wide range of compound drugs—the 1764 catalog of Tongrentang described 352 compound drugs treating all complaints from head to toe—but did not disclose the actual formulas in the catalog. The rhetoric of piety and humanity (*ren*) notwithstanding, the intention of such publications was still to get customers into their store rather than that of a competitor.

Compared to elite shops with connections to imperial agents, up-and-coming pharmacists elsewhere found other strategies to achieve business success. In 1790, a new pharmacy named Jingxiutang (Hall of Respectful Cultivation) opened for business in the city of Canton, the designated port for trade with European merchants. The pharmacy was founded by Qian Shutian, a silk dealer who hailed from Cixi County, a town near the port of Ningbo known for its lineages of pharmaceutical merchants (see map 0.2). During his sojourn in Canton, Qian reportedly cured the son of a wealthy man. The patient's family invited him to stay and provided him with funds to open his own shop.[73] In 1804, Qian Shutian decided to promote his brand by issuing a printed catalog, which he titled *Jingxiutang yao shuo* (*Discourses on the Drugs of Jingxiutang*).

Overall, the catalog was no match for the impressive repertoire of Tongrentang and Heniantang. Qian's pharmacy could only produce up to seventy compound drugs, yet he customized a few of his best-selling "tried and true" (*jingyan*) remedies and advertised them aggressively. Another major difference was that Qian Shutian listed the price for each compound drug, suggesting that he expected the catalog to directly bring in new orders from customers. In his preface, Qian mobilized the familiar rhetoric of using authentic (*daodi*) ingredients and labor-intensive pharmaceutical procedures that were "expertly handled to perfection." In particular, Qian boasted that his special cures were so efficacious that they could be compared with "refined gold, deployable as one wishes."[74] For smaller and newer enterprises like Jingxiutang, pharmacists often sought to establish themselves with a few effective secret remedies—comparable to the "patent drugs" popular in the nineteenth-century world—and gradually acquired the capacity to concoct a wider range of regular compound medicines.

Qian Shutian's entrepreneurial career took off from the interregional trade of unrelated merchandise, not necessarily from a medical background. A copy of Jingxiutang's catalog was discovered in the Qing imperial collection, indicating that Qian's remedies successfully gained the attention of the imperial pharmacists. Despite their distinct regional origins, Qing pharmacists found common ground via their connections to an integrated domestic marketplace. All over the empire, new shops modeled themselves after each other, imitating each other's products and evoking the same language of authenticity, piety, and ingenuity.

In this chapter, I have sketched out the changing roles of the marketplace and the urban pharmacies in China's early modern medical scene. The division of labor between physicians, who prescribed without dispensing medicine, and pharmacists, who were connected to a national market and manufactured compound cures, became an important indicator of urban living in Qing China by the end of the eighteenth century. The communities of wholesale dealers, brokers, shop owners, and their apprentices replaced the small-scale operation of medical households in earlier times. In Angela Ki-Che Leung's words, the disappearance of the state-designated medical institutions around the sixteenth century marked the beginning of the decline of "organized medicine." We see in Qing China a *new* organized model of healing that hinged on the commodification of pharmacy without state supervision.

This new "organized medicine" that was featured prominently in Qing urban landscape paintings—and later, in the literary and photographic travelogues of foreign visitors—derived its coherence not from centrally designed institutions and standardized examinations, but rather from access to an integrated domestic market. The challenge of understanding this phenomenon, however, lies in the fact that most participants to this trade were constantly on the move and stayed largely outside official purview. The sea change they brought to the socioeconomic fabric of both their native places and their new homes can only be fathomed through indirect evidence and retrospective accounts from later generations. For instance, local officials were held responsible for banditry or robbery cases that affected the security of traveling merchants; numerous reports in the Qing state archive therefore recorded the victims' names, extent of loss, and itineraries.[75] More so than the native sons who migrated to faraway places, the local gazetteer of Zhangshu commemorated dozens of virtuous women (*lienü*) whose husbands died while doing business in southwestern provinces such as Hunan, Guangxi, and Yunnan.[76] In one incident, a young woman traveled all the way from Guangxi to the town of Zhangshu and introduced herself as having married a merchant who had now died. The story had a happy ending as the bereaved stranger was accepted by her husband's extended family and lived the rest of her life there.[77]

Modern accounts of Qing business organization, on the other hand, overcorrected the lack of official records by granting the origin stories almost sacrosanct status. Tongrentang is a case in point, as the official history of the pharmacy was beholden to the interests of the modern-day company that descended from the original shop. The longevity of the company has been cited as proof of the Yue family's virtue and business prowess, and successful figures such as Yue Pingquan (1810–80) and his wife Xu Yefen (1827–1907) have become celebrated figures in popular culture today, including TV dramas based on the Yue family's stories. As TCM acquired a nationalistic aura over the twentieth century, Tongrentang's professed commitment to manufacturing "ancient recipes" gained extra political appeal.[78] Similarly, the celebrated pharmaceutical companies (*yaobang*) of Zhangshu were documented as if the town had been destined for great success since time immemorial.[79] The rich potential of this literature has yet to be carefully mined for telling details, such as the existence of separate guilds where shop owners, accountants, storage keepers, and apprentices socialized within their own groups.[80] We also learn from oral histories that in early twentieth century a young pharmacy apprentice would receive a stipend to shave his head three times a month, in addition to tips from customers, and was typically allowed to drink tea and smoke with his coworkers. Everybody in the trade learned to recite two primer pharmacy texts popularized by seventeenth-century authors.[81] A little song popular among Zhangshu apprentices conveyed a sense of optimism and mobility:

> Carrying a bundle and an umbrella
> A boy goes out and becomes a boss;
> Having left with naked arms and bare ass
> He returns in long robes and a smart vest.[82]

The prospect of upward mobility was complicated, however, by violent treatment from bosses and conflict with native laborers where they traveled.[83] All caveats notwithstanding, these sources together suggest the *organized* nature of the mercantile community and the development of a rich subculture of their members.

Reviewing the general features of economic life in Qing China, historian William T. Rowe remarked that toward the end of the eighteenth century, "virtually anything that could be defined, packaged, and sold, was."[84] An integrated marketplace necessarily connected the mercantile community and the customers they served, and it is only reasonable to expect vocabularies of the tradesmen to enter that of the literati. In the next chapter, we will follow the footsteps of the pharmaceutical merchants to new frontiers of the Qing dominion, where they established shops and transformed residents into willing business partners with the lure of profit. We shall start with the question of knowing exotica.

6

Eating Exotica

IN 1784 (QIANLONG 49), the Tongrentang pharmacy in Beijing received two unusual customers. Introducing themselves as students from the Ryukyu Kingdom, the two young men produced an album of plant drawings with dried specimens tucked inside. One by one, they asked three leading pharmacists to help them identify fifty plants that grew on their island. A letter from their teacher, a senior scholar named Wu Jizhi, explained that the album and the native species it contained had been compiled so that experts in Qing China could help them identify which ones could be used as medicine. The students, who were selected to study in designated lodges in Fuzhou, would bring the album to local scholars and healers and record whatever they might learn. During the single trip on which they were allowed to tour the imperial capital, the only interlocutors they engaged there were the Tongrentang pharmacists.[1]

Eight years later, the Ryukyu scholars had accumulated several albums annotated with records of conversations with Chinese experts, in addition to information supplied by Chinese merchants and other travelers who had visited the island kingdom. On some occasions, additional pictures or specimens were sent with envoys to China in order to ascertain the identity of a plant. The entire set of correspondence was eventually compiled in an illustrated treatise aptly titled *Shitsumon Honzō / Zhiwen bencao* (*Questions on the subject of Materia Medica*; see figure 6.1). The work was published with the sponsorship of the lord of the Satsuma Domain, the southernmost territory of Tokugawa Japan. In fact, modern scholars have ample grounds to suspect that samurai-physicians in the Satsuma Domain were in fact responsible for making the album and sending the Ryukyu students to China, and there never existed a real person named Wu Jizhi.[2] For the Satsuma elite,

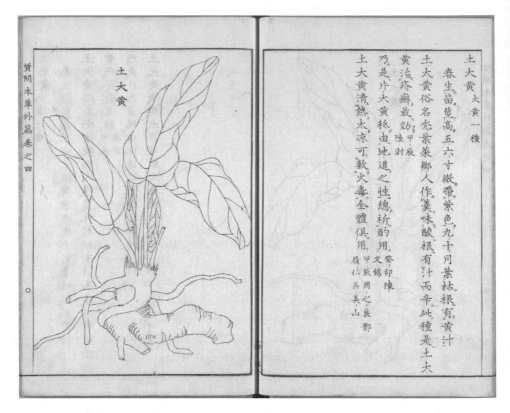

FIGURE 6.1. Page from Wu Jizhi, *Shitsumon honzō*, on "native rhubarb" (*tu dahuang*).
Courtesy of the National Diet Library of Japan.

surveying native plants of the islands was an important part of expanding
Japanese influence in Ryukyu. The process of Japan's geopolitical expansion
would culminate in the annexation of Ryukyu as Meiji Japan's Okinawa Prefecture in 1879.

Quite unlike the Qing court's decision to patronize nonmedical natural
history and treat pharmacy as a narrow and isolated field, the holistic appeal
of *Honzō / Bencao*, which combined descriptive and prescriptive elements,
prospered in Tokugawa Japan.[3] We may be tempted to see the divergence of
scientific cultures of China and Japan toward the end of the early modern era
as a harbinger of their fates later in the nineteenth century. Yet to do so risks
reducing the complexity and dynamism in each place to nationalistic stereo-
types. Like the late Ming literati, the Japanese elite samurais' pursuit of bencao
was also influenced by Zhu Xi's teaching about nature. As advisors to the Sho-
gun and domainal lords, their knowledge exerted far greater sway on domestic

policy than Confucian scholars in eighteenth-century China. More importantly, the different positions of the two countries in regional and international trade at the time prompted Tokugawa leadership to directly intervene in the exploitation of native medicinal resources, in order to find substitutes for authentic materia medica imported from China. In contrast, the Qing state deftly manipulated mercantile agents to profit from an export-oriented economy of manufactured goods, of which the State held little direct supervision and knowledge.

Rather than seeing *Shitsumon Honzō* as evidence of an opportunity that Qing China failed to pursue, we could instead use the text to reveal a *vernacular* realm of knowledge teeming with scholars, healers, pharmacists, and merchants drawn together by their curiosity about novelties. In their responses, the Tongrentang pharmacists consulted the *Bencao gangmu* and earlier medical sources, demonstrating a certain pride in their trade.[4] Whereas some physicians and scholars in Fujian saw no need to know the exact identity of "wile grass and idle flower" (*yecao xianhua*), others readily supplied names of local medicinal plants that did not count as daodi authentic but could be useful as cheaper substitutes. Some were more audacious in trying new remedies, while others warned of potential adverse effects and advised caution.[5] Overall, Qing informants were willing to defy their designated roles in society and venture guesses about something they had never seen before. It was this curiosity that gave rise to the possibility of reinventing bencao for a new audience.

Critiques of the longing for exotica had a long history in the Chinese political tradition. In their crusade against state abuses of local tribute, Ming gazetteer editors repeatedly warned against the overvaluing of extraordinary things (*yiwu*), praising instead objects of everyday use (*yongwu*). Taking up the binary distinction between state and popular consumption, Ming civil officials railed against the perceived tendency of emperors to pursue frivolous pleasure and inflate the value of luxury goods.[6] Yet they were also writing against a popular culture that relentlessly spread enticing information about foreign lands and the exotic peoples who lived there.[7] When the Qing conquest took place in the mid-seventeenth century, the divide between luxury consumption for the elite and plain utility for the populace had become blurred. If the widening availability of daodi medicine from afar is any indicator of the extent to which the market economy penetrated into everyday life in late Ming times, we can continue to observe the development of consumer culture in Qing China from the vantage point of pharmacies, as well as their connection to the wider world.

In his classic study of exotica in medieval China, *The Golden Peaches of Samarkand*, Edward H. Schafer noted the stark disjuncture between the "age of imports, the age of mingling, [and] the golden age" up to the mid-eighth century under the Tang dynasty and a belated "peak of literary interest in the exotic" fueled by nostalgia for that bygone age.[8] In other words, exoticism in Tang literature peaked only after exotic merchandise and foreign traders receded to the backstage of social and economic life. The situation of High Qing times was different: as the exchange of goods accelerated following the opening of maritime trade in designated ports, so did the coproduction of literary and scientific discourses. At times, it became impossible to tell whether reality led to imagination or the other way around. For someone residing in an urban center with ready access to the marketplace, exotic objects were not just something one might have heard of or read about, but tangible specimens to collect, examine, and (in many cases) ingest. In this chapter, we follow one author's journey through the Qing world of goods to shed light on new directions in the bencao tradition. Toward the end of the chapter, I will discuss the political significance of this vernacular sphere of knowledge and the double-edged meaning of curiosity.

A Life Adrift

Zhao Xuemin's life was typical of many educated men in eighteenth-century China. Growing up in the populous urban environment of Hangzhou, Zhao possessed neither connections nor wealth to launch an official career. Well educated but without an examination degree, Zhao took on temporary jobs as family tutor or private secretary to local officials around Hangzhou. He befriended renowned book collectors as well as practicing herbalists, gleaning much information from private libraries and banquet chatter. In his youth, Zhao took a special liking to the art of medicine but never practiced as a physician. In addition, he also claimed deep knowledge in subject matters such as fireworks and horticulture, composing treatises in those fields that were never published in his lifetime. His life resembled that of Shen Fu, a contemporary of his who also lived a peripatetic life at the fringes of officialdom and devoted much passion to crafts, bonsai, and garden design.[9] Due to their marginal status in the Qing cultural scene, their written works received little notice in their lifetimes, and their lives went unmentioned in local gazetteers. In Shen Fu's case, his moving memoir, *Six Accounts of a Life Adrift*, only came to be discovered in Suzhou's flea market decades after his death. Similarly, Zhao Xuemin's life only became known to us through his writings that were posthumously published in the nineteenth century.[10]

It was in 1765—a few years before Zhao would embark on a lifetime of temporary employment as a private secretary—that he wrote a preface to mark the completion of an ambitious work he titled *Bencao gangmu shiyi* (*Supplement to Systematic Materia Medica*, hereafter *Shiyi*). Anticipating possible criticism from readers, Zhao composed a hypothetical dialogue between himself and a visitor, for whom Li Shizhen's *Bencao gangmu* represented the pinnacle of bencao learning. According to the visitor, the pharmacopeia tradition derived from imperial prestige, for which "no effort and cost were ever spared" (*buxi gongfei*). He imagined that Li Shizhen could "interview physicians from all over the country" and inquire into the various local customs (*tusu*). How could an ordinary scholar go about making it even better? To this question, Zhao Xuemin replied in the following way:

> Sure, yes—but not quite! Binhu [Li Shizhen]'s book is indeed very erudite. However, things do proliferate in kind and category after living long enough. The folk customs today value curiosities, hence marvelous and extraordinary things all assemble.[11]

It was in fact imperative, argued Zhao, that his knowledge be recorded at the present moment, lest it might be forever lost to future generations. In the manuscript, Zhao described a total of 921 new drugs in addition to Li Shizhen's *Bencao gangmu*.

Although Zhao called his bencao a mere "supplement" to Li Shizhen, their working methods were quite different. Whereas Li Shizhen carefully arranged quotes from previous authorities, subsuming his own medical experience in layers of commentary, Zhao Xuemin's bencao consisted of strings of quotations from contemporary sources, ranging from local herbalists' recipes to travelogues from the Qing empire's newly conquered frontier regions. In the 1770s, the Qianlong emperor bestowed a complete set of the imperial encyclopedia *Gujin tushu jicheng* to a Hangzhou book collection, in return for the latter's generous donation to the *Siku quanshu* project, and Zhao Xuemin eagerly gleaned much new information from it. Among the sources he quoted most were Fang Yizhi's *Notes on the Principle of Things*, a high Manchu official's miscellaneous notes taken during his tenure in many different provinces. His bencao gave voice to the expanding intellectual and material horizons of the Qing world, as well as the verifiable excitement and confusion that surrounded it.

In addition to his broad reading, Zhao continued to add notes to the un-published manuscript until as late as in 1803, drawing from his personal experiences as well as reports from his acquaintances. Unlike Li Shizhen, who saw his pharmacopeia going to press, Zhao Xuemin's meandering inquiries led him further and further away from the plan he started with. His unfinished manuscript ended up in a local physician's possession, and was not published in print until the 1860s. Through Zhao's eyes, we now turn to the ways in which the quickening pulse of economic exchange reshaped pharmaceutical object-hood in Qing China.

From the Mountains, into the Towns

In the summer of 1787, while working in Fenghua County near Hangzhou, Zhao Xuemin saw mountain village people (*shancun ren*) carrying bundles of dried herbs for sale in urban markets (*chengshi*). He bought a bundle with one hundred copper coins, thinking that it looked like dried mint. Named Sixth-Month Frost (*liu yue shuang*), the herb made a very good cup of tea that also improved digestion. Zhao tried it himself and experienced immediate relief from summer heat.[12]

Throughout *Shiyi*, Zhao paid acute attention to such boundary-crossing actions and documented his own interaction, as a consumer, with those who brought over (*dailai*) the novel remedies from the wilderness, imperial frontiers, and foreign lands. The commercial exchange of medicinal ingredients was by no means limited to organizations and individuals dedicated to the trade of pharmaceuticals. The timber traders (*ban ke*) of Fujian, so he learned, regularly carried a bitter chestnut produced in the Far South, a drug undocumented in previous bencao literature but now ubiquitous in local pharmacies, for it was said to be a good purgative and a cure for hemorrhage.[13] Wool traders (*yang rong ke*) from Shaanxi were known to possess a popular cure for sores.[14] Traders who plied the coastal ports in the Ningbo area prepared and peddled new delicacies such as sago flour (*zhu er fen*).[15] Faced with the well-established daodi authenticity of "mainstream" herbs, Qing traders often sought to challenge and disrupt the status quo by establishing their unique authority over novel cures and opening up new markets.

As a native of Hangzhou and frequent traveler to the countryside, Zhao Xuemin took an avid interest in the new products that came from the wilderness (*yesheng*). He considered it unacceptable that some of the most famous regional varieties in his lifetime, such as *Bai Zhu* from Yuqian County—

a mountainous region west of Hangzhou—received no mention in Li Shizhen's *Bencao gangmu*. His investigation even went below the county level and reached the sites of harvest. The most superior kind of wild Bai Zhu, noted Zhao, came from Crane Hill, a place where the herb allegedly "has [the] long neck, wings and claws of a crane; the skin is thin with yellow hues. If you cut it open, there are vermillion-colored dots in the texture." Echoing other contemporary authors, Zhao Xuemin dismissed the bulk supply of cultivated Bai Zhu as useless and possibly contaminated with fertilizers. He hastened to add that the roots of cultivated herbs looked nothing like the neck of a crane.[16] The notion that domestic cultivation would somehow impart an "impure quality" to a medicinal plant was unseen in previous bencao, and wilderness came to be increasingly associated with the image of the pure and pristine.

Fascination with the wild knew no end. Zhao soon found out that the commercial success of the Yuqian variety had quickly exhausted the sources of wild Bai Zhu there and, in turn, incentivized the exploitation of similar plants elsewhere. In 1791, a visitor gave Zhao a batch of natural grown (*tian sheng*) Bai Zhu from Qingtian County, a place further south down the coast near the border between Zhejiang and Fujian. He was told that this freshly harvested herb grew not in soil, but on the surface of a particular rocky cliff; only 20–30 jin of the plant was made available every year. He noted that the dried root also had an elegant curve resembling a crane's neck, a desirable feature that reminded him of Crane Hill. Samples of wild Bai Zhu reached him from other sources near and far, and Zhao would cut them open, gaze at their texture and color, and record their taste. One especially successful variety found near Hangzhou was marketed as "fragrant and sweet" and recommended for casual chewing in order to alleviate thirst and aid digestion. Importantly, wild Bai Zhu became a choice tonic for those who could not afford ginseng.[17]

From a consumer's perspective, the pursuit of pure, authentic products did not necessarily prevent one from delighting in the wide range of options made available by intense competition. Blood orange peels (*juhong*) from Huazhou, a place located at the border between Guangdong and Guangxi, had long been considered to be the daodi authentic variety of this cooling drug. Zhao Xuemin heard that oranges growing on one old tree in front of the prefectural government office were especially coveted. Since the tree only grew "one fruit per month," substitutes and fakes flooded the market. Quoting a contemporary herbalist's recommendation, Zhao described visual cues to tell the authentic Huazhou orange peels from others. At the same time, he was also delighted to report that a market town near his home in Hangzhou had recently begun to sell a new variety of sweet orange jam. Pleasant to taste and less pungent than the Huazhou variety, noted Zhao, it might be more suitable for delicate southerners.[18]

The most famous substitute drugs in eighteenth-century China were no doubt the increasingly popular Japanese (*Dongyangshen*) and American ginseng (*Xiyangshen*).[19] Prior to the arrival of these products, however, Qing consumers like Zhao Xuemin were already sampling from a great variety of "ginseng-like" products produced domestically. In *Shiyi*, Zhao Xuemin described his own experience using ginseng (*shen*) from the Zhaotong Prefecture (at the Yunnan-Guizhou border), the You River in Guangxi, the Qiongzhou Prefecture (Hainan Island), Tibet, and "Mountain Dong territory in Guangxi" (*Guangxi shan Dong*).[20] He concluded that many of these products were, in fact, quite different from the most expensive Korean and Liaodong ginseng. Less palatable for him was the blatant attempt by some merchant groups to sell their local herbs as "ginseng." For instance, Fujian merchants brought an unknown plant from the "red-haired" (*hongmao*) foreigners, and it looked "nothing like ginseng."[21] The coastal province Fujian now had its own local variety of "ginseng," which in turn was transplanted to Henan, probably carried by merchants moving between the two provinces. Zhao complained that virtually everywhere now claimed to have a "local" (*tu*) variety of ginseng. "Day in and day out, people search for curiosities," wrote Zhao, to the extent that they would comb through "remote rocks and barren valleys" looking for any obscure herb, hoping to earn some profit by selling it as a cheaper substitute.[22] The problem was that no one could speak with certainty for a novel product's medicinal efficacy.

The Song pharmacopeia first used the term "wild grown" (*yesheng*) in a negative light: the editors warned that plants such as *wild* sesame, garlic, eggplant, and lettuce should be used with caution, as they might be poisonous compared with the more reliable domesticated varieties.[23] Sixteenth-century bencao authors such as Li Shizhen and Chen Jiamo further admonished physicians to distinguish "wild" from "homegrown" types of plants. Li Shizhen wrote that while wild yam (*shuyu*) was used regularly as a medicine, homegrown yam had less potency and was better eaten as food.[24] Chen Jiamo in his abridged bencao warned against mixing different sources of the same herb in one's practice and composed a rhyme on this topic for his disciples to memorize.[25] In general, both Li and Chen were interested in the different qualities of "wild" and "cultivated" varieties of the same plant, yet held no clear preference for one over the other.

The seventeenth century, however, witnessed a remarkable interest in "wild" medicinal plants. Lu Zhiyi, a native of Hangzhou, dismissed the ubiquitous plum trees planted around the city and recommended harvesting plum fruits instead from "the wild-grown trees, or those whose branches had not yet been grafted."[26] Zhang Lu, a Suzhou native proud of locally produced basil and other fragrant herbs, was also opinionated about the common medicinal plant Bai Zhu. The "cultivated and irrigated" (*zaiguan*) varieties commonly seen in shops, noted Zhang, were inferior to a new variety "grown in the wilderness," which possessed "purer *qi*."[27] Wu Yiluo (ca. 1704–66), a Jiangnan physician who claimed to update Wang Ang's popular bencao while "conforming to new standards (*congxin*)," complained about the quality of aconite sold in shops:

> Aconite in Sichuan previously grew in the wild; the harvest was rare, the price was high, and its power was quite strong. Recently, it has come to be cultivated; the harvest is more abundant, but the price has dropped and its power has become quite thin. Local people preserve it with salt, which further weakens it.[28]

Wu Yiluo's complaint reflected the substantive expansion of interregional trade in his own times and the psychological effect elicited by increased supply. This new preference for the wild over the homegrown would have startled Li Shizhen and Chen Jiamo less than two centuries earlier.

The Taming of Wilderness

The process of "bringing over" new medicines from the wilderness, however, was by no means peaceful and free of tension. One intriguing feature of *Shiyi* and the sources it cited was a conspicuous willingness to elaborate on the danger, violence, and human cunning that were necessary to obtain exotica. When traveling along the Zhejiang coast, Zhao Xuemin learned that people from Xianju County had formed a group of professional mountain foragers, who specialized in picking delicate fungi from steep rocks on high cliffs. Carrying their special tools, the company performed their own rituals upon beginning their ascent up the mountains; every year, someone would die from this risky yet lucrative trade.[29] Elsewhere in Guangxi Province, people discovered a rare kind of "golden fruit olive" (*jin guo lan*) tree, which was originally grown in northern Vietnam. Zhao's father once obtained twenty pieces of the precious fruit, which was picked by local people (*turen*) from the bottom of deep valleys.[30] The fact that people risked their lives to obtain these products only served to increase their market value and perceived efficacy.

In the winter of 1790, a man named Li Jinshi stopped by a butcher shop outside the Western gate of Lin'an County and watched the butcher cut open the stomach of a goat. A strange object emerged from the goat's viscera; it looked "like duck egg yolk, perfectly round, shiny and smooth, when put in a basin of water it would float." The butcher identified it as "hundred-herb elixir" (*baicao dan*) and told Li that he had only seen such a thing three times in more than thirty years of his practice. Intrigued, Li purchased the object from the butcher and brought it to Zhao Xuemin, who was then living in the vicinity as a private secretary. Together they examined it and compared it with ox bezoars.[31]

On four other occasions, Zhao identified the same Li Jinshi as a man from Penglai, a county that sits at the northern coast of the Shandong peninsula. From him, Zhao heard vivid tales of how local fishermen hunted for seals (*haigou*, "sea dogs"). According to Li, the only opportunity to kill these agile creatures would be during the coldest months of the year, when river mouths were frozen, and many sea dogs emerged from the deep sea to lie on the ice, bathing under the sun. And then,

> [hunters] quickly jump into the water, hit the seadog's waist with a wooden stick, and only in that way can they get it. Otherwise, if the ice cracks, or one makes the slightest sound with footsteps, or if the seadogs are not asleep, it would be impossible. But every year many people are drowned to death while "hitting the dogs." As the profit is high, they are willing to risk their lives.

The body fat of sea dogs was of special interest to Zhao Xuemin. He had seen coastal residents put a few drops of the precious liquid into the sea, which instantly illuminated the turbid water, revealing eels and sea cucumbers that hid in the depths. Someone had also brought some sea dog fat to Zhao "from East of the Pass"—that is, the Manchu homeland that ordinary traders should have been forbidden to enter. Examining the substance, Zhao described it as a "dry, greenish paste." Learning that locals used it as an ointment for cold sores, Zhao concluded that this proved the "hot and fierce" (*re lie*) nature of this mysterious cure.[32]

An abundance of such hunting stories made such a lasting impression on Zhao Xuemin that he recorded them in *Shiyi*. A student of his once told him about the hunting of large ravens that lived in the mountains of eastern Zhejiang. Again, the birds became desirable to "local people" because of the alleged medicinal virtues of their bile. According to hunters' lore, the bird's gallbladder was always empty during the day and full of bile at night. Hunters would wait patiently until a raven fell asleep, quickly cut open its abdomen with a sharp knife, and snatch the gallbladder intact with no liquid spilled.[33] Tiger meat was a famous remedy said to be able to prevent smallpox, and so hunters would release a stray dog and entice a tiger to kill it, which allegedly made the tiger "drunk" and unable to flee. Following the trail of dog blood, they would capture the immobile tiger, harvesting its meat, fat, and bones for medicinal use.[34] Ever since deer fetus (*lu tai*) came to be mentioned as a powerful remedy in Zhang Lu's seventeenth-century bencao treatise (Li Shizhen said nothing about it in *Bencao gangmu*), hunters began to go after fawns and pregnant does.[35] Although animal drugs had always held a secure place in the bencao tradition, never before had so many vivid depictions of people tricking, subjugating, and then killing animals found their way into the genre. Those stories seemed to celebrate human cunning itself as part of the efficacy for those medicines.

Once "brought over" from the wilderness and transformed into consumable objects, exotic drugs of animal origin remained in the possession of common households, eliciting further curiosity and awe. Zhao Xuemin once knew a man named Wang Yitang, who kept a piece of "lion feces" at home in an iron box. Nourished (*yang*) with bits of iron, the substance became hard as metal, and developed a reddish hue (probably from iron rust). Wang told Zhao that this made an excellent remedy for malignant sores (*e chuang*) on the lower body and the removal of scabs.[36] In 1796, another friend of Zhao surnamed Shao obtained a small amount of "lion fat," a purported remedy for urological dysfunctions. Uncertain about whether he should try the exotic drug or not, Shao gave it to a townsman, who then sold it on to a third person for a high price. That night, the buyer took one "half kernel" of the substance and was found dead in the morning. Fearing an official investigation, the intermediary seller also killed himself. Tragic stories like this, however, did not lead Zhao to question the efficacy of the drug itself, but rather to conclude that the potency of lion fat was probably "too harsh" for human bowels.[37]

Butchers, fishermen, and seal hunters knew what it was like to cut open an animal's body, and the toil and cunning required to maintain such a livelihood.

What is truly remarkable is that Zhao Xuemin, an educated and urbane literatus, took great care to interview these tradesmen and acknowledged their authority in his bencao. In this process of transmission, these kinds of stories became an organic part of what wilderness meant to Qing consumers, fueling their fantasy about the exotic places where such specimens were procured. The wilderness was no empty space but was populated with "fierce" creatures, as well as the enterprising "local people" who risked their lives to hunt them. There was a sense of ruthless pleasure in the ways in which Zhao Xuemin related these stories. The animals here were not, in Martina Siebert's words, the "text animals" that philologists joyously pursued on paper.[38] Neither were they allegorical animals like those which appeared in the writings of neo-Confucian teachers to illuminate the potential and limitations of human nature. Their fierce appearances instead elicited human desire to subjugate them, possess them, and (if possible) consume them.

The commercial operations that extended far into the wilderness had largely evaded official attention, except for the common complaints in local gazetteers that the drive for profit among desperate people (*qiongmin*) would quickly exhaust the natural resources of a place. Whereas late Ming officials could petition for the conversion of local tribute burdens, Qing magistrates wielded little power with which to confront commercial operations that extended far beyond their jurisdiction.[39] It was only in the aftermath of the Great White Lotus Rebellion that Qing officials paid attention to the sprawling plantations (*chang*) of medicinal plants in the so-called tri-province area between Shaanxi, Sichuan, and Henan. Yan Ruyu (1759–1826), a former private secretary who eventually rose up the official ranks owing to his deep knowledge of the rebellious region, reported that Golden Thread and magnolia barks (*houpu*) were two of the most famous daodi authentic medicines that merchants sought to cultivate and sell to faraway places (*xingyuan*). Contrary to popular belief, Yan pointed out that these drugs were, in fact, all cultivated in the deep mountains:

> The ancient woodlands having been cleared long ago, the Golden Thread and Magnolia barks that are produced here are hardly wild. Magnolia saplings are planted on plain slopes and patchy terrain, and they are as thin as a brush pot. The trees grow to the diameter of a cup or a bowl in several to a dozen years, and they then yield good quality bark. As for Golden Thread, it is cultivated in the hollows and valleys of cleared mountain land. Merchants buy an enclosure with a circumference of several tens of

li, and plant the herb all over. Since it takes up to ten years for the plant to grow, they rent the land to "shed people" (*pengmin*) to take care of the herbs, and on each yard there are several dozen households. In general, the quality of medicine is the best when the mountain is high and the valley is deep.[40]

Yan Ruyu's astute observation reveals the dubious status of categories like "wild" and "homegrown" in Qing commercial parlance, for the plants labeled "wild" may well have been grown artificially. Yan Ruyu's sensitivity to the instrumental role of "shed people" is, in a sense, comparable to Zhao Xuemin's close observation of traders and hunters. Despite their upbringing as educated men, they could not live a life aloof from practical concerns. Instead, their placement among the informal retinue of government compelled them to pay attention to different walks of life in order to survive.

Culinary Transformations

Captured and tamed, new remedies often required further expertise in order to prepare them for consumption. In this regard, little guidance could be found in previous bencao literature, and the division between pharmaceutical and culinary processes quickly became blurred. Since exotic ingredients often could not fit easily into previously used medicinal formulas, they were more frequently folded into the regular course of preparing a meal at home.

Building on previous literatures on dietetic bencao, Qing authors grappled with the new ingredients and tried to form a consensus wherever possible. American ginseng was cold in nature; Japanese ginseng less so. Too much sweetness caused congestion, and excessive heat generated phlegm. Statements about the nature of drugs were almost always accompanied by methods of moderating their pernicious effects: the cool-natured American ginseng, for instance, could be rendered mild and agreeable by steaming it over rice.[41] The Tibetan wonder drug "Summer herb, winter worm," which was held to be warm in nature, was paired in several recipes with cool-natured duck meat, steamed "through the entire body of the bird" to make a nourishing food for convalescing patients.[42] Other popular "base" ingredients that were often prepared together with medicinal ingredients included chicken and animal viscera, which arguably might well have been the principal nourishments of the dish.[43] Eating and cooking thus became sites of *experimentation* for Qing consumers, in the sense that *experience* gathered this way, and articulated in a formulaic fashion, would then be counted as valid information to share with others.

The Japanese scholar Shinoda Osamu is quite right to suggest that the "modernization of dietetic life" (*shokuseika ni okeru kindaika*) took place across the Ming-Qing transition.[44] In the late sixteenth century, Li Shizhen noted the good taste of shark fin, but made no comment on its medicinal virtues; two hundred years later, it had become a "regular favorite" of banquets, and Zhao Xuemin quoted multiple sources recommending it for "enhancing core strength" (*zhang yao li*).[45] Dozens of accounts described the delicacy known as "swallow's nest" (*yanwo*) but disagreed over its true nature. What did the swallows look like? What kind of food did they eat? Some said small fish, some said powdery rock salt, some said small shellfish. There was also disagreement over how to prepare it for banquet: some recommended it sweetened, some scolded against eating it as a dessert.[46] Notably, both shark fin and swallow's nest were essentially by-products of the late Ming maritime trade into the South China Sea and Southeast Asian countries, where the hunting of sharks became more prevalent. The exploitation of the coastal habitat in these regions gave rise to the specialized, highly risky trade of collecting swallow's nests from rocky cliffs. Both substances were also recommended as possessing the medicinal virtue of "opening up the appetite" (*kai wei*). The consumption of these foods, in other words, facilitated yet more consumption.

Poisoning from eating unfamiliar foods was quite common, and Zhao collected personal testimonies from his acquaintances to ascertain whether a plant was safe to eat. A friend named Zhou told him about a night spent in panic, after carelessly consuming the colorful flower of autumn crabapple (*qiuhaitang*), which was supposed to be toxic. When he found himself still breathing normally at daybreak, Zhou concluded that the poisonous reputation of the plant must have been false.[47] In another personal story, Zhao Xuemin recalled a young servant of their household, who had suffered from chronic intermittent fever for many years. One day, he "accidentally ate chili pepper sauce" and never lapsed back into fever again.[48] No one had mentioned the antimalarial properties of the popular condiment, noted Zhao. In the absence of an authoritative opinion, he gathered anecdotal testimonies from over two hundred individuals, many of whom were private tutors like him.

We might recall how Chen Jiru, the celebrity author who dabbled in late Ming dietetic bencao, announced that the matter of everyday eating and drinking was "something that I could govern myself." Writing in the long tradition of dietetic treatises that advised temperance and decried gluttony, Chen joked that reading the bencao made him waggle his tongue and remember to restrain his appetite. The various ways in which Zhao Xuemin and his eighteenth-century sources explored food and medicine, however, placed less emphasis on the innate properties of things than on how culinary methods might render exotic substances edible, wholesome, and even pleasant. Zhao wrote with appreciation about the new delicacies he encountered at shared meals with his colleagues. From 1788 to 1791, Zhao worked in Lin'an for Magistrate Liu, nephew of the high official and renowned scholar Liu Yong (1719–1805). At one of the magistrate's banquets, Zhao tasted a delicious clam that he had never seen before, which had been delivered fresh from Liu's hometown on the northern coast.[49] He referred to the sumptuous parties offered by the wealthy salt merchants of Yangzhou, which always started with shark fins, swallow's nest stews, and lavish amounts of wild game.[50] While Zhao was clearly familiar with the admonition against excessive consumption in older bencao, throughout Shiyi he voiced little protest against the conflation of medicinal and culinary procedures. Rather, he took obvious pleasure in the extent to which people could manipulate nature for their own benefit.

One rather extreme set of examples of this manipulative tendency mobilizes other living creatures as the instruments of pharmaceutical processing. Zhao Xuemin wrote about a man named Zhu Qiuting, who spent "a thousand taels of silver" to buy a secret recipe from traders to prepare a very bitter herb into a satisfactory substitute for authentic Liaodong ginseng. He shared it with Zhao Xuemin begrudgingly: Take five ounces of the bitter herb, mix and rub with powdered aconite. Find a fresh egg, empty the egg white and yolk, put five ounces of the herbal mixture into the shell, and seal it back intact. Let a hen sit on the fake "egg" (marked with a circle) along with her other eggs. When the latter all hatch, take the fake egg out and let her sit on it again, repeat seven times, after which the herbal mixture will acquire the tonic quality of authentic ginseng.[51] A similar method of artificial fashioning (rengong zhizao) came from another friend. This involved tricking wild cranes to hatch cooked eggs, repeating the process three times, and using the eggshell as a drinking vessel, which allegedly carried various health benefits. According to Zhao, this rare object could command a very high price at the local market.[52] In both cases, it was believed that intimate contact with the mother bird's body would imbue the bitter and dead substance with miraculous efficacy.

What might have driven someone to buy such a recipe for a thousand taels of silver? Like hunting stories, the elaborate procedures and deceptions that went into the methods constituted an important aspect of the market value of the end result. The complex processes resonated with contemporary pharmacists' pledge to piously reproduce ancient recipes without sparing material expense or labor. But it was, in fact, all this additional labor that inflated the end product's market value. In other words, labor and effort could transform dead matter into gold.

Souvenirs of Empire

In 1788 (Qianlong 53), Zhao Xuemin received a package from his son, who also worked as a private secretary in faraway Xuzhou Prefecture (map 0.2). Enclosed in the letter was a specimen that Zhao had requested: the so-called Chicken Blood Vine (*jixueteng*), a plant whose woody stalk oozed crimson-red resin reportedly curing any injuries immediately. His son explained that he had obtained the plant from the indigenous ruler (*tusi*) of the Jinsha River. Holding the piece of dried resin in his hand, Zhao recalled another recent occasion where an official, who had once served in Yunnan, showed him a piece of Chicken Blood Vine: it was similar in appearance but with an altogether different texture inside. The riddle was still not resolved three years later, when an official returning from Yunnan gave Zhao another piece of Chicken Blood Vine resin to treat his joint pain. This one looked still different from the previous two samples. After examining the samples with his son, who was visiting home at the time, Zhao could not reach a conclusion over what the true appearance of the plant should look like. "If only I could be there myself (*qinli qi di*)," Zhao noted with some frustration, "and check on these things carefully!"[53]

Qing emperors and their ministers were not the only ones who could claim authority in frontier matters and spread new knowledge. Middle-tier bureaucrats serving in frontier posts wrote travelogues and memoirs upon returning home; so did their secretaries and technical assistants. Aside from repeating the official lines that touted the benefits of civilization under Qing rule, these writings also documented the extensive process of cultural domestication via gift exchange and consumption of tangible objects. The multiple specimens of Chicken Blood Vine, which Zhao asked his son to inquire about at the southwestern frontier, served essentially as souvenirs of the frontier experience for many visitors from the provinces. One returnee told Zhao Xuemin that soldiers stationed in Tengyue, a strategic location near the Qing-Burmese border, regularly went into deep valleys to harvest the crimson-red resin to use as gifts or sell to dealers.[54] From a vice-prefect who had sojourned in the Western border territories (*xichui*), Zhao learned about a leafless plant growing in the deep mountains of Barköl (*Balikun*), where the Kazakhs lived. Again, it was the "horse-herding soldiers" who knew and harvested the stalks, reduced the juice into a paste, and sold it to "guest merchants from afar" (*yuanke*).[55] The gift economy between members of the bureaucracy and their extended kin inevitably fueled the commodification of frontier products. Their additions to the existing range of pharmaceutical offerings were an unintended consequence of Qing imperial expansion throughout the eighteenth century.

The influx of new frontier products to central China during the eighteenth century took place before any learned consensus over their uses could be consolidated, let alone regulated. Taken from their native habitats, the exotic cures offered new promise for alleviating familiar maladies. One predominant therapeutic appropriation revealed a deep-seated anxiety over the deadly scourge of smallpox among young children. Tibetan incense, for instance, was promoted in earnest as a preventive measure for households with young children. Zhao expressed some doubt about the soundness of the idea, yet nevertheless asked for the recipe for the expensive incense from an old man who once worked for Cao Yin (1658–1712), the powerful bondservant and confidant of the Kangxi emperor.[56] Another frontier product that acquired anti-pox fame was the so-called Divine Yellow Beans, brought in from Yunnan and Sichuan. According to Zhao's description, the dried beans produced a pleasant sound when one tapped or shook the pod. A visitor once showed him a sample from Yunnan. A popular recipe dictated that the beans should be prepared half-raw and half-baked, and consumed together with cilantro water: the cure worked wonders for dissipating the "pox poison." If one started the regimen early enough, a child might even be spared from going through the ordeal of smallpox altogether.[57] By passing on remedies that invoked the "divine" (*shen*) power of the novel cures, Zhao Xuemin effectively acknowledged the occult nature of their efficacy that, in part, derived from their exotic origins in the empire's latest frontier.

Layers of Foreignness

Though he repeatedly quoted Fang Yizhi's work, Zhao Xuemin did have a small disagreement with the great scholar over the true nature of white pepper. From "Cantonese ships" (*Guang bo*), Fang heard that "jade-colored" peppercorn had a particularly pungent taste versus the dark-colored ones. A hundred years later, Zhao Xuemin claimed that white peppercorns were sold "in abundance" at the "foreign goods shops" (*yanghuodian*) in Ningbo, a major port of maritime trade. Moreover, a merchant friend had learned from his foreign business partners that white peppers were prepared by removing the skin of the peppercorns before sun-drying the fruits and therefore were of essentially the same kind (*zhong*).[58] Although Zhao Xuemin did not do business directly with foreigners, foreign merchandise like white pepper was very much present and accessible to him and constituted objects of intense interest. He expected exotic and exciting products to be "brought over" (*dailai*) from "foreign ships in Canton and Macau" (*Yue Ao yangbo*), such as essential oils, benzoin resin (*anxi xiang*), and ambergris (*longxian xiang*).[59] In 1800, another family member brought him some cinchona branches from eastern Guangdong, and taught him a recipe transmitted by "Macau barbarians" (*Ao fan*), in which one treated all kinds of malaria with a decoction of cinchona and cinnamon.[60]

Zhao Xuemin deployed a complex and nuanced terminology in *Shiyi* to describe foreigners and foreignness. He continued to use the geographical terms "Western Seas" (*xiyang*) and "Eastern Seas" (*dongyang*) seen in earlier geographical literature. Meanwhile, he frequently used the term "yang" to describe objects associated with maritime trade. Business vessels docking in Canton and Macau were "foreign ships" (*yangbo*), and Chinese-run groceries that carried imported goods in Ningbo were "foreign goods shops" (*yanghuodian*). Things that were yang were well within his range of consumption, as exemplified by his mention of "foreign painting" (*yanghua*), "foreign cloth" (*yangbu*), and "foreign sugar" (*yangtang*; refined sugar prepared according to foreign/new methods). In *Shiyi*, Zhao recorded a recipe for preparing a confectionary snack using fresh oranges dipped in "pure white foreign sugar," a delicacy that could improve digestion and dissipate phlegm.[61] Overall, the attribute of yang foreignness was presented as nonthreatening and even positive, if still a somewhat rare treat.

Another term, *fan*, however, presented a different kind of otherness. It referred to people residing in territories closer to home, especially in the Far South, such as "Macau indigenes" (*Aofan*) as mentioned earlier. "Fan" was also a popular term in Qing governmental parlance to refer to indigenous people who were nominally under Qing rule but followed their own customs. From the time of the Qing Conquest in 1683, the distinction between "raw" and "cooked" indigenous people (*shengfan/shufan*) in Taiwan was an influential context for the spread of the terms. "Western indigenes" (*Xifan*), a term that had been in use since earlier times to refer to the Tibetan cultural region, continued into the Qing when it became increasingly common to use the modern-day term *Zang*, or *Xizang*. In *Shiyi*, Zhao Xuemin displayed a deep fascination with Tibetan lamas, the elite clergy who resided in Beijing and performed rituals for the Qing court. In 1792, Zhao Xuemin obtained "several dozen" mani pills, a remedy that had been blessed by the monks and reportedly could be used as a panacea. From family and friends, Zhao received detailed instruction on the storage (in glassware) of those pills and their upkeep ("feed" the pills with Tibetan saffron). He also heard vivid stories of the ritual during which the lamas in Beijing had gathered to pray and bless the pills, which could behave as if they were alive: larger pills could procreate by self-division and generate smaller ones, or fly around in the air. A popular gift for Qing aristocrats and high officials, the pills also found their way into ordinary households in the south. According to a tale told by an itinerant physician, Zhao learned that a local deaf man had miraculously regained his hearing by taking just three mani pills, only to lose it again after spending a night at a prostitute's home.[62] Through such cautionary stories of self-medication, strange objects from Tibet found a place in the domestic moral imagination of High Qing Jiangnan.

The more predominant usage of "fan" in this text, however, extended to objects associated with lands and peoples in and beyond the South China Sea and closely connected to home by the junk trade. For instance, when referred to as *fanbo*, business vessels were related to Batavia (Sunda Kalapa, *Halaba*) or other trading outposts in today's Southeast and South Asia.[63] Through Zhao Xuemin's carefully gathered quotes and stories, we see how the category of fan mediated the long process of introducing and domesticating new crops that came into China via Southeast Asia throughout the seventeenth century, from as far away as America. A seventeenth-century source first documented "foreign bananas" (*fanjiao*) that reportedly came from the Ryukyu Kingdom.[64] Similarly, the term "fan" was applied to the naming of chili pepper (*fanjiao*), peanuts (*fandou*, "foreign bean"),[65] and sweet potato (*fanshu*, "foreign yam").[66] Plants that were unique to Taiwan presented themselves as "foreign/indigenous garlic" (*fansuan*) and "foreign/indigenous ginger" (*fanjiang*).[67] Here, the image of the indigene plant overlapped with the image of the indigene person, slowly being transformed into part of the familiar spheres of Qing rule. Fan was, for Zhao Xuemin, foreign in a nonthreatening, even mysterious way.

Lastly, the term *yi* was perhaps the only word of foreignness in *Shiyi* that carried a rather strong pejorative connotation. Zhao Xuemin quoted earlier sources that employed the term with reference to "barbarian ships" (*yichuan*) that encroached upon the Ming coast in the late sixteenth century,[68] "Japanese barbarians" (*Woyi*), and erotic tales of "barbarian women" (*yifu*) in Burma who transformed wondrous insects into love potions.[69] Early Qing governmental compendia referred to "barbarian territory" (*yifang*) in remote frontiers of Yunnan.[70] Yet the occurrence of the pejorative "yi" (28) in *Shiyi* is far less frequent than the more positive or neutral terms of "yang" (95) and "fan" (79), and Zhao almost never used "yi" in his own commentary, which was narrated in the first person. Unlike many of the authors he quoted, it seems that he found the term neither particularly useful nor relevant for his purposes. This attitude, in my mind, poses a stark contrast with the prevalent use of "yi" as a "super sign" in Qing governmental documents that set the tone for foreign policy in the nineteenth century.[71] The Qing official insistence on using the denigrating term "yi" was also a political statement aimed at a domestic audience who, like Zhao Xuemin, might very well have become used to foreign things—yang or fan—as a familiar presence in their life.

From a pharmacist's perspective, then, there was no a priori, binary distinction between Chinese things and foreign things. Not only did the foreign exist in various terminologies and shades of strangeness, the processes of trade themselves yielded unexpected products that possessed medicinal efficacy. The most extreme examples of impromptu appropriation took place again in the Canton Bay, where foreign ships docked. After inspections were performed by Qing officials, and the merchandise was unloaded and stored at one of the Chinese-run factories, locals came to the ships to harvest the so-called Foreign Ship Membrane (*yangchuanpu*), a type of algae attached to the protruding keel of the vessel. According to local recipes, the substance made an excellent remedy for stomach pain.[72] In another entry, Zhao documented that ships coming from Malacca were equipped with a special kind of torch made with an ignitable resin produced there. Local Chinese healers sought out the unburned remainder resin from the torches, calling it "foreign horse whip" (*fan da ma*). They would grind it into powder, mix it with mercury, and prepare an ointment that became a popular remedy against syphilis.[73] Iron wires that Europeans produced and brought to China were usually rusted when they reached Canton; the oxidized rust was carefully scraped off to treat skin sores.[74] Flint stones sourced from Canton and Macau were attributed to the "Red-Haired Nations" (*Hongmao guo*), and after the foreigners (*fanren*) sold the inner cores, the "white, chalky" skin of the stones was removed and given away for free, becoming a popular remedy for minor wounds.[75] Such wondrous creations were, in a sense, by-products of foreign trade itself. Their attraction expressed not the commonly supposed Chinese xenophobia, but an abiding popular interest in exchanges with afar.

Finally, here is one last example of High Qing pharmaceutical fantasy that combined a fascination with the exotic and the pleasures of artificial processing. Again, Zhao Xuemin will be our guide:

> The so-called "foreign beetle" (*yang chong*) came from the outer seas (*wai yang*), and was introduced to China in the late Ming; or, as it is said, the bugs came from the Great Western Sea (*Da Xiyang*), and only appeared in the Kangxi reign. Their shape is like that of a rice weevil, and the young larvae look like little silkworms, and then turn black like fermented beans. There are male ones and female ones; nowadays, people keep them in bamboo boxes, and feed them with grains. They are vulnerable to cold, and in winter must be kept on the lap, or inside the sleeve, and put under the beddings at night, otherwise they will die. They live on human breath (*renqi*), and reproduce quickly. If you feed them shredded *fuling*, saffron, or Vietnamese cinnamon, their shells will turn a lovely, lustrous red color. They are extremely good as medicine.[76]

Zhao Xuemin quoted a very long list of recipes and recommended ingesting the insects alive with different drinks such as wine, mint water, orange water, and ginger soup. The tiny insect allegedly could treat a variety of illnesses ranging from sleep disorders to the common cold, from strokes to malaria. (One might observe that the many different ingredients and decoctions that were taken *with* the beetle might in fact have been the real medicine.)

In the end, the possibility of a "foreign beetle" craze lay precisely in the open-ended pleasure of raising a little creature at home. By keeping the box in his lap and sleeping by it at night, the owner of the strange and tiny pets cultivated their curative power by imparting his own vitality and human breath (*renqi*). One could imagine it to be either an expensive pastime or a relatively accessible hobby, depending on how much one decided to invest in its upkeep. Arguably, the alleged medicinal efficacy of the "foreign beetle" was not rooted in any cosmological speculation about its nature, but rather in the amount of time and care spent cultivating the communion between oneself and the beetle, which served as a depository of vitality that could later be returned to the self. Here the intricate correlative cosmology of yin/yang and the five phases did not apply; all that mattered was the karmic chain of feeding and being fed, an endless stream of pulsating, bare life.

Threats of the Unknown

The sudden popularity of foreign beetles may also have been a kind of substitute phenomenon, as the earlier fad of consuming "human drugs" had fallen out of favor. Qing laws deemed any mutilation of corpses to be illegal and punishable by the severest sentences. Writing in the eighteenth century, Zhao Xuemin found the use of human body parts as medicine so repelling that he eliminated "humans" as a category of medicine that had been present in all previous bencao.[77] Yet the law did not prevent the continuation of another kind of fetishistic fascination with the human body that hinged not on its own nature but on its existence as a *medium* for receiving and imparting human vitality. These practices involved proximity to dead bodies.

One such example documented in *Shiyi* involved rosin and wax that had been customarily used in northern China to seal coffins where lacquer was not available. When it came the time to relocate a grave to a new site, the decaying coffin was dug out, and local people (*turen*) would scratch off the rosin and wax to make a poultice used to treat wounds. According to Zhao, the material was so valued because of the "remnant *qi* of blood and flesh" it contained.[78] Zhao also quoted contemporary sources and an old servant's eyewitness testimony to describe the illicit trade in "human aphids" (*renya*)—small insects that fed on corpses and were collected by mortuary keepers who drilled holes in coffins and retrieved them. The worms, "steamed into existence" from the dissipated vital energy of the dead, were then used by "magicians" (*fangshu jia*) and folk healers to treat wounds of those who had been beaten during official trials. One could imagine a macabre economy revolving around a prison—the remnant vitality of executed convicts transferred, through those insects, to heal the tortured and battered bodies of other inmates.[79] The functioning of law and order was sustained through the dark efficacy of magic healing.

In his memorable account of Qing China's sorcery scare in 1769, historian Philip A. Kuhn pondered the strange tale of sorcerers sneaking up behind people to cut their queued hair and steal their souls. Using archival documents generated from the Qing state's herculean effort to locate and persecute the elusive sorcerers, Kuhn noted how, for a while, princes and peasants alike all dreaded the threats from "persons unknown and forces unseen."[80] Yet even without the mass hysteria fueled by such extraordinary events, was it not the case that the everyday fabric of Qing lives would have been unimaginable without the presence of the occult? In his book, Kuhn discusses the charms and rituals performed by carpenters and builders who came under suspicion due to their perceived supernatural powers. On a more general level, however, the inexplicable—yet widely accepted—pharmaceutical efficacy of exotic commodities revealed a deeper-seated vulnerability in the Qing psyche. In good times, curiosity begat prosperity; but in bad times, orthodox piety could transform into heterodox sedition. If someone like Zhao Xuemin accepted the plausibility of human aphids as a miraculous medicine, he already came quite close to falling under the influence of sorcerers.

The remarkable success of the commodification of pharmacy in Qing China thus also posed an "unseen threat" to the rulers, who wielded great purchasing power but did not really know where their remedies came from. The transregional network of trade could easily be appropriated to spread politically subversive messages. Pharmacists, for example, played a crucial role in the notorious "bogus memorial" case in the 1750s. A fake memorial, full of slanderous criticism of the Qianlong emperor, was discovered at a courier station in remote Guizhou in 1751. Presaging the pattern of the soulstealer case eighteen years later, the Qianlong emperor furiously directed his provincial officials to hunt down the culprit, only to get lost in a labyrinth of parallel investigations and fake accusations. Officials in Guizhou homed in on a small-time trader named Tan Yongfu, who had carried the bogus memorial while traveling from Sichuan to Yunnan to sell the medicinal herb Golden Thread. Relaying the information back east, neighboring provinces eventually traced Tan's source to a pharmacy shop named Tianyitang in Jiangxi, likely with connections to the "medicinal wharf" of Zhangshu. The case was brought to a close after the conviction and execution of a former military officer in Jiangxi, who had allegedly authored the bogus memorial.[81] Without the extensive interregional network of pharmaceutical merchants, the slanderous material could not have spread so quickly to the southwest provinces. And yet even at the height of his power, the Qianlong emperor remained incapable of monitoring the merchants' minds and deeds, even though he had gone to unprecedented lengths in censoring political speech among the educated men of the empire.

Individuals constituting the very lowest strata of the pharmaceutical trade had little to lose and much to gain by playing up their access to potent substances and wielding semimagical powers. Healing was frequently cited as among the single most attractive means of recruitment for heterodox religious sects in the eighteenth and early nineteenth centuries. The leaders of these shadowy groups often gained credibility by performing healing rituals using a range of methods including tea leaves, massage, meditation, and, in some cases, actual medications.[82] On one occasion, the outsized ambitions of such a leader came into direct conflict with the imperial presence. In 1779 (Qianlong 44), the emperor's retinue was returning from a visit to the Qing ancestral tombs outside Beijing when a young man showed up by the side of the road and presented a letter full of lunatic prophecies that predicted the current reign to last no more than fifty-seven years, essentially foreboding Qianlong's death date. The letter-bearer, an illiterate man named Zhang Jiuxiao who had worked all his life as a hired laborer (*yonggong*), confessed that he was merely delivering the letter on behalf of another man named Zhi Tianbao, who was also promptly arrested and rigorously interrogated.

Zhi Tianbao turned out to be a former pharmacist practicing in Qizhou (map 0.2), where a centralized medicinal marketplace was taking shape around that time. The great pharmacies of Beijing, such as Tongrentang, made purchases in Qizhou at the annual market fair, which would eventually rival the stature of Zhangshu during the nineteenth century. Due to bad fortune, Zhi had lost his shop and made a living instead by coming to Qizhou only during the market fairs, setting up a stand selling medicinal poultices. Unable to make ends meet, he traveled around nearby counties with no stable home, and eventually conjured up an astrological prophecy that enabled him to gather a small group of followers. Notably, both Zhi and laborer Zhang were married at the times of their arrest, indicating that the tiny sect was doing well enough for the leaders. During his interrogation, Zhi confessed that he had hoped that by claiming spiritual communication with the deceased emperor Yongzheng, he would receive wealth and status (*fugui*) in return. Authorities searched his home, only to find some old and tattered (*jiupo*) books on medicine and astrology, which Zhe likely inherited from his father.

Strangely enough, the Qianlong emperor seemed to believe some elements of Zhi's prognostication. When officials recommended the most severe punishment—death by a thousand cuts (*lingchi*)—the emperor wrote a lengthy response that seriously engaged with Zhi Tianbao's prophecy of the end date of his rule, saying that he would in fact be content enough to reign for as many as fifty-seven years. Yet he still took offense at Zhi's pretentious claim to have had spiritual contact with his deceased father. In the end, Zhi Tianbao received a death penalty by immediate beheading (considered more lenient than a slow death). The whole case was summarized in a brief report in an official gazette that praised the emperor's sagacity.[83] Again, in this case, we see a common belief in miraculous prophecy shared by both the emperor and the poor pharmacist alike. Qianlong did not doubt the existence of spiritual mediums; he merely took offense that anyone *other than himself* might claim access to the souls of his ancestors.

A final case that epitomized the problematic nature of the pharmaceutical trade occurred in 1791, only a few years before the aging emperor abdicated his throne after ruling for sixty years. Reviewing a letter sent from the Ryukyu Kingdom's envoys, Qianlong noticed that they had requested to purchase a long list of goods, including a large quantity of medicinal rhubarb (*dahuang*) and outer sea (*waiyang*) commodities such as "foreign" ginseng (*yang shen*) and sappanwood (*sumu*). It was several years since Qianlong decided to punish the unruly Russians by temporarily shutting the border trade outpost in Kiakhta (map 0.2) and imposing an embargo on rhubarb, a commodity that the Russians seemed unable to live without. (In reality, the Russians were merely intermediaries supplying Chinese rhubarb to the European market). Imports of Russian fur were also banned at the southern port of Canton, for fear that rhubarb might be smuggled out in transactions with Russians. The large quantity of rhubarb that the Ryukyus requested thus raised alarm for the emperor: Might they have been seeking illicit profit by reselling the rhubarb back to the Russians?

Upon investigation, it turned out that the Ryukyus made their purchases in Fujian, where they were allowed to stay, but "all sorts of medicine" they bought had, in fact, been "transported from the town of Zhangshu in Jiangxi." Furthermore, the rhubarb in Zhangshu was originally "assembled" by wholesale merchants in Jingyang county in northwestern Shaanxi, where the herb was produced (map 0.2). Ryukyu envoys also testified that all their medicines had been purchased from local officials in Fujian, including "several hundred, or one thousand *jin* of rhubarb," for use back in their own country. As for the purchase of American ginseng and sappanwood, the Ryukyu envoys claimed that it was difficult for them to trade with Europeans and Siamese merchants who would not necessarily dock their ships in Ryukyu, making it easier for them to buy from Chinese traders with ready access to the Canton market.[84] Upon receiving the report, Qianlong let the matter drop.

This report nicely illustrates the multilayered process by which rhubarb became a commodity: the plants were first assembled in bulk (*chengzhuang*) at a primary marketplace (Jingyang), then shipped via waterways downstream to Zhangshu, where the northwestern plant was redistributed to traders hailing from all parts of the country. Qing China (through Canton) commanded a much higher place in market exchange than smaller countries, such as the Ryukyu kingdom, and so one could obtain the best price for foreign (*yang*) merchandise such as American ginseng and sappanwood. European, American, and Siamese merchants not only purchased goods manufactured in China but also participated in the supply of consumer goods *to* Qing China, thus linking their operations with those of domestic pharmaceutical wholesalers frequenting Zhangshu and Qizhou. The blurring of boundaries between domestic interregional and maritime trade was treated as a reality by the Qing state as well as by other players.

The Qianlong emperor's assumptions about the familiar and the exotic turned out to be wrong. By the turn of the nineteenth century, opium produced in the subcontinent would enter China via the same routes through which Zhao Xuemin had received his exotica, albeit in much more abundant quantities. In 1791, Qing authorities could not prevent the Ryukyu envoys from buying medicine in China; five decades later, they could hardly use their laws to keep opium out of the waters of Canton. The newly organized medicine was built on curiosity and mercantile knowledge instead of official purview or medical orthodoxy, and hence remained opaque to both. The world of goods built by Qing pharmacists and consumers would prove to be more tenacious than the rivaling schools of medical theory and outlast the dynasty itself.

Epilogue

I combine the grand volumes of *Bencao*, forge and refine them into a book. To lift up the dead and return them to life, I must first enliven the rotten matter of herbs, wood, metal, and stones. For the likes of Licorice and Golden Dendrobium, I dress them in costumes of the theater, and they sing, dance, laugh, and cry onto the paper. With the power of the living drugs, none of the dead will fail to swiftly rise again. Even if we do not use these living drugs every day, how could we ever forget them? Let us dance and sing merrily, so that everyone will know these remedies—that is to say, know their natures.

—GUO TINGXUAN, PREFACE TO *A CHRONICLE OF HERBS*, C. 1804

FIERCE, TOXIC TROOPS of foreign origin descend on the Central Kingdom. Licorice, the venerated minister, tries to negotiate peace, but rhubarb, the fearless general, advocates fighting back. The enemy captures chrysanthemum, licorice's beautiful daughter; gardenia, the swift-legged messenger, relays her call for help back home. Golden Dendrobium, the brash youthful warrior, rescues chrysanthemum and marries her. In the end, ginseng, emperor of all medicine, hosts a grand banquet to honor the newlyweds and his faithful officials. The plot of this short play written by Guo Tingxuan (fl. 1804), a physician practicing in central China, reenacts human dramas with characters drawn from the pharmacopeia. Departing from previous "pharmaceutical dramas" composed by literati authors, Guo intended for his didactic show to reach as wide an audience as possible. The anthropomorphized medicinal drugs "sing and dance merrily" on stage, their lively performance encouraging viewers to reflect on their own natures.[1]

The making of the bencao pharmacopeia had long faded from the government-sponsored cultural stage, but the power of pharmaceutical object-hood endured in less centralized expressions. As late as the early twentieth century, Guo's play remained popular with many local adaptations preserved in hand-copied manuscripts.[2] The urgency of Guo's moral message took on new meanings during the second half of the nineteenth century as the Qing state, resembling more or less the metaphorical kingdom reconstructed in the play, faced serious challenges from both internal and external threats. The popularization of pharmaceutical culture mirrored the efforts of local communities' efforts to reclaim moral agency in the wake of the traumatic Taiping Wars (1852–64) and the Arrow War (1856–60).[3] Pharmacists joined forces with resident gentry, clergy, and a growing contingent of Confucian activists to rebuild local society and reshape national politics. The struggle for authority over the nature of drugs continues to shed light on the complex interplay among knowledge, power, and ethics in modern China; pharmacy remains a good vantage point from which to observe the perennial search for consensus over the political administration of human nature.

On August 24, 1844, a French delegation arrived in Macau in the wake of Qing China's defeat by Great Britain during the First Opium War (1839–42). Following the Sino-British Treaty of Nanjing, the French negotiated with Qing officials and signed a comparable Treaty of Whampoa in October that year, which granted France privileges of trading and residing in the newly opened treaty ports. During the delegation's visit to some of these ports, including Ningbo and Shanghai, the accompanying physician, Dr. Melchior-Honoré Yvan (1803–73), visited local pharmacies there and, upon his return, published an account of the pharmaceutical trade according to his observations. The Chinese pharmacist, observed Yvan, plays a crucial role in Chinese society "as man of science, as merchant" and occupies a place "of importance with this civilization." Yet, in Yvan's eyes, this civilization remained so "stationary" that a small shop could contain the "complete specimen of what exists in all the extent of the Celestial Empire."[4] Writing in 1847, when Europe herself was about to be swept into another round of revolutionary zeal, Yvan was keen to use this publication on China to secure his own status as a man of science.

By now, I hope this book has made a compelling case for the usefulness of pharmacy in "scientific, industrial, and social" life in Chinese history. Our assumptions today, however, differ from Yvan's in that we learn much more by seeing that civilization as a dynamic process, not static entities. Yet even so, Yvan's report brims with revealing details that should, I hope, sound familiar at this point. The "enormous consumption of drugs" in China that he witnessed in the pharmacies of Ningpo—establishments that matched in their exquisite service the "grandest shops of droguerie" in contemporary France—would have been familiar to Zhao Xuemin, who had inquired after the nature of white pepper in that city only a few decades earlier. Yvan also noted that Chinese pharmacies from Ningpo to Malacca in Southeast Asia shared the same "provisions and mode of arrangement," confirming the interregional and overseas extension of Chinese mercantile networks.[5] The Chinese entrepreneurs he encountered in Singapore boasted secret techniques for cultivating the shrub gambier and extracting the tannin-rich substance known as catechu, a profitable venue of trade.[6] Were they not peers of the owners of "plantations" in China's own hinterland, where magnolia barks and Golden Thread were cultivated as "wild" medicine? Are these all but manifestations of a motionless civilization, frozen in time? Looking back at the miniature model of the Chinese pharmacy presented at the beginning of this book (figure 0.1), one might now have a different answer.

The people of Zhangshu, the modest town that established itself as the important "medicinal wharf" beginning in the late sixteenth century, would have been familiar with the world of trade described by Yvan. Throughout the turbulent history of the nineteenth century, Zhangshu merchants and their counterparts in different merchant companies fared quite well overall. Up to the 1930s, market fairs held in Zhangshu and Qizhou enjoyed attendance of 70,000–80,000 customers, and the extensive operations of foreign interests, in fact, helped local pharmacists set up shops in the treaty ports and expand their foothold in Hong Kong, Southeast Asia, and all over the world.[7] Their newfound fortunes suggest a less defeatist narrative of China's late imperial era than is commonly assumed. Despite the carefully constructed tales of "tradition" in today's Zhangshu, the story of its people belongs to a modern history of global medicine as much as the grand hospitals being erected in cities at the turn of the twentieth century. In war and in peace, China continued to supply large quantities of raw pharmaceutical materials to the world, much of which had been harvested from the former empire's frontier regions.[8] Though this is a story yet to be told, I hope that the present study has served to anchor the merchants, physicians, and scientists of contemporary China in a lively political and scientific tradition.

In this book, I have traced the trajectory of change in Chinese knowledge of pharmaceutical objecthood between 1500 and 1800. We began when the processes of cultural reproduction no longer looked to an imperial center for guidance, and witnessed the amazing variety of expressions this decentralizing process unleashed in late Ming times. We followed the most zealous attempts to reinvent bencao and establish a reliable science of nature that could, in turn, serve as a basis for moral action. We saw the defeat of literati amateurism by both dynastic crisis and resistance from the medical marketplace. Finally, we parsed the contingent processes through which the High Qing state forcefully reclassified knowledge and delegated pharmaceutical matters to mercantile actors. Beginning in mid-Qing times, two divergent paths developed, each leading to different futures in which the phantoms of bencao pharmacopeia would be called back to life.

One of these paths led to a revival of science-based activism in the figures of modern scientists and medical professionals who insisted that their own privileged understanding of nature justified their paths to power. In 1930, the first modern pharmacopeia was published under the supervision of the Harvard-trained doctor and Minister of Health of the Republic of China, Liu Jui-heng (1890–1961). According to his vision, the pharmacopeia was to include only substances congruent with the international standard of the day.[9] This approach exemplified the attempt on the part of scientists and medical doctors to establish a new unity of knowledge and power from the high altars of the republican government and the modern universities, a universalist move rooted in the neo-Confucian search for morality in the investigation of things.

Swept along in this spirit, a new generation of scientists vowed to modernize Chinese materia medica with the modern tools of chemical analysis. Zhao Yuhuang, a young pharmacologist trained in Japan, visited the annual market fair in Qizhou (where the hapless Zhi Tianbao had once hatched his astrological prophecy) and attempted to ascertain the botanical and chemical identities of medicinal substances on sale there.[10] Zhao was actively involved in the patriotic rush to manufacture pharmaceuticals using native botanical resources during the 1930s and 1940s. This lineage of scientific transformation of tradition continues today. Professor Zheng Jinsheng, a leading scholar on Chinese materia medica research and the bencao literature was, in turn, trained by one of Zhao's students in the 1970s.

Following a second path and resisting the all-encompassing power of science, defenders of native medical orthodoxy quickly rallied around the ontological difference between "Chinese" and "Western" drugs—a statement that amounted to a particularist reading of human nature. The discourse of onto-logical divergence first appeared in late Qing synthesizers (*huitong*) of Chinese and Western medicine and picked up momentum in the aftermath of the first Sino-Japanese War and surging nationalism during the 1911 Revolution.[11] Mo-bilizing nationalist sentiments, the modern traditionalists argued that Chinese people must never be severed from Chinese remedies steeped in Chinese cul-ture. Pharmacists toed a cautious line by posing themselves as representatives of a modernized, yet quintessentially Chinese, business.[12]

The first open clash between advocates of Chinese medicine (*Zhongyi*) or national medicine (*guoyi*) against Western medicine (*xiyi*) took place in the late 1920s and 1930s, and in the end the reform-minded leaders within the nationalist government could not prevail over the defenders of tradition. A compromise was reached in which the two systems of medical practice, along with their pharmaceutical repertoires, would coexist and coevolve in the state-building process of modern China, a result that historians have dubbed "mon-grel medicine."[13] The Chinese Communist Party, winning the civil war in 1949 under a strong anti-American nationalist platform, espoused the efficacy of tradition. In 1963, the People's Republic of China revised its official pharma-copeia to include, for the first time, traditional materia medica (*zhongyao*) in a separate volume from "Western drugs" (*xiyao*).[14] As recently as in 2013, China consolidated its regulatory offices into one Food and Drug Administra-tion (CFDA). The task of defining and regulating the dual system of health care remains logistically challenging and politically complicated.

Since the 1970s, the institutionalized form of TCM in China has gained more and more international recognition amid much controversy.[15] Practice-oriented interests all over the world have rejuvenated the academic study of the Chinese medical tradition as an alternative mode of therapeutics to bio-medicine. Somewhat parallel to the late Ming publishing market, a large num-ber of previously obscure texts, many of which dated to Ming-Qing times, were discovered and republished thanks to a robust demand from TCM advocates. This study has benefited, to some extent, from that publishing boom. At the same time, enhanced publicity also made TCM notorious for ethical issues involving the abuse of toxic substances, animal abuse, and other environmen-tal concerns.[16] Today, each time a debate over the status of TCM erupts in real life or online, the exchanges quickly escalate into political disagreements along the fault line between universalism and cultural nationalism. If we can now agree that there was no monolithic scientific tradition in any one civilization— Chinese or otherwise—then the goal of investigating these many pasts and many traditions is to create new norms, protocols, and narratives for the future.

Like Guo Tingxuan, I "forge and refine" the "grand volumes of bencao" to compose the present book, but not for didactical purposes. The present is no time for nostalgia of any kind: I do not wish to call for a twenty-first-century replica of the Tang-Song state-sponsored pharmacopeia, nor indulge in speculations as to whether China could have had a scientific revolution in the seventeenth century had the Qing conquest not been successful. It may be apparent by now that I do, after all, have a position to take: compared to the stern-faced admonitions of the *Doctrine of the Mean*, I find more consolation in the empowering message of *Great Learning*, which is to believe that a person's innate capacity for moral action must be grounded by knowledge gleaned from the investigation of things. More importantly, this knowing person can be anyone who applies themselves to this journey, not just a preordained few. By activating the full spectrum of positions that motivated this history of pharmaceutical objecthood, I hope to avoid thinking in terms of the false dichotomy between Chinese tradition and (Western) modernity. To know our remedies is to know ourselves.

APPENDIXES

1. Dates for Dynasties and Ming-Qing Reign Periods Discussed in This Book (up to 1800)

Han	206 BCE–220	Jingtai	1450–56
Three Kingdoms	220–65	Tianshun	1457–64
Northern and Southern		Chenghua	1465–87
Dynasties	386–589	Hongzhi	1488–1505
Sui 581–618		Zhengde	1506–21
Tang	618–907	Jiajing	1522–66
Northern Song	960–1127	Longqing	1567–72
Southern Song	1127–1279	Wanli	1573–1620
Jin 1115–1234		Taichang	1620
Yuan	1271–1368	Tianqi	1621–27
Ming	1368–1644	Chongzhen	1628–44
Hongwu	1368–98	Qing	1636–1912
Jianwen	1399–1402	Chongde	1636–43
Yongle	1403–24	Shunzhi	1644–61
Hongxi	1425–25	Kangxi	1662–1722
Xuande	1426–35	Yongzheng	1723–35
Zhengtong	1436–49	Qianlong	1736–95

2. Ming-Qing Chinese Measures and Currencies
(*equivalencies are approximate*)

Weight/currency:
  1 *jin* (catty) = 605 grams = 16 *liang*
  1 *liang* (ounce / tael) = 37.8 grams = 10 *qian*

Length and distance:
  1 *li* = 0.5 kilometer
Area: 1 *mu* = 0.077 hectare

CHINESE CHARACTER GLOSSARY

Personal and place names commonly found in standard references are omitted; original characters for authors and book titles cited in the notes are provided in the bibliography.

Anguo 安國

baicaodan 百草丹
Balikun 巴里坤
ban ke 板客
Baozhi gangmu 保治綱目
ba xiang 八象
bianyan yaocai 辨驗藥材
buxi gongfei 不惜工費
buyi 布衣

Cai Chen 蔡沈
Caishikou 菜市口
cai song zhi ren 采送之人
Cao Yin 曹寅
chang 廠
Changshu 常熟
Chen Cheng 陳承
Chen Jiru 陳繼儒
Chen Mei 陳枚
cheng yijia zhi yan 成一家之言
chengze 成則
cheng zhuang 成莊
chuai er zi qiu zhi 揣而自求之
chuanbo 蹯駁
chixin 侈心
Chuan-Guang 川廣
chuchan difang 出產地方
Cixi 慈溪
cong shi shan qu 從實刪去

cunmu 存目
cuping 粗評

Daguan bencao 大觀本草
Dai Xian 戴銑
Dashilan 大柵欄
daode zhi tu 道德之途
daodi yaocai 道地藥材
Deng Yuanxi 鄧元錫
dianmu qiuran 電目虯髯
dijiao 地椒
Ding Yuanjian 丁元薦
dingzi yao 錠子藥
Dong Qichang 董其昌
Dupian xinshu 杜騙新書

e ban 額辦
e chuang 惡瘡

faming 發明
fan da ma 番打馬
fan dou hua 番豆花
fangke 坊刻
fangshiren 坊市人
fangshu jia 方術家
fan jiao 番蕉 / 番椒
fan ze huo 繁則惑
fa xiang 法象
Feng Chuzhan 馮楚瞻
Fuchuntang 富春堂

187

Gao Panlong　高攀龍
Ge Nai　葛鼐
gewu zhizhi　格物致知
guoben　國本
Guo Tingxuan　郭廷選

haigou　海狗
haiwai zhuyi　海外諸夷
Halaba　哈喇叭
hanyang shenglei　涵養生類
haoqi　好奇
Heniantang　鶴年堂
Hesihen (Ch. Heshiheng)　赫世亨
Hongmao guo　紅毛國
houzao　猴棗

jiangzhi　降志
Jiang Zhushan　蔣竹山
Jianqiao　繭橋
jianwu　簡誤
jian zhushu zhi quan　僭著述之權
jiazu　甲族
jiena　解納
Jigu ge　汲古閣
jinfang　今方
jin guo lan　金果欖
jinxing　盡性
jixueteng　雞血藤
jundao　君道
junxu　軍需

kaiwu　開物
ke sheng zhu　客勝主
Kong Zhiyue　孔志約
kugao　枯槁

laotao　老饕
licai　理財
Li Gao　李杲
Li Jianyuan　李建元
Li Jinshi　李金什
limu　吏目
Li Ping'er　李瓶兒
liri zhizhang　曆日紙張

li yi fen shu　理一分殊
liuyueshuang　六月霜
Liu Yunhong　劉雲鴻
Lu Fu　盧復
Lüjunting　綠君亭
lunsi　論思
Luo Qinshun　羅欽順
Luo Wenying　羅文英
lutai　鹿胎

mai shou changwu　埋首場屋
Mao Fengbao / Mao Jin　毛鳳苞 / 毛晉
Meng Rui　孟銳

Nanling　南陵
neiwufu　內務府
neizhao　內照
Ni Yuanlu　倪元璐

pengmin　棚民
pianse　偏塞
piansheng/pianjue　偏勝 / 偏絕
pin bu ji li　貧不計利

Qian Qianyi　錢謙益
Qian Shutian　錢樹田
Qian Weiqi　錢蔚起
Qian Yunzhi　錢允治
Qingming shanghe tu　清明上河圖
qinli qi di　親歷其地
Qintianjian　欽天監
qiong min　窮民
Qiu Ying　仇英
quyong zhu junzi　取用諸君子

rengong zhizao　人工製造
rentu zuogong　任土作貢
ren ya　人蚜
Riyong bencao　日用本草
rulin shangda　儒林上達
ru zhe hao zi zhangda　儒者好自張大

shancun ren　山村人
Shandong yuanban　山東原板

Shang Lu   商輅

shang zhi chaoting   上之朝廷

shan ma   善罵

shengfan / shufan   生番 / 熟番

shengxi yinliang   生息銀兩

shengxue   聖學

shengyaoku   生藥庫

shengyao yinpian   生藥飲片

she xu jiu shi   捨虛就實

shi dao   市道

shi jie   十誡

shi min yong   示民用

shishang   士商

shiyi   世醫

shizi   師資

shuaixing   率性

shuyao wansan   熟藥丸散

Siming   司命

suiban yaocai   歲辦藥材

suke   俗刻

Su Qian   蘇乾

suyi   俗醫

Suzhou pian   蘇州片

Taiyiyuan   太醫院

Tanyangzi   曇陽子

Tianyitang   天一堂

tianxia zhujun   天下諸郡

tiren   體認

tongdu dayi   通都大邑

tongshe   同社

tui chen zhi xin   推陳致新

tuo   鼉

tusu   土俗

waike yangyi   外科瘍醫

waiyang   外洋

Wang Ji   汪機

Wang Lü   王履

Wang Lun   王倫

Wang Qiu   王秋

Wang Yitang   王怡堂

wei'ai   違礙

weigao   偽稿

wuchan   物產

wuhuo   物貨

wuliao   物料

Wulin zhu junzi   武林諸君子

Wu Mianxue   吳勉學

wu ti xing qing   物體性情

wuze   物則

xiafang yuanyi   遐方遠裔

Xia Liangxin   夏良心

xianhao   賢豪

xiang yang xiang sheng   相養相生

xihuo   細貨

Ximen Da   西門達

Ximen Qing   西門慶

xing chenmo   性沈默

xingwo   行窩

xingyuan   行遠

xinlie   辛烈

xiongzhen   雄鎮

Xue Ji   薛己

yang chuan pu   洋船璞

yang chong   洋蟲

yang huo dian   洋貨店

yangrongke   羊絨客

yao chu zhoutu   藥出州土

yaolu   藥露

yao matou   藥碼頭

yaopu yiren   藥舖醫人

yaoshi   藥室

yaoshi yixing   藥市異形

yaoxing   藥性

yaoxu   藥墟

ya ren   牙人

yecao xianhua   野草閒花

yesheng   野生

yi bu bei yao   醫不備藥

yidi   夷狄

yigong   醫工

yihui   醫會

yijian   易簡

Yimen falü   醫門法律

yipu   醫舖

yiren shushi   藝人術士

Yisheng weilun   頤生微論

yitiaobian fa   一條鞭法

yiwu / yongwu   異物 / 用物

yi yao bu yi bing   議藥不議病

Yizong bidu   醫宗必讀

yonggong   傭工

Yuanfeng jiuyu zhi   元豐九域志

Yuan Jie   原傑

Yue Ao yangbo   粵澳洋舶

Yue Fengming   樂鳳鳴

Yue Pingquan   樂平泉

Yue Zunyu   樂尊育

Yu Dingzhi   于定志

Yugong   禹貢

Yuqian   於潛

Yuwen Xuzhong   宇文虛中

yuyaofang   御藥房

zaiguan   栽灌

Zhang Cunhui   張存惠

Zhangming   彰明

Zhangshu   樟樹

zhang yao li   長腰力

Zhang Yu   張瑜

Zhang Yuansu   張元素

Zhao taicheng jia   趙太丞家

zhengsuo   徵索

zhengxue   正學

zhese   折色

zhi liangzhi   致良知

Zhi Tianbao   智天豹

zhi xing he yi   知行合一

zhi yao bu zhi yi   知藥不知醫

zhongren yi shang zhi zi   中人以上之資

zhuangke laoban   莊客老闆

zhuanmen zhi shi   專門之士

zhu er fen   珠兒粉

Zhu Youcheng   朱祐樘

zhuyou ke   祝由科

Zhu Zhenheng   朱震亨

zhuzhi canhu   主治參互

ziben   資本

zihao   字號

ziran zhi dao   自然之道

zuanji bing shuhua   纂輯並書畫

zungu paozhi   遵古炮製

zuoban / paiban   坐辦 / 派辦

zuofang   作坊

zuogu   坐賈

NOTES

Introduction

1. Fang Yizhi, *Wuli xiaoshi*, 1:12b.

2. See discussion in chapters 3 and 4.

3. Schafer, *The Golden Peaches*, 2.

4. The formulation and enforcement of novel regulations for pharmacy became an indispensable episode in the historiography of modern American medicine and the professionalization of pharmacy in the United States. The modern profession of pharmacists, now reconstituted as an allied sub-subfield of biomedicine, proudly presented itself as an embodiment of progress and standardization against quackery and the peddlers of patent medicines. See, for instance, Kremer and Urdang, *Kremer and Urdang's History of Pharmacy*; Anderson, *Making Medicines*; Young, *The Toadstool Millionaires*; Liebenau, *Medical Science and Medical Industry*; Barzansky and Gevitz, *Beyond Flexner*. For the grounding of medical history in therapeutic practices, see a more recent attempt to overcome the Whiggish overtones of earlier histories in Rosenberg, "The Therapeutic Revolution"; Warner, *The Therapeutic Perspective*. For more recent takes on the history of modern pharmaceuticals in the United States, see Greene, *Generic*; Janik, *Marketplace of the Marvelous*, among many others.

5. Sivin, "A Multi-Dimensional Approach." For the intersection between the historiography of medicine and general Chinese history, see Li Jianmin, *Lüxingzhe*.

6. Rawski, "The Qing Formation"; see also the variety of positions taken in the same edited volume, and Struve, ed., *Time and Temporality*.

7. Elman, *From Philosophy to Philology*; Peterson, *Bitter Gourd*; Henderson, *The Development and Decline*; Handler-Spitz, *Symptoms of an Unruly Age*.

8. Pomeranz, *The Great Divergence*. See also essays in So, *The Economy of Lower Yangzi Delta*, in which the authors take a variety of positions toward the characterization of Ming-Qing China's economic development. For institutions and social practices developing around business enterprises, see Zelin, *The Merchants of Zigong*; Hamashita, *China, East Asia*. Also related to economic modernity in the nineteenth century is the periodization of environmental historians; see Perdue, *Exhausting the Earth*; and the modern chapters in Marks, *China: Its Environment and History*.

9. For a critique of the imposition of European experience on the study of China, see Wong, *China Transformed*. For major discussions and developments in global history in which historians of China took a prominent part, see, among others, Brook, *Vermeer's Hat*; Pomeranz,

"Areas, Networks"; Clunas, "Modernity Global and Local"; Elman, *On Their Own Terms*; Crossley, *What Is Global History*.

10. For a recent discussion and summary of the field, see Meyer-Fong, "Conference Note."

11. Harper, *Early Chinese Medical Literature*, 98–109. Compare with Totelin, *Hippocratic Recipes*, 141–96. For the ideas, practices, and archival formations of Canonic medical texts, see Unschuld, *Huang di nei jing*; Kuriyama, *The Expressiveness of the Body*; Brown, *The Art of Medicine*; Yamada Keiji, *Chūgoku igaku*.

12. Fan Jiawei, *Liuchao Sui Tang yixue*; Stanley-Baker, "Drugs, Destiny and Disease"; Liu, "Toxic Cures." The influence of Buddhism at this time also dramatically changed the healing traditions of medieval China. The impact of Buddhist ideas on pharmacy is a rich topic beyond the scope of this book. See Salguero, *Translating Buddhist Medicine*.

13. Shang et al., *Lidai zhongyao*, 44–50.

14. BCTJ, 1.

15. See Cipolla, *Public Health*; Cook, *The Decline of the Old Medical Regime*; Park, *Doctors and Medicine*; Welch and Shaw, *Making and Marketing*.

16. BCTJ, 1. See also ISK, 10.58–59.

17. Hinrichs, "Governance through Medical Texts"; Goldschmidt, *The Evolution of Chinese Medicine*, 107–22 passim; Sivin, *Health Care*; Fan Jiawei, *Bei Song jiaozheng yishuju*.

18. BCJJZ, 32–33.

19. XXBC, 12.

20. Zimmermann, *The Jungle and the Aroma of Meats*, viii.

21. For an account of *pulu*, an equally venerable tradition of creating literary catalogs of objects of interest, see Siebert, *Pulu*.

22. In 1870, Bretschneider published a short account of Chinese botanical works (*On the Study and Value of Chinese Botanical Works*), followed by a two-volume study in 1882. See Bretschneider, *Botanicum Sinicum*. He would later write a history of "European botanical discovery" in China in 1898.

23. Stuart, *Chinese Materia Medica*. The study was revised from an unfinished manuscript by British medical missionary Frederick Porter Smith (1833–88).

24. Read worked for the Henry Lester Institute in Shanghai in the late 1930s and was imprisoned by the Japanese from 1941 to 1945. See Read and Liu, *Bibliography of Chinese Medicinal Plants*. For natural studies in 1920s and 1930s China and its close connections to the study of past texts, see Jiang, "Retouching the Past."

25. Okanishi, *Chugoku isho honzō kō*; see also the works by Mayanagi Makoto; Unschuld, *Medicine in China*; Shang, et al., *Lidai zhongyao wenxian jinghua*. For another trend of using a cultural historical approach to study bencao in Japan, see Yamada Keiji, *Mono no imēji*.

26. Needham, *The Grand Titration*; SCC6.1, 220–29. Having dealt with the botanical content of bencao, Needham planned a section on pharmacology, following that on medicine, in *Science and Civilisation in China*, but was never able to finish it.

27. SCC6.1, 308–21, 322–29. Compare with Arber, *Herbals*; Stannard, *Herbs and Herbalism*.

28. For a representative account that offset late imperial stagnancy against the early onset of a technological renaissance in Song times, see Elvin, *The Patterns of the Chinese Past*.

29. Shang et al., *Lidai zhongyao*, 419–90.

30. Okanishi, *Chugoku isho honzō kō*, 309–10; Unschuld, *A History of Pharmaceuticals*, 169–204.

31. Shapin and Schaffer, *Leviathan and the Air-Pump*; Pickering, *Science as Practice and Culture*.

32. SCC6.4. See also Métailié, "Concepts of Nature" and "The *Bencao gangmu* of Li Shizhen." Métailié's rejection of the Needham question echoes a similar move by Nathan Sivin in the late 1990s of not completing the planned section on medicine according to Needham's instructions.

33. Nappi, *The Monkey and the Inkpot*; Schäfer, *The Crafting of 10,000 Things*; Sivin, "Why the Scientific Revolution." For a recent review of Needham's legacy, see Hsia and Schäfer, "History of Science."

34. Elman, *On Their Own Terms*; for equally excellent accounts with slightly different assumptions, see Sakade, *Chūgoku kindai*; Han Qi, *Zhongguo kexue jishu*.

35. Marcon, *The Knowledge of Nature*; Suh, *Naming the Local*. For early modern European research on Chinese herbals, see Barnes, *Needles, Herbs*, 100–106. For recent monographs on Jesuits as intermediaries of knowledge in early modern world, see Hsia, *Sojourners in a Strange Land*; Hart, *Imagined Civilisations*; Zhang, *Making the New World*; Jami, *Emperor's New Mathematics*; Cams, *Companions in Geography*, among others.

36. Chemla and Fox Keller, *Cultures without Culturalism*. For a survey of different approaches to knowledge available within the Chinese tradition, see Allen, *Vanishing into Things*.

37. My motivation for an integrated approach to early modern knowledge has been inspired by works such as Grafton, Shelford, and Siraisi, *New Worlds, Ancient Texts*; and essays in Park and Daston, *The Cambridge History of Science: Vol. 3 Early Modern Science*. This methodological move, however, aims at mutual comparison and comprehension, and not at making conjectures to predict future success or failure.

38. Bol, "The Localist Turn"; Schneewind, *Shrines to Living Men*; Szonyi, *The Art of Being Governed*; Faure, *Emperor and Ancestor*.

39. Leung, "Organized Medicine"; Bray, "Chinese Literati." For belief in cosmic unity, see Bol, *Neo-Confucianism*, 194–217. For Ming state-sponsored industry, see Schäfer and Kuhn, *Weaving an Economic Pattern*.

40. Another aspect of Ming history that was selectively forgotten was military culture. See Robinson, *Martial Spectacles*. For ways in which late Ming sentiments colored the literati elite's historical consciousness, see Brook, *The Confusions of Pleasure*.

41. Levenson, *Confucian China*, vol. 1, 16, and see the full chapters in 3–43.

42. Legge, *Lun yu*, 4.

43. Yang Xiong, *Fayan* 12.17, 216–17. Michael Nylan translates *ru* as a "classicist," which was how Confucians were generally perceived in early Chinese context.

44. Chen Yuanpeng, *Liang Song*. For a Northern Song polymath's epistemic positions, see also Zuo, *Shen Gua*.

45. Furth, *A Flourishing Yin*; Furth et al. eds., *Thinking with Cases*. For a thoughtful discussion of amateurism and expertise in late imperial art, see Cahill, *The Painter's Practice*.

46. Chow, *Publishing, Culture, and Power*; He Yuming, *Home and the World*; McDermott, *A Social History*. Robert Hegel's work in particular traces the remarkable *discontinuity* of illustrated

vernacular novels in Ming-Qing China, pointing out important reasons why the novels looked so different in the Qing and how they might have catered to a different, but wider, range of readers. See Hegel, *Reading Illustrated Fiction*, 327–36. For the growing influence of mercantile interests on the cultural scene, see Clunas, *Superfluous Things*; Brokaw, *Ledgers of Merit and Demerit*. For the mobilization of this public arena for political ends, see Zhang, *Confucian Image Politics*.

47. Ko, *Teachers of the Inner Chambers*.

48. Meyer-Fong, *Building Culture*; Ko, *The Social Life of Inkstones*; Wu, *Reproducing Women*.

49. Rowe, *Saving the World*; Dunstan, *State or Merchant?*; Will, *Bureaucracy and Famine*.

50. Ko, *The Social Life*, 15; Wu, *Luxurious Networks*; Schlesinger, *A World Trimmed with Fur*; Akçetin, "Consumption as Knowledge"; Finnane, "Furnishing the Home"; Waley-Cohen, "Food and China's World of Goods," and other essays in the edited volume.

51. Appardurai, *The Social Life*; Morton, *The Poetics of Spice*. For more recent object-oriented works with a global coverage, see Findlen, *Early Modern Things*; Gerritsen and Riello, *The Global Lives of Things*. For studies of specific commodities in Qing China, see Benedict, *Golden-Silk Smoke*; Jiang, *Renshen diguo*; and Zhang, "Timber Trade."

52. Guy, *The Emperor's Four Treasuries*; Spence, *Treason by the Book*; Elman, *Classicism, Politics, and Kinship*.

53. Naquin and Rawski, *Chinese Society*, 236; Skinner, *The City in Late Imperial China*; Brokaw, *Commerce in Culture*.

54. See the essays in Johnson et al., *Popular Culture*. For a study of popular publishing sectors, see Brokaw, *Commerce in Culture*. Compare with Burke, *Popular Culture in Early Modern Europe*; Thompson, *Customs in Common*; Medick, "Plebeian Culture in the Transition to Capitalism."

55. See a recent study of miners, carvers, and female artisans in the general "craft of *wen*" in Ko, *The Social Life of Inkstones*. Compare with Cook, *Matters of Exchange*; Harkness, *The Jewel House*; Smith, *The Body of the Artisan*; Newman, *Atoms and Alchemy*; Moran, *Distilling Knowledge*; Eamon, *Professor of Secrets*; Roos, *The Salt of the Earth*; Bentancor, *The Matter of Empire*; Fors, *The Limits of Matter*.

56. To be sure, my experience in handling pharmaceuticals cannot compare to White's intimate knowledge of gardening. White, *Onward and Upward in the Garden*.

Chapter 1: The Last Pharmacopeia

1. MS, 188.4972; Huangfu Lu, *Huang Ming jilüe* 1:15b–16a.

2. He Qiaoyuan, *Mingshan cang* 19:9a.

3. The original Ming copy of the pharmacopeia was stolen from the palace in the early twentieth century and was rediscovered in Hong Kong in the 1950s. For the work's transmission and extant copies, see Na Qi and Liu Zhengxiong's essay in BCPHJY-CP, vol. 2, pp. 1–79; Unschuld, *Yü-chih pen-ts'ao p'in-hui ching-yao*; Unschuld, *Medicine in China*, 142–145. For the influence of palace bencao manuscripts on paintings of flora and fauna, see Zheng, *Yaolin*, 207–22.

4. He Qiaoyuan, *Mingshan cang* 68:22a–24a; Wang Shizhen, *Yanshantang bie ji*, vol. 6, 94, pp. 4141–43 (1a–2a). Liu was accused of having caused discord between Wang Shu (1416–1508) and Qiu Jun (1421–95).

5. Shen Defu, *Wanli yehuo bian*, suppl. 3:887–88; Wang Shizhen, *Yanzhou shiliao*, qianji, 13:15a–16b. See also Zhu Guozhen, *Yongzhuang xiaopin* 25:584–85.

6. Shen Defu, *Wanli yehuo bian*, suppl. 3:887–88.

7. Ditmanson, "Imperial History;" Huang, *1587*, 1–41; Fisher, *The Chosen One*.

8. BCPHJY, 37.

9. See a similar discussion of textual communities in late Ming Buddhism, Wu, *Enlightenment in Dispute*, 249–56.

10. ISK, 10.53–55. Manuscript fragments of *Bencao jing jizhu* and *Tang bencao* were excavated in Dunhuang and Turfan. See Wang Shimin and Mayanagi Makoto's essays in Lo, *Medieval Chinese Medicine*, 293–305, and 306–21; also see Rong, *Eighteen Lectures*, 420–22.

11. ISK, 10.59. Chen reportedly descended from a family of officials. He was later assigned to work on the compilation of *Hejiju fang* (The Medical Bureau's formula for compounding). See Goldschmidt, *Evolution*, 123–40.

12. ISK, 11.66–67. Kou's bencao commentary was printed with the funding of his nephew, who was also an official with the rank of local magistrate. The text had no pictures but was circulated as a short commentary to the Song pharmacopeia. See BCYY-1879.

13. ISK, 10.60–61. For Huizong's close involvement in medical learning as a part of his ambitious cultural projects, see Goldschmidt, "Huizong's Impact"; Ebrey, *Emperor Huizong*, 190–94. For modern editions of the original two-part Song pharmacopeia, see JYBC and BCTJ.

14. Zhao Yushi, *Bin tui lu*, 3:37.

15. Yuwen Xuzhong's epigraph, in ZLBC, 662; ISK, 10.61. Caught in between two regimes, Yuwen eventually chose to serve in office under Jin rule and was murdered in a political intrigue. His biography in dynastic histories documented his wrongful death, claiming that the wealth of books (*tushu*) in his collection were cited as evidence for treasonous intent. See Tuotuo et al., *Song shi* 371.11526–28; Tuotuo et al., *Jin shi* 79.1791–93. For the pursuit of literary culture under Jurchen rule through examinations, see Xin Wen, "The Road to Literary Culture."

16. The Southern Song pharmacopeia is only extant as a manuscript in Japan. See ZLBC, appendix 12–13; ISK, 10.64–65.

17. For a sample examination question that asked candidates to discuss principles of prescription with reference to a bencao pharmacopeia, see He Daren, *Taiyiju zhuke chengwenge*, 3:9a–12b passim.

18. At least three editions of the *Daguan bencao* were published in 1185, 1195, and 1221, funded by various scholar-officials but not commissioned by the court. See ZLBC, appendix, 11.

19. ISK, 10.61–63. For Pingyang as a center for cultural activities during the Jin and Yuan dynasties, see Ye Dehui, *Shulin qinghua*, 4:89–90. For a discussion of the pictorial elements in the Pingyang edition, see Bussotti, "Woodcut Illustration," 469–76.

20. *Daozang*, vols. 58–60, 535–50. When Daoists lost to Buddhist monks in competition over Mongol patronage, the Khan ordered the destruction of the Daoist canon, which later resurfaced in the early fifteenth century. For more detailed information regarding the Jin-Yuan Daoist revival and medical works in the Daoist canon, see Schipper and Verellen eds., *The Taoist Canon*, vol. 1, 28–37, 338–43, and especially Catherine Despeux's discussion of the *Bencao* text in vol. 2, 765–70. For an early Qing anecdotal suggestion of how bencao entered the Daoist canon, see Zhu Yizun, *Pushuting ji*, 55:1b–2b. Also see Lucille Chia, "The Uses of Print in Early Quanzhen Daoist Texts."

21. *Yuan shi* 13.271, 315.

22. Hinrichs and Barnes, *Chinese Medicine and Healing*, 97–128.

23. ISK, 13.81; De Weerdt, *Competition over Content*; Leung, "Medical Instruction and Popularization."

24. Ulrike Unschuld's translation of *faxiang* was "regularities and manifestations." See Unschuld, "Traditional Chinese Pharmacology," 229–31.

25. Despeux, "The System of the Five Circulatory Phases"; Angela Ki-Che Leung, "Medical Learning from the Song to the Ming."

26. Zhu Xi, *Zhuzi yulei*, 4:1a–8a. For more discussions of Zhu Xi's doctrines of nature, see Munro, *Images of Human Nature*; Kim, *The Natural Philosophy*; Yamada Keiji, *Shushi no shizengaku*.

27. Zhu Xi, *Zhuzi yulei*, 4:15b.

28. ISK, 13.82–83.

29. Furth, "The Physician as Philosopher of the Way"; Boyanton, "The Treatise on Cold Damage." For an overview of medicine in this period, see Leung, "Medical Learning."

30. Shinno, *Politics of Chinese Medicine under Mongol Rule*, 2–3; Hymes, "Not Quite Gentlemen?"; Chao, *Medicine and Society*, 25–52.

31. Wang Lü, *Su Hui Ji*, 1, preface paginated outside of chapters. See also Liscomb, *Learning from Mount Hua*, 85–92.

32. See Dai Yuanli and his disciple's biographies in MS, 299.7645–47.

33. ISK, 13.85.

34. The 1523 reprint of the 1468 edition included a total of 1,340 woodblocks. See ZLBC, appendix, 19. Shang won first place in all three rounds of civil service examination, a feat that was never again accomplished by anyone in the Ming dynasty. See Elman, *Civil Examinations and Meritocracy*, 78–80.

35. ZLBC, appendix, 19–21.

36. Ye Dehui, *Shulin qinghua* 7:180.

37. Dennis, *Writing, Publishing, and Reading Local Gazetteers*, 197–205.

38. See Clunas, *Screen of Kings*, 175–80, also note 203. Clunas discussed a 1577 edition of the *Zhenglei bencao* published by a Ming princely household.

39. See the text in Zhu Su, *Jiuhuang bencao*, and discussions in chapter 4.

40. Zhou Hongzu, *Gujin shuke*, upper part, page 3c (Imperial Academy in Beijing, "*Bencao* recipes"), 7b (Imperial Academy in Nanjing, Daguan reign), 12a (Yingtian Prefecture, Southern Song imprint), 14a (Ningguo Prefecture, Daguan reign), 19a (Fujian bookshops, Daguan reign), 40a (Shandong, Provincial Judge's office, *Zhenglei bencao*), 49b (Guangzhou Prefecture), and 53a (Guizhou Provincial Financial Commissioner's office).

41. The publishers even adapted the book title in order to cater to a wider range of readers: *Complete Map Guides, including Treatment of Common Symptoms, the Daguan edition of Materia Medica.*

42. Feng Menglong, *Xingshi hengyan*, 38:863–64.

43. Several decades later, the carved woodblocks of the pharmacopeia appeared in a chief eunuch's record as property of the inner court. Liu Ruoyu, *Zhuoz hong zhi*, 18:5a. "Re-printed *Zhenglei bencao*, 10 books. 1,345 folios."

44. Dennis, *Writing, Publishing, and Reading*, 213–48.

45. *Nanling xianzhi* [Jiaqing], 9:3a and 17a.

46. Zhu Yizun, *Pushuting ji*, 55:3b–4a; Yang Shoujing, *Riben fang shu zhi*, 148–49; ISK, 10.64.

47. Wang Daxian's colophon can be found in ZLBC-1577.

48. Zhu Chaowang's preface to the 1600 reprint of Wang Qiu's edition. ZLBC, appendix 13–15.

49. The title is *Baoqing bencao zhezhong* by Chen Yan, and the only copy surviving today was printed during the Yuan Dynasty, under the sponsorship of two officials. In fact, we only know of the existence of other similar works during the Southern Song thanks to a bibliography listed in Chen's treatise. See Zheng Jinsheng, *Song dai bencao shi.*

50. ISK, 13.84. The earliest commercially published version was in 1602 by Liu Longtian in Jianyang.

51. ISK, 13.85. For a study of Wang Ji's medical cases, see Grant, *A Chinese Physician.*

52. For commercial publishing of medical works from Jianyang, see Chia, *Printing for Profit*, 314. For the rise of Nanjing as a major publishing center, see Chia, "Of Three Mountain Street."

53. *Kuaiji xian zhi* (Kangxi), 26:7.

54. Zhang Zhibin, "Ming 'Shiwu bencao.'"

55. ISK, 13.86–87.

56. The list of benefactors includes a prince, a grand secretariat, and numerous high ministers. Xu Chunfu, *Gujin yitong daquan*, vol. 94–95.

57. Engelhardt, "Dietetics in Tang China"; Lo, "Pleasure, Prohibition, and Pain"; Buell and Anderson, *A Soup for the Qan.* For medicine in the culture of the Mongol Eurasian empire, see Allsen, *Culture and Conquest*, 141–60.

58. See editor's preface in SWBC-1643, 4–7; Li Shizhen reviewed some of the earlier dietetic texts in BCGM, 1.

59. Wang Wenjie, *Taiyi xianzhi*, first documented opium (*yapian*) prior to *Bencao gangmu*; Yu Ruxi, *Xinkan Leigong*; Yu Yingkui, *Taiyiyuan buyi.* See a summary of these texts in Li Chunxing, *Zhongyao paozhi*, 88–89.

60. Zheng, *Yaolin*, 155–94; Zhang and Guan, "Leigong paozhi lun."

61. Shen Gua, *Mengxi bitan* 4.32; Hong Mai, *Rongzhai suibi*, part 4, 3.663–64. See also Zuo, *Shen Gua's Empiricism*; Hansen, *Changing Gods.*

62. Allen, *Vanishing into Things*, 210–34.

63. Anon., *Buyi Leigong paozhi bianlan.* The manuscript emerged out of a private collection and wasn't published until the 1990s.

64. Métailié, "The *Bencao gangmu* of Li Shizhen"; Nappi, *The Monkey and the Inkpot*, 12–49. For Li's son serving as magistrate in Sichuan, see *Pengxi xian zhi* [Kangxi], juan shang 29a.

65. Qian Yuanming et al., *Li Shizhen.*

66. Berg, *Women and the Literary World*, 28–52.

67. Wang Shizhen, *Yanzhou xu gao*, 10:9b.

68. Dong Qichang, *Rong tai ji*, 1:1–3. Also see Ditmanson, "Imperial History," 35–36.

69. BCGM, 1; Hammond, "Wang Shizhen and Li Shizhen."

70. BCGM-CP, 27–29.

71. BCGM-CP, 24–26. Historians have noted that despite the higher quality of its carvings, the Jiangxi edition is less accurate in the depiction of plants.

72. Dong Qichang, *Rong tai ji*, 1:1–3. The Huguang officials maintained that since Li Shizhen

was a native of the Chu lands, it was only natural for the local Chu people to have an edition of the text to themselves. Again, it echoes the regional sentiment of official publishing.

73. Biography of Xia Liangxin, in *Jiangnan tongzhi*, 150:44.

Chapter 2: Converting Tribute

1. *Longqing zhi* (1549), 3:13b.

2. The official Xie Tinggui was punished for having written "too many memorials" protesting his demotion. Reduced to the status of registered commoner (*bianmeng*), Xie used the gazetteer to reassert his cultural authority. See Xie's 1475 postscript in *Longqing zhi* (1549).

3. Remarkably, his father, Su Ming, earned the same highest degree later than his son in the next metropolitan exam held in 1505. See *Longqing zhi* (1549), 5:7b–8a. Su organized a small group of local literati to complete the revision in forty days. Plagued by Mongol raids, Longqing officials did not manage to publish the revised gazetteer until the following year in 1549. See Su's postscript in *Longqing zhi* (1549).

4. Li Xian, *Da Ming yitong zhi*, 5:18b.

5. Bray, "Utility and Essence"; SCC, 6.4, 113–18.

6. *Longqing zhi* (1549), 3:18ab. As a subprefecture, Longqing was also in charge of Yongning County, which had a separate quota of tribute medicine consisting of half the amount of Longqing's.

7. *Longqing zhi* (1549), 3:18b.

8. Huang, *Taxation and Governmental Finance*; Atwell, "International Bullion Flows." Note that silver never became the sole currency of China but played a different role from that of copper coins. For a longer view of Chinese monetary policy, see von Glahn, *Fountain of Fortune*. Liu Zhiwei mentioned it briefly in *Zai guojia*, 149. For a revisionist critique against using the year 1436 as the conventional starting point of converting grain tax in silver, see Grass, "Imperial Silver Laundering."

9. Brook, *The Confusions of Pleasure*; von Glahn, "The Enchantment of Wealth"; Clunas, *Superfluous Things*; Ariel Fox, "Southern Capital."

10. For local administrations in Ming times, see Nimick, *Local Administration*; Schneewind, *Shrines to Living Men*; Fei, *Negotiating Urban Space*. For the socioeconomic background to fiscal reform and local responses to central directives, see Fu Yiling, *Ming Qing shehui*; Heijdra, "Socio-Economic Development"; Faure, *Emperor and Ancestor*; Liu Zhiwei, *Zai guojia*; Szonyi, *The Art of Being Governed*.

11. Chittick, "The Development of Local Writing," 67. Hu Baoguo, *Han Tang jian*, 159–85, surveyed the multiple origins and tendencies of local writing in the early medieval period.

12. *Shang Shu: Xia Shu-Tribute of Yu*. For broader discussions of the significance of *Shang Shu*, see Kern and Meyer, *Origins of Chinese Political Philosophy*.

13. Du You, *Tongdian*, Compendium on Food and Commodities (*shihuo*), 6:112–25.

14. Zhao Yushi, *Bin tui lu*, 10:132–36. Zhao's source was the *Yuanfeng jiuyu zhi* (*Gazetteer of the Nine Domains during the Yuanfeng reign*, 1080).

15. Sun Simiao, *Qianjin yi fang*, 1:11–15. The phrase "bukan jin yu" indicates that the patient belongs to a higher social status and hence should not be presented with inferior drugs. See also Chen, *Shenfen xushi*.

16. Wang, Tao, *Waitai miyao*, 18:59b, 31:59a, and 37:13b. Note that in some formulas the physician explicitly noted that the *zhoutu* of certain ingredients "does not matter."

17. Li Fang et al., *Taiping yulan*, 983:4485–1.

18. *Lin'an zhi* (Xianchun), 58:15a–17a. The bencao documented common mica (*yunmu*), Chinese lovate (*gaoben*), Skimmia (*yinyu*), and vegetable turtle seeds (*mubie*). The tribute items were Chinese foxglove (*dihuang*), Achyranthes (*niuxi*), and dried ginger.

19. Lin, "The Local in the Imperial Vision."

20. Du You, *Tongdian*, Compendium on Food and Commodities (*shihuo*), 6:112.

21. See my discussion of Song-Yuan public pharmacies in the introduction.

22. MHD, 224:2963–68.

23. MSL-Xuande, 10/2/26, 2:59–60.

24. MHD, 224:2968–71.

25. MHD, 224:2969–71. A prefecture or subprefecture in the "metropolitan areas" was not subordinate to a provincial administration but instead reported directly to the capital ministries.

26. The *Ming History* attributed the heavy land tax on Jiangnan to Zhu Yuanzhang's revenge on the area, which his rival Zhang Shicheng held as his base for a long time. See MS, 78:1896–1901.

27. Brook, *The Confusions of Pleasure*, 23–27, 36–56; Kawakatsu Mamoru, *Min Shin kōnōsei*; Hoshi Ayao, *Min Shin Jidai*, 156–61. Kawakatsu argued that state demand for tribute items directly triggered the rise of urban economy in Ming-Qing times, whereas Hoshi's case study of safflower questioned the assumption that state demand necessarily triggered production and commercialization.

28. MS, 78:1901–02.

29. An early example recorded a conversation between the newly enthroned Hongxi emperor and Yang Shiqi, the grand secretariat in chief, in which the emperor ordered Yang to draft an edict of tax reduction on the spot, against the latter's proposal to consult the Ministries. MSL-Hongxi, 1/4/3, 9:277.

30. MSL-Xuande, 8/4/19, 101:2271; See also Tianshun, 1/1/21, 274.5801.

31. *Huizhou fu zhi* [Hongzhi], 3:65a–66a; compare with *Huizhou fu zhi* [Jiajing], 8:1a–8a, esp. 6ab.

32. MSL-Hongzhi, 17/L4(leap month)/7, 211.3933. For the original memorial, see Chen Zilong et al. eds., *Ming jingshi wenbian*, 79:12b.

33. MSL-Hongzhi, 10/5/3, 125:2225–26. For an earlier censorial petition in the Chenghua reign, see Xu Sanzhong, *Caiqin lu*, 3:11–12.

34. MSL-Hongzhi, 1/10/18, 19:452. For a comprehensive study of the oversight and remonstrations performed by Ming censors, see Hucker, *The Censorial System*.

35. For the date of the memorial, see MSL-Hongzhi, 16/10/27, 204:3805. The full memorial is reproduced in a modern gazetteer of Dai's hometown, see [*Chongxiu*] *Wuyuan xianzhi* (1925), 64:22a–32b. The proposal for local tribute reform is on page 31a–b. For Dai's biography in local sources, see *Huizhou fu zhi* [Jiajing], 16:23a. For the Ministry of Revenue's response to Dai's memorial, see MSL-Hongzhi, 18/9/3, 5:155.

36. MS, 188:4976.

37. Chen Li, *Shu jizhuan zuanshu*, 2:1a.

38. Ma Duanlin, *Wenxian tongkao*, vol. 22; the quote comes from Ma's preface, 4–5.

39. Qiu Jun, *Daxue yanyi bu*, 22:2. See also Brook, *The Confusions of Pleasure*, 101–3.

40. Qiu Jun, *Daxue yanyi bu*, 22:28a.

41. Qiu Jun, *Daxue yanyi bu*, 22:17a.

42. Qiu Jun, *Daxue yanyi bu*, 22:29a.

43. Qiu Jun, *Daxue yanyi bu*, 21:11b.

44. Zhan Ruoshui, *Gewu tong*, 76:8a–9b.

45. MS, 78:1894–95.

46. *Gusu zhi* (Zhengde), 15:14b.

47. Fuling (Poria cocos) was known as China Root, sometimes conflated with *Tu-fu-ling* (native fuling), *Smilax glabra*. See Hu, *Enumeration*, 31 and 145. *Zhejiang tong zhi* (Jiajing), 17:5a.

48. Cangzhu (Ts'ang-shu) remained an important trade item well into the nineteenth century. Regional varieties were identified to the botanical genus *Atractylodes*. Hu, *Enumeration*, 137.

49. *Liuhe xian zhi* (Jiajing), 2:15a.

50. *Yizhen xian zhi* (Longqing), 6:7a.

51. Various Fujian prefectural gazetteers documented this internal solution. See, for example, *Zhangzhou fu zhi* (Wanli), 5:9a.

52. MS, 78:1902. The dynastic historians even acknowledged that monetization reduced the burden on the populace despite soaring tax rates at the time.

53. Wu Zun, *Chu shi lu*, 21a.

54. See another similar list from an earlier time period in *Shanxi tongzhi* (Chenghua), 6:1a.

55. [*Chongxiu*] *Taiping fu zhi* (Jiajing), 5:1a.

56. *Haizhou zhi* (Longqing), 3:15a.

57. *Shunchang yi zhi* (Zhengde), 8:1b.

58. *Laiwu xian zhi* (Jiajing), 3:5a.

59. *Anqing fu zhi* (Jiajing), 12:1a.

60. *Changsha fu zhi* (Jiajing), 3:26a.

61. *Haizhou zhi* (Longqing), 2:19b.

62. *Chaoyi xian zhi* (Zhengde), manuscript, page 16.

63. *Yingshan xian zhi* (Wanli), 3:11ab.

64. *Dongxiang xianzhi* (Jiajing), 34a.

65. *Dengzhou zhi* (Jianjing), 10:32b–33a.

66. Regional and commercial varieties of *huangqi* have been identified with the botanical genus *Astragalus*. Hu, *Enumeration*, 44–45.

67. *Chunhua xian zhi* (Longqing), 5:26a.

68. *Wangjiang xian zhi* (1594), 4:38a.

69. *Yongfeng xian zhi* (Jiajing), 3:7a.

70. For a recent informative review essay that presents a much more nuanced and dynamic account of Ming-Qing China's relationship with neighboring rulers, see Perdue, "The Tenacious Tributary System."

71. He did cite the mid-fifteenth-century dynastic geographical survey (*Da Ming yitong zhi*) twenty-five times but mostly for documentations of exotica (tribute items from "barbarians").

As we have seen in the case for the Longqing Subprefecture, the *Yitong zhi*'s list of local products did not align well with local perceptions.

Chapter 3: The Nature of Drugs

1. Li also requested a preface from a popular former magistrate, who took a much more encouraging tone toward his interest in pharmacy. See Ma Yinglong's Preface, BCYS, preface 1a–3a. For Ma's career in Qi County, see *Qi xian zhi* (Qianlong), 9:47a, 10:7a, 14:19a, 21ab.

2. Luo Wenying's preface, BCYS, 1.

3. BCYS, 1:1a.

4. Shang Zhijun et al., *Lidai zhongyao*, 297–99; Zhang and Zhang, *Bencao yuanshi*; Métailié, SCC6.4, 192–200. Note that Métailié, following Okanishi Tameto in 1977, misidentified this Li Zhongli with a different man of the same name. The other Li Zhongli was a native of Songjiang and nephew of Li Zhongzi, a medical author we will examine later in this chapter. He obtained a jinshi degree and high offices, whereas the Li Zhongli of Qi County did not rise above the juren degree.

5. See Brook, "Rethinking Syncretism"; Wu, *Enlightenment in Dispute*.

6. Zhu Xi, *Zhuzi yulei*, 4:1a–1b.

7. Zhu Xi, *Zhuzi yulei*, 4:2a–2b.

8. Schäfer, *The Crafting of 10,000 Things*, 16.

9. De Bary, *Neo-Confucian Orthodoxy*.

10. For a suggestive comparison with the spectrum of interpretations of Aristotelian metaphysics, see Bloch, *Avicenna and the Aristotelian Left*, xviii–xix passim.

11. Zhan was later criticized for proposing an inconsistent and cumbersome idealism. See Huang Zongxi, *Mingru xue'an*, 37:876–77.

12. Bloom, *Knowledge Painfully Acquired*, 65–70, 157–58, 171–72. Also see Bloom's discussion of the term, 38–42.

13. Ong, "The Principles Are Many."

14. For a study of the relationship between cosmology and phonology in Ming times, see Vedal, "New Scripts."

15. Deng Yuanxi, *Han shi*, 81:16b–17a. The digest of bencao took up the bulk of the chapter, 16b–83a.

16. Deng Yuanxi, *Han shi*, 80:78ab.

17. Dong Qichang, *Rong tai ji*, 1:1a–2a.

18. For a comparison with European aristocratic women's pharmaceutical investment, see Rankin, *Panaceia's Daughters*.

19. Cahill, *The Painter's Practice*, 36.

20. Gao Lian, *Zunsheng bajian*, 7.273.

21. Clunas, *Superfluous Things*.

22. Chen, *Yangsheng yu xiushen*.

23. By the famous general Qi Jiguang (1528–88). For Qi's life and career, see Huang, *1587*, 156–88. Ge and his brothers built a rich collection of ancient and recent texts, boasting as many as 30,000 fascicles in their possession. They regularly reissued rare texts and anthologies known as "Ge woodblocks," frequently with inserted commentary by him. See Wu Han, *Jiangzhe*, 205.

24. Ge Nai, preface, BCYS-1638.

25. Dardess, *Blood and History*, 1; see also Xie, *Ming Qing zhi ji*, 1–37.

26. For literati leadership in late Ming charitable enterprises, see Handlin Smith, *The Art of Doing Good*.

27. Zhao Nanxing, *Shangyi bencao*.

28. Bian, "Documenting Medications." Compare with recipe-sharing in early modern England, as depicted in Leong, *Recipes and Everyday Knowledge*.

29. Shen Defu, *Wanli yehuo bian*, 22.560–61; Wang Yingkui, *Liunan suibi*, 6.112; *Zhaowen xian zhi* (Yongzheng), 8:15a.

30. *Changxing xian zhi* (Tongzhi), 31:56ab.

31. Qian Qianyi, "Preface to *Bencao bacui*," in *Qian Muzhai quanji*, vol. 5, 716–18.

32. *Changxing xian zhi* (Tongzhi), 26:11b–12a.

33. Bian, "Documenting Medications," 115–16.

34. Unschuld, *Medicine in China*, 249.

35. Wang Kentang, *Zhengzhi zhunsheng*, preface 2a–b.

36. Wang Kentang, *Yugang zhai bi zhu*, 2:41b.

37. Already in Miao and Wang's time, other authors disagreed with their approach and insisted on a much more integrated curriculum of medicine. Zhang Jiebin (1563–1640), for instance, always discussed bencao under the rubric of formulaic prescription (*fang*), which was based on the basic physiological and pathological doctrines of medical classics. One could read Zhang's approach as an alternative way of establishing virtuosity, comparable to my discussion of Li Zhongzi. See Zhang Jiebin, *Zhang Jingyue yixue quanshu*, 1565–74.

38. Such was the opinion of eighteenth-century editors of *Siku quanshu*. Miao Xiyong, *Xianxingzhai guang biji*, "Summary" (*tiyao*). The editors also pointed out that Miao's name was not in the extant version of the list they had seen, probably as a result of factional politics.

39. Miao Xiyong recommended Mao Fengbao's father to Yang Lian for an official appointment. Yang sent a letter of mourning of Mao's father in 1624 right before his arrest and death. See Qian Dacheng, "Mao Zijin nianpu gao," 11–12.

40. MS, 236:6156–57; 243:6311–14. See Dardess, *Blood and History*, 9–149; Xie, *Ming Qing zhi ji*, 38–58.

41. For the occasion of Miao's return, see Qian Qianyi, *Qian Muzhai quanji*, vol. 5, 716–18.

42. BCJS, prefatory matter, 2. BCJS-1625, preface–3b. Mao's studio name then was *Lüjunting* (Pavillon of the Green Lord).

43. Miao Xiyong, "Author's Preface," in BCJS, prefatory matters, p. 3; BCJS-1625, preface–1b.

44. BCJS, prefatory matter, 3; BCJS-1625, preface–1b.

45. Qian Qianyi, *Qian Muzhai quanji*, vol. 5, 716.

46. BCJS, prefatory matter, 4; BCJS-1625, "Note to readers (*fanli*)," p. 1a. See also Elman, *On Their Own Terms*, 227–36.

47. BCJS, prefatory matter, 3; BCJS-1625, preface–1a.

48. BCJS, 1.

49. BCJS, 153.

50. BCJS, 153; BCJS-1625, 10:16b–18a.

51. BCJS-1625, 8:1b–2b.

52. BCJS-1625, 1:32a–32b.

53. BCJS-1625, 1:4b. On the issue of poison in medieval pharmacy texts, see Liu, "Toxic Cures."

54. Unschuld, *Huang Di nei jing su wen*, 22–58, 284–312.

55. Unschuld, *Huang Di nei jing su wen*, 307.

56. Wang Bing ed., *Chongguang buzhu Huangdi neijing suwen*, 22.30b–31a.

57. The theory was accepted and recorded in bencao pharmacopeias. See "Loss of Balance with the Five Flavors" (*wu wei pian sheng*). BCGM, 31.

58. See the OEB entry for idiosyncrasy (n.): c. 1600, from French *idiosyncrasie*, from Greek *idiosynkrasia* "a peculiar temperament," from *idios* "one's own" (see idiom) + *synkrasis* "temperament, mixture of personal characteristics," from *syn* "together" (see syn-) + *krasis* "mixture" (see rare [adj. 2]). In English this was originally a medical term meaning the particular physical constitution of an individual.

59. Cf. Murdoch, "The Analytic Character," 8.

60. Qian Qianyi, *Qian Muzhai quanji*, vol. 5, 716; vol. 2, 870–71.

61. Li Zhi, "Preface," in Miao Xiyong, *Xianxingzhai guang biji*.

62. BCJS, prefatory matter, 2. BCJS-1625, preface–3b.

63. Dardess, *Blood and History*, 150–70; Xie, *Ming Qing zhi ji*, 59–97, 119–66.

64. Qian, "Mao Zijin nianpu gao."

65. Ni Yuanlu's preface, BCHY, 1–5. Ni Yuanlu referred to Ni Zhumo as his "grandnephew" (*zhisun*).

66. *Renhe xian zhi* (Kangxi 26), 21:15b.

67. BCHY, "Notes to the reader" (*fanli*).

68. See BCHY-2005. The list of names was taken out in the 1645 edition.

69. *Qiantang xian zhi* (Kangxi), 26:20ab, 35:7a. Note that Lu Fu's biography appeared in the chapter on physicians and formulaic arts, whereas Lu Zhiyi's appeared in the chapter of "hermits" (*yinyi*). See also a biography of Lu Zhiyi in Hang Shijun, *Daogu tang wenji*, 29:10a–12a.

70. BCSYBJ, 21. One of the frequent lecturers was the retired official Wang Shaolong (jinshi 1589), another mentor of Ni Zhumo.

71. BCSYBJ, 217. The three quotes on bamboo appear on the same page.

72. For this reason, he named his bencao manuscript *Quadruple Refinement* (*Shengya*), an explicit reference to the ancient dictionary *Erya*.

73. BCSYBJ, 38.

74. BCSYBJ, 30.

75. These publishers, *Zhijin tang* and *Sheyuan tang*, were both located in the Huizhou Prefecture. Personal communication with Zheng Jinsheng, June 20, 2019.

76. Qian Yunzhi, preface, *Shiwu bencao*, 1621 edition. Falsely attributed to Li Gao, the Jin-dynasty master physician.

77. Volkmar, "The Physician and the Plagiarists."

78. SWBC-1643, 4–6.

79. SWBC-1643, 2–3.

80. Qian also published the collected works of the celebrity art critic Li Rihua (1565–1635), *Si liu quan shu*, in 1640.

81. Qian Weiqi's preface to the Hangzhou edition of *Bencao gangmu*. BCGM-CP, 20.

82. His father's name is Li Shanggun. See *Songjiang fu zhi* (Chongzhen), 34:24a; *Songjiang fu zhi* (Jiaqing), 61:26ab; *Shanghai xian zhi* (Qianlong), 10:1852–54 (Airusheng database pagination). The gazetteer biography documented that Li treated celebrities, including Wang Kentang in his old age and a Ming prince.

83. Li Zhongzi, *Li Zhongzi yixue quanshu*, 701. The content is derived from Li Shizhen's *Bencao gangmu*.

84. Li Zhongzi, *Li Zhongzi yixue quanshu*, 556.

85. Li Zhongzi, *Li Zhongzi yixue quanshu*, 555.

86. Li Zhongzi, *Li Zhongzi yixue quanshu*, 79–283.

87. *Jiading xian zhi* (Kangxi), 3:38ab.

88. Schäfer, *The Crafting of 10,000 Things*.

89. Li Zhongzi, *Li Zhongzi yixue quanshu*, 643.

Chapter 4: Virtuosity and Orthodoxy

1. *Zhongyong*, 1.

2. Peterson, "Advancement of Learning," 515–28; Peterson, *Bitter Gourd*, 12–17.

3. Fang Yizhi, *Wuli xiaoshi*, 1:16a.

4. Fang Yizhi, *Wuli xiaoshi*, 1:16ab. For instance, Fang was puzzled by the fact that the hawthorn fruit is sweet and sour in taste but was not documented as such in bencao.

5. Fang Yizhi, *Wuli xiaoshi*, 5:15a and 5:4b.

6. Fang Yizhi, *Wuli xiaoshi*, 5:6b–7a; Yu, *Fang Yizhi wanjie kao*, 275–77. For the centrality of the pharmacy metaphor in Fang's Daoist commentary, see Xing Yihai, *Fang Yizhi Zhuangxue*, 7–22.

7. Fang possessed a "pharmaceutical chamber" in one of his dwellings in exile. Yu, *Fang Yizhi wanjie kao*, 91–101.

8. Zuo, *Shen Gua*, 171–200.

9. *Qiantang xian zhi* (Kangxi), 29:10a. The widow, née Shen, earned more posthumous celebration than her husband. Shen was only nineteen when her husband died. She raised their son on her own and served her mother-in-law diligently through war and famine.

10. Hang Shijun, *Daogu tang wenji*, 29:11b–12a. Also see *Hangzhou fu zhi* (Qianlong), 99:31b.

11. Mao Jin, *Yewai shi*, 4b–5a.

> Piling up like mountains, the commentaries and books were unable to be read
> Master Zhongchun glared at this, deeply angered
> He spoke bluntly on the pros and cons [in the use of drugs], startling the guests
> And his teachings continued from the ancient sages, what a wonderful thought!
> He ordered me to cut the jujube wood, and carve it into a book
> Just as clouds dispersing from the sun's shines, the text radiates precious light

12. See prefaces by Zhang Chaolin, Wu Sichang, and others in BCGM-CP, 3–19. For *Bencao gangmu*'s popularity in Qing commercial publishing, see Brokaw, *Commerce in Culture*, 428–38.

13. BCS, prefatory matter, 2b.

14. Pu Shizhen, *Xi'an du bencao*, 520. Pu identified himself as a follower of Li Zhongzi, who wrote a preface for his bencao and disparaged Miao Xiyong's work.

15. For a successful case, see *Jiading xian zhi* (Kangxi), 3:38ab. Li's last bencao is titled *Bencao tongxuan* (*Comprehending the Subtlety of Pharmacy*).

16. Zhao et al., *Qing shi gao*, 502:13868–69.

17. Yu Chang, *Yuyi cao*, preface.

18. Yu Chang, *Yuyi cao*, preface.

19. Yu Chang, *Yuyi cao*, 1:1a–2b.

20. In 1651, Qian Qianyi wrote a poem to honor Yu Chang, praising him as a "comprehensive Confucian" and devout monk. Qian Qianyi, *Qian Muzhai quanji*, vol. 4, 4.135–36.

21. Yu Chang, *Yimen falü*, preface.

22. *Wuxian zhi* (Kangxi), 56, 6b–7a.

23. "Author's Preface (*zixu*)," in Zhang Lu, *Zhang Luyu*, 5; Zhao et al., *Qing shi gao*, 502:13869–70.

24. BJFY, preface, 1b–2a.

25. BCGMSY, preface.

26. BJFY, preface, 1a.

27. For Wang Ang's career as publisher, see Widmer, "The Huanduzhai of Hangzhou and Suzhou."

28. BCBY, "Author's Preface."

29. BCBY, "Notes to Readers." Wang marketed his bencao textbook with another bestselling title of his, *Rhymes for Decoction Starters* (*Tangtou gejue*), which adapted common prescriptions into simple songs.

30. *Bencao beiyao* is still held as a useful introductory text for students of TCM today. See Chang Hsien-che, "The *Pen-Ts'ao Pei-Yao*."

31. Li Chunxing, *Zhongyao paozhi*, 88.

32. Zhang Rui, *Xiushi zhinan*, 1a–b. The text was "reviewed" (*ding*) by Hu Zuomei (1653–1718), a civil official in the Kangxi court. Hu's specific role in the compilation of this text is unclear.

33. Zhang Guangdou. *Zengbu Leigong*, preface.

34. Schonebaum, *Novel Medicine*, 73–121.

35. Compare with Blair, *The Theater of Nature*.

36. Zhang Lu, *Zhang Luyu yixue*, 1.

37. MS, 299.7653.

38. For more information on the Imperial Publishing Office, see Yang Yuliang, "Wuying dian."

39. "Memorial (*biao*)," in BCPHJY-KX, 1a–5a.

40. Giles, *An Alphabetical Index*, xvii; Pei Qin, *Gujin tushu jicheng yanjiu*, 27–42 (process of compilation); 97–140 (list of gazetteers cited).

41. Giles, *An Alphabetical Index*, xii; appendix 2. The rise of nonmedical natural history could be traced back to Song-Yuan-Ming works. See Siebert, "Making Technology History."

42. Hanson, "The Golden Mirror," 112.

43. Guy, *The Emperor's Four Treasuries*. For collectanea in private scholarly circles, see Bian, "Recollecting the Glorious Age."

44. *Qinding Siku quanshu zongmu*, 91.1ab.

45. Ji Yun et al. *Qinding Siku quanshu zongmu*, vol. 3, 103:35b–38a, 104:10a–11a, 32ab, 36b–37a, 42a–43a.

46. Ji Yun et al. *Qinding Siku quanshu zongmu*, vol. 3, 105:11b–12a.

47. Ji Yun et al. *Qinding Siku quanshu zongmu*, vol. 3, 105:4a–7b, 43b. The editor Zhou Yongnian (1730–1791) provided the originals of Huang's published corpus.

48. Zhang Zhicong, *Lüshantang*, 96–97.

49. The medical collectanea was titled *Yilin zhiyue* (1764–1777) and edited by Wang Qi.

50. See the "Three-Character Primer for Medicine" by Chen Nianzu, *Chen Xiuyuan yixue quanshu*, 816–17. For Zhang's biography, see Zhao et al., *Qing shi gao*, 502:13871–72.

51. See, for instance, the New Text school described in Elman, *Classicism, Politics, and Kinship*.

52. See the summaries of Xu's works in Ji Yun et al., *Qinding Siku quanshu zongmu*, part 3, 104:51b–55a.

53. *Wujiang xian xuzhi* (Guangxu), 21:6b–7a.

54. Xu Dachun, *Shennong bencaojing baizhong lu*. For Xu's discussion of medical ethics, see Paul Unschuld's translation in Xu, *Forgotten Traditions*.

55. Xu Dachun, *Yixue yuanliu lun*, juan shang: 57–59a.

56. Xu Dachun, *Shen ji chu yan*, 14b.

Chapter 5: The Marketplace and the Shop

1. Semedo, *History*, 11.56. Semedo later returned to China and remained there until his death in 1658 (in Canton).

2. Nakagawa Tadahide, *Shinzoku kibun*, book 1, 2.109–11. For illustrations of pharmacy tools, see Tadahide, *Shinzoku kibun*, book 1, illustrations, 120–22.

3. Von Glahn, *An Economic History*, 295–347; Fan, "Long Distance Trade."

4. Ren Fang, *Ming Qing Changjiang*; Xiao Fang, "Ming Qing shidai."

5. Rowe, *Hankow*, 56–61, 206–8; Tang Tingyou, *Zhongguo yaoye shi*.

6. Zhang Ji, *Zhang Siye ji*, 7:5.

7. Liu Zongyuan, *Liu Hedong ji*, 17.304–5.

8. Shiba Yoshinobu, *Commerce and Society*.

9. Meng Yuanlao, *Dongjing menghua lu*, 2.164, 3.268.

10. The official title of "defense general" (*fangyu*) seems to have been a popular title for doctors in the Northern Song. An anecdote told of how a "doctor of the marshes" (*caoze yi*) gained the title as a reward for curing the empress dowager's cataract. See Hong Mai, *Yi jian zhi*, 7:7b–8a.

11. Zhou Mi, *Wulin jiushi*, 6:6.

12. Tao Gu, *Qing yi lu*, juan shang: 14a.

13. Wu Yuan, "An Account of the Benevolent Pharmacy," in *Suzhou fu zhi* (Tongzhi), 22:53a. See also *Bamin tongzhi* (Hongzhi), 61:12b.

14. See Tang Tingyou, *Zhongguo yaoye shi*, 75–77. Anecdotal sources include Cai Tao, *Tieweishan cong tan*, 6:14a; Zhuang Jiyu, *Jilei pian*, juan shang, 29ab; Lu You, *Laoxue an biji*, 6:12a.

15. Yang Tianhui, "Zhangming fuzi ji."

16. *Lin'an zhi* (Xianchun), 58:15b.

17. A horticultural treatise dated to the fourteenth century described the planting and harvesting of less than twenty species. "Treatise on the Cultivation of Medicine (*zhong yao shu*)," in Hunan manshi, *Shuibian linxia*, 701–4.

18. Bian, "Shui zhu yao shi," 49–52.

19. Liu Chun, *Liu Chun yixue quanshu*, 468–69. Liu Chun's father was a disciple of Zhu Zhenheng, thus establishing a credible line of transmission. Liu also alleged that he only shared the "ten commandments" at the repeated request of a civil official, who promised to sponsor the printing of his medical works.

20. *Wugong xian zhi* (Zhengde), 2:3b.

21. A literary critic boasted in a letter about his ability to guess the name of a poet from glancing over their works, since each person practiced a distinct style, just as regionally produced silk had specific daodi patterns. See Yan Yu, *Canglang shihua*, appendix, 235. In colloquial Chinese today the word "daodi" ("routes and places," or didao, another version of the same word) still means "authenticity" of commodities, and sometimes the intentions of people.

22. *Jiangyin xian zhi* (Chongzhen), 2:73b.

23. Tang Xianzu, *Mudan ting*, 34:169–70; Tang Xianzu, *Yuming tang quan ji*, 1:9b.

24. BCSYBJ, "Notes to Readers," 27–28.

25. BCMQ, prefatory matter, 2–3.

26. Feng Menglong, *Xingshi hengyan*, 38.861–62.

27. The late sixteenth century was the time when the original Song Dynasty Qingming scroll emerged from private collections in the south, making it possible for anonymous artists to study and copy it, in the process grafting many contemporary Suzhou scenes into the painting. See Laing, "*Suzhou Pian.*" The painting I refer to is in the collection of the Liaoning Provincial Museum. See Qiu Ying, *Qingming shanghe tu*.

28. BCGM, 43.1002–3. The position of the tuo in the representation of a Chinese apothecary posed an intriguing parallel with another reptile on the opposite side of the globe: compare with the crocodile specimen in the museum of the Neapolitan apothecary Ferrante Imperato (c. 1525?–1615). See image in Findlen, *Possessing Nature*, 39.

29. Wang, "Guoyan fanhua."

30. Xiaoxiaosheng, *Jin Ping Mei*, 1.12.

31. Modified translation from Roy, *The Plum in the Golden Vase*, vol. 1, 16.322.

32. See Shang, "The Making of the Everyday World."

33. Modified translation from Roy, *The Plum in the Golden Vase*, vol. 4, chapter 67, 208–9. Roy's translation of Xiajiang as "the Yangtze Gorges" is mistaken, as I will explain below.

34. Brook, *Geographical Sources*, 24–27; Yang Zhengtai, *Mingdai yizhankao*, appendix.

35. Xiaoxiaosheng, *Jin Ping Mei*, 17.243–47, 19.270.

36. Xiaoxiaosheng, *Jin Ping Mei*, appendix, Cihua edition, 54.1939–40.

37. Xiaoxiaosheng, *Jin Ping Mei*, 54.728–30, 55.732. See also Cullen, "Patients and Healers," 136.

38. "Raising the Price and Losing the Profit," in Zhang Yingyu, *Dupian xinshu*, 2:14a–15b. The story is not included in the recent translation by Christopher Rea and Bruce Rusk.

39. See also Lufrano, *Honorable Merchants*, 132–39.

40. *Qingjiang xian zhi* (Qianlong), 24:28a.

41. *Qingjiang xian zhi* (Tongzhi), 8:66b; Sun and Huang, *Zhangshu zhongyiyao*, 62–64. In local lore, Hou was remembered as the "sixth generation medicine king" (*di liu dai yaowang*). Hou's biography likely only appeared in nineteenth-century gazetteers because of the business community's need for an ancestor-like figure in local history.

42. Although it is hard to believe that merely moving the market downstream 30 li and across the river could have made all the difference. See Guan Daxun, "Discourse on Setting up a Tax-Collecting Bridge in Zhangshu," in *Qingjiang xian zhi* (Chongzhen), 8:163ab.

43. *Qingjiang xian zhi* (Chongzhen), 1:7b–8a.

44. The temple was rebuilt in 1540. *Qingjiang xian zhi* (Chongzhen), 8:120b–121b.

45. "Local Products," *Qingjiang xian zhi* (Chongzhen), 3:35ab.

46. Yang Zhengtai, *Mingdai yizhankao*, appendix, 268–71.

47. Wang Shixing, *Guang zhi yi*, 4.85.

48. Xiong Hua, "An Account of the Town of Zhangshu," in *Qingjiang xian zhi* (Chongzhen), 8:147a–149a. Xiong was a native of Qingjiang County.

49. The gazetteer credited the local magistrate for standing up to the imperial agents and restoring order. "Biography of Zhang Rulin," in *Linjiang fu zhi* (Tongzhi), 17:16ab.

50. An annual tax of at least 2,000 taels of silver was collected from Zhangshu. "Market Towns," *Qingjiang xian zhi* (Chongzhen), 1:25.

51. *Qingjiang xian zhi* (Chongzhen), 1:25b.

52. "Local Customs," *Qingjiang xian zhi* (Chongzhen), 1:34b.

53. Guan Daxun, "Discourse on Setting up a Tax-Collecting Bridge in Zhangshu," in *Qingjiang xian zhi* (Chongzhen), 8:163ab. Referring to an example in a nearby town, Guan pointed out that trade in the entire region stalled because of a new bridge built there to extract levies. Worse, the bridge itself had recently been destroyed by flood.

54. Many local literati warmly received the former scholar-in-exile and wrote poems to commemorate the occasion. *Qingjiang xian zhi* (Qianlong), 6:8b, 29:1a–b.

55. Fang Yizhi, *Wuli xiaoshi*, 5:35a.

56. Memorial by Li Ripeng in 1651. Database of Ming and Qing Grand Secretariat, Taipei, no. 089132–001.

57. *Xuancheng xian zhi* (Jiaqing), 24:9–12.

58. Yuan Liangyi, *Qing yitiaobian fa*.

59. QHD-KX, 78.6, and 161.19.

60. For provincial tribute items, see He Xinhua, *Qingdai gongwu*, 23–53. For Qing court medicine, see Guan Xueling, *Qingdai gongting yixue*, 108–39,176–201.

61. Aricanli, "Diversifying the Center," chapter 2; Guan Xueling, *Qingdai gongting yixue*, 8–35.

62. For Qing imperial fiscal practices during the Qianlong reign, see Lai Huimin, *Qianlong huangdi*. For changing distribution of "regular" domestic customs (*changguan*) from Ming to Qing, see Ni, *Customs Duties*; Xu Tan, "Changing Configurations." For the evolution of Qing policy toward maritime trade, see Zhao, *Qing Opening to the Ocean*.

63. See Xu Menghong, *Beixin guan zhi*, 13.182–84; Anon., *Zhe hai chaoguan zhengshou shuiyin*

ze li, 14–18. For a survey of Qing China's pharmaceutical trade with Tokugawa Japan, see Habu Kazuko, *Edo jidai*, 123–31. The most popular merchandise included ginseng, licorice, aconite, rhubarb, and ephedra.

64. Jiang, *Renshen diguo*, 51–147; Kim, *Ginseng and Borderland*.

65. Yue Chongxi, *Bainian Tongrentang*, 110–14. According to memoirs by Tongrentang's descendants, the temple fair at Qizhou would hold all transactions until agents of Tongrentang arrived at the scene.

66. Yu Hui, "Cong Qingming jie".

67. Xu Yang, *Gusu fanhua tu*.

68. Also known as "transmission of pharmaceutical skills but not medical knowledge" (*chuanyao bu chuanyi*). Zhang Peiyu et al., *Beijing Tongrentang shi*, 1–11; for the shop's status as a purveyor for the Imperial Household, see 12–27; for the Yue family's loss of ownership, see 28–35. Yue Chonghui, a descendant of the Yue family, claimed that after the generation of Yue Pingquan, the managers themselves knew very little about medicine. See Zhuo Zunhong et al., *Yue Chonghui*, 41.

69. Yue Fengming, "Preface," in *Tongrentang yaomu*, Guangxu edition (1889).

70. Liu and He, "Wanquan tang." The original documents of Wanquan tang came into the hands of Deng Tuo (1912–66), who was chief editor of the *People's Daily* during the 1950s. Deng was interested in using the pharmacy as a case study of economy and labor during the Qing, but this project was interrupted by his subsequent political marginalization and eventual suicide during the Cultural Revolution. For the lack of clear evidence indicating the existence of similar pharmacies prior to the seventeenth century, see Tang Tingyou, *Zhongguo yaoye shi*, 309–13.

71. Four of them had jinshi degrees, and the prefaces were printed in different calligraphic styles to impress the reader.

72. Wang Jikui's preface in *Heniantang zhiyao mulu*; Yue Chongxi, *Bainian Tongrentang*, 81.

73. See company website http://www.jxt.com.cn/index.html, accessed Feb. 6, 2014.

74. Preface and table of contents in Qian Shutian, *Jingxiutang yaoshuo*.

75. Memorial by Cui Yingjie, the governor-general of Fujian and Zhejiang, Qianlong 34, Archive of the Grand Secretariat, no. 090536–001; For instance, see the memorial by Zhang Shicheng, the governor of Fujian, in Jiaqing 16, Archive of the Grand Secretariat, no. 115100–001, Also see the memorial by Wang Shaolan, the governor of Fujian, in Jiaqing 19, Archive of the Grand Secretariat, no.122979–001.

76. Tang Tingyou, *Zhongguo yaoye shi*, 115–30, 250–53. Mostly these women were praised for promising never to remarry and remaining filial daughters to their in-laws. *Qingjiang xianzhi* (Qianlong), 19:11–12, 15a, 16b, 17b, 22b, 24a, 25b, 34a, 35a, 37b, 38a.

77. *Qingjiang xianzhi* (Qianlong), 19:28a.

78. Cochran, *Chinese Medicine Men*, 21–24; for a range of complex voices gleaned from oral history interviews of Tongrentang's early twentieth-century employees, see Ding, *Geren xushu*.

79. Sun and Huang, *Zhangshu zhongyiyao*, 17–25, 149–51.

80. Sun and Huang, *Zhangshu zhongyiyao*, 51–52, 128–29.

81. Sun and Huang, *Zhangshu zhongyiyao*, 81–86, 127.

82. Sun and Huang, *Zhangshu zhongyiyao*, 105.

83. Sun and Huang, *Zhangshu zhongyiyao*, 132.

84. Rowe, "Political, Social, and Economic Factors," 44.

Chapter 6: Eating Exotica

1. The three pharmacists in Tongrentang were Deng Lüren, Zhou Zhiliang, and Wu Meishan (none of them were related to the owner's family). For Ryukyu students in China and their activities in Fuzhou, see Hukazawa Akihito, *Kinsei Ryūkyū Chūgoku kōryūshi no kenkyū*, 29–58, 161–194.

2. For more detailed description of the work see Higashionna Kanjun, "Shitsumon Honzō."

3. Marcon, *The Knowledge of Nature*.

4. Deng, Zhou, and Wu's response letters, in ZWBC, *Nei pian*, 1:20ab.

5. ZWBC, *Wai pian*, 4:5ab, for local rhubarb (*tu dahuang*).

6. *Weinan xian zhi* (Jiajing), 3:8a.

7. He, *Home and the World*, 202–44.

8. Schafer, *The Golden Peaches*, 32–35.

9. Chen, "*Craft*."

10. The arguments in this section are condensed from a previously published article. For more detailed information on Zhao's life and methods of work, see Bian, "An Ever-Expanding Pharmacy."

11. BCGMSY, prefactory matter, 5a.

12. BCGMSY, 4:8b. Zhao found that the herb had been documented as an antidote in the Song dynasty *Zhenglei bencao*, but not as a digestive drink.

13. BCGMSY, 5:27a.

14. BCGMSY, 5:18b.

15. BCGMSY, 8:31ab.

16. BCGMSY, 3:16b–19b.

17. BCGMSY, 3:16b–19b.

18. BCGMSY, 7:62b–65b.

19. See Nappi, "Surface Tension"; Jiang, *Renshen diguo*, 170–235.

20. BCGMSY, 3:9b.

21. BCGMSY, 3:11a.

22. BCGMSY, 3:16a.

23. ZLBC-1249, 24.2a (sesame), 27.20a (bitter lettuce).

24. BCGM, 27.711.

25. BCMQ, 1.1a.

26. BCSYBJ, 5:51b–52a.

27. BJFY, 1:60a. For modern nomenclatures of the variety, see Hu, *An Enumeration of Chinese Materia Medica*, 82–83.

28. BCCX, 4:2b–3a.

29. BCGMSY, 8:64b–65a.

30. BCGMSY, 4:26ab.

31. BCGMSY, 9:69ab.

32. BCGMSY, 9:55ab.

33. BCGMSY, 9:38a.

34. BCGMSY, 9:50b–51a.

35. BCGMSY, 9:52a–53a.

36. BCGMSY, 9:48a.

37. BCGMSY, 9:47b–48a.

38. Siebert, "Animals as Text."

39. *Yingjing xian zhi* (Qianlong), 3:10ab.

40. Yan Ruyu, *Sansheng bianfang*, 9:15b.

41. BCGMSY, 3:5b.

42. BCGMSY, 5:25b.

43. BCGMSY, 3:8ab.

44. Shinoda, *Chūgoku shokumotsushi*, 299–300. Shinoda also suggested that the divide between medieval and early modern should not be placed at the Tang-Song transition as his generation had been led to believe; rather, the modern (*kinsei*) had begun in the mid-Ming after the consummation of Song-Yuan culture took place. It should be obvious by now that my analysis in this book confirms his periodization.

45. BCGMSY, 10:18b.

46. BCGMSY, 9:31a–34a.

47. BCGMSY, 7:47ab.

48. BCGMSY, 8:73ab.

49. BCGMSY, 8:77b–78a.

50. For instance, Tong Yuejian, *Tiao Ding ji*; Waley-Cohen, "Food and China's World of Goods" (mostly focusing on court banquets); Shinoda, *Chūgoku shokumotsushi*, 274–301; Spence, "Ch'ing."

51. BCGMSY, 3:4ab.

52. BCGMSY, 9:27b–28a.

53. BCGMSY, 7:1a–4a.

54. BCGMSY, 7:3b.

55. BCGMSY, 5:73b.

56. BCGMSY, 2:25a–26b. See also Spence, *Ts'ao Yin and the K'ang-Hsi Emperor*.

57. BCGMSY, 8:38a–39b.

58. BCGMSY, 6:11b.

59. BCGMSY, 6:7a–8b.

60. BCGMSY, 6:44ab.

61. BCGMSY, 8:18ab.

62. BCGMSY, 5:20b–23a.

63. BCGMSY, 9:1a.

64. Xie Zhaozhe, *Wu za zu*, 10:21b–22a; BCGMSY, 5:62a.

65. BCGMSY, 7:76ab. Zhao went to great lengths in ascertaining whether peanuts were pathogenic. Some popular advice, for instance, forbade people from consuming peanuts together with cucumber, and Zhao noted that when many people took the risk of trying the combination and felt no discomfort, new advice emerged to prohibit eating peanuts with yellow cantaloupe. Zhao himself witnessed the son of a magistrate who collapsed into paralysis apparently as a result of craving peanuts. However, he also heard that a respectable nun had once

cured a wealthy matron of chronic cough with a long-term diet of peanuts, of which she consumed a total of twenty jin.

66. BCGMSY, 8:54a.

67. BCGMSY, 8:86a, 8:72a.

68. Tellingly, the quote came from a late Ming source, Zhu Guozhen's *Dazheng ji*. BCGMSY, 10:7b.

69. BCGMSY, 10:40b.

70. BCGMSY, 5:55b.

71. Liu, *The Clash of Empires*, 31–69.

72. BCGMSY, 9:23ab. See also Van Dyke, *The Canton Trade*.

73. BCGMSY, 9:1a–4a.

74. BCGMSY, 2:35ab.

75. BCGMSY, 2:60ab.

76. BCGMSY, 10:46ab.

77. Snyder-Reinke, "Afterlives of the Dead"; Cf. Sugg, *Mummies, Cannibals and Vampires*.

78. BCGMSY, 9:4.

79. BCGMSY, 10:68.

80. Kuhn, *Soulstealers*, 223.

81. For more on the bogus memorial case, see Kuhn, *Soulstealers*, 60–63; Liu Wenpeng, *Shengshi beihou*.

82. Zhuang Jifa, *Zhenkong jiaxiang*, 491–512.

83. Zhang Jiuxiao got off with "death penalty awaiting autumn assizes," which frequently was commuted to prison time. Zhi's wife was sold into servitude; his books burned to ashes. See the record of QL 44.05.19–20 in BnF Chinois 2216. I thank Emily Mokros for sharing this source with me. For Qianlong's edict, see also QSL-Qianlong, 44.532–33.

84. QSL-Qianlong, 57.538.

Epilogue

1. Jia and Yang, *Qingdai yaoxing ju*.

2. See the manuscripts collected by Paul Unschuld in Unschuld and Zheng, *Chinese Traditional Healing*, vol. 1, 175–84.

3. Meyer-Fong, *What Remains*, 21–64.

4. Yvan, *Lettre sur la Pharmacie*, 6–7. For an account of botanical explorations associated with this expedition, see Bretschneider, *History of European Botanical Discoveries*, 518–25.

5. Yvan, *Lettre sur la Pharmacie*, 6, 16–17.

6. Yvan, "Extrait d'un travail sur Singapore."

7. Sun and Huang, *Zhangshu zhongyiyao*, 105–8, 130–32.

8. A Japanese report from Shandong in 1922 quoted a 1914 survey conducted by the Republican government of China, which stated that Yunnan Province alone supplied up to 6,500,000,000 jin of raw medicine, amounting to seventy-seven percent of the total domestic production. See Kindō, *Kita Shina*, 237–38.

9. *Zhonghua yaodian* (1930). For the colonial origin of state-centered approaches to public health, see Rogaski, *Hygienic Modernity*.

10. Zhao Yuhuang, *Qizhou yao zhi*.

11. Andrews, *The Making of Modern Chinese Medicine*.

12. Cochran, *Chinese Medicine Men*, 16–37.

13. Lei, *Neither Donkey nor Horse*.

14. *Zhonghua renmin gongheguo yaodian* (1963). This revision departed from an earlier pharmacopeia the PRC issued in 1953, which was largely identical to Liu Jui-heng's 1930 pharmacopeia in content and structure. Part I includes 446 kinds of Chinese materia medica and 197 compound medicines; and part II includes 667 kinds of chemical, antibiotic, and other compounds used in Western medical practice.

15. Sivin, *Traditional Medicine in Contemporary China*; Scheid, *Currents of Tradition in Chinese Medicine*; Farquhar, *Knowing Practice*; Zhan, *Other-Worldly*. For an excellent recent English translation of the earliest bencao text for practitioners, see Wilms, *The Divine Farmer's Classic*.

16. For similar attention to the pharmaceutical dimension of contemporary healing traditions in Tibet, see Saxer, *Manufacturing Tibetan Medicine*; Craig, *Healing Elements*.

BIBLIOGRAPHY

Abbreviations

ISK Taki Monotane. *Yiji kao (I seki kō)* [A Bibliographical Study of Medical Texts], Beijing: Xueyuan chubanshe, 2007.

MHD Shen Shixing et al. *Da Ming huidian* [Statutes of the Great Ming]. 1587. Academia Sinica, *Hanji quanwen ziliaoku (Scripta Sinica)* database.

MS Zhang Tingyu et al. *Ming shi* [History of the Ming]. Beijing: Zhonghua shuju, 1974.

MSL *Ming shilu* [Veritable Records of the Ming]. Academia Sinica, *Hanji quanwen ziliaoku (Scripta Sinica)* database.

QSL *Qing shilu* [Veritable Records of the Qing]. Academia Sinica, *Hanji quanwen ziliaoku (Scripta Sinica)* database.

SCC6.1 Needham, Joseph, with the collaboration of Lu Gwei-Djen and a special contribution by Huang Hsing-Tsung. *Science and Civilisation in China, Vol. 6: Biology and Biological Technology, Part 1: Botany.* Cambridge: Cambridge University Press, 1986.

SCC6.4 Métailié, Georges. *Science and Civilisation in China, Vol. 6: Biology and Biological Technology, Part 4: Traditional Botany: An Ethnobotanical Approach.* Cambridge: Cambridge University Press, 2015.

SKQS *Wenyuange Siku quanshu* [Complete Library in Four Sections, Wenyuange copy]. Taipei: Commercial Press, 1983.

XXSKQS *Xuxiu Siku quanshu* [Supplements to *Siku Quanshu*]. Shanghai: Shanghai guji chubanshe, 1995–99.

Major Works of *Bencao*

BCBY Wang Ang 汪昂. *Bencao beiyao* 本草備要. Expanded edition. Huanduzhai: Kangxi 33 [1694]. Accessed through Academia Sinica, *Hanji quanwen ziliaoku* (Scripta Sinica).

BCCX Wu Yiluo 吳儀洛. *Bencao congxin* 本草從新. N.p. preface 1757. Reprint, XXSKQS, vol. 994.

BCGM Li Shizhen 李時珍. *Bencao gangmu* 本草綱目. Based on the Jinling edition (1st edition). Beijing: Zhongyi guji chubanshe, 1994.

BCGM-CP Li Shizhen. *Bencao gangmu.* Shanghai: Commercial Press, 1954.

BCGMSY Zhao Xuemin 趙學敏. *Bencao gangmu shiyi* 本草綱目拾遺. N.p. 1871. Reprint, XXSKQS, vols. 994–95.

BCHY Ni Zhumo 倪朱謨. *Bencao huiyan* 本草彙言. Dacheng zhai, 1645. Reprint, XXSKQS, vol. 992.

BCHY-2005 Ni Zhumo. *Bencao huiyan*. Edited by Zheng Jinsheng 鄭金生. Beijing: Zhongyi guji chubanshe, 2005.

BCJJZ Tao Hongjing 陶弘景. *Shennong bencaojing jizhu* 神農本草經集註. Edited by Shang Zhijun 尚志鈞 et al. Beijing: Renmin weisheng chubanshe, 1994.

BCJS Miao Xiyong 繆希雍. *Shennong bencaojing shu* 神農本草經疏. Edited by Xia Kuizhou. Beijing: Zhongguo zhongyiyao chubanshe, 1997.

BCJS-1625 Miao Xiyong. *Shennong bencaojing shu*. Changshu: Lüjunting, 1625. Reprint, *Yingyin Xiulu xiancang hanchuan shanben congkan*. Edited by Wang Yunwu. Taipei: Commercial Press, 1973.

BCMQ Chen Jiamo 陳嘉謨. *Bencao mengquan* 本草蒙筌. N.p. Renshoutang, 1572. Reprint, XXSKQS, vol. 991.

BCPHJY Liu Wentai 劉文泰 et al. *Bencao pinhui jingyao* 本草品匯精要. Edited by Cao Hui. Beijing: Huaxia chubanshe, 1994.

BCPHJY-CP Liu Wentai et al. *Bencao pinhui jingyao*. Shanghai: Commercial Press, 1937. Reprint, with a research essay by Na Qi and Liu Zhengxiong. Taipei: Nantian shuju, 1983.

BCPHJY-KX Wang Daochun 王道純 et al. *Bencao pinhui jingyao xuji* 本草品匯精要續集. Beijing: 1702–3. Reprint, *Gugong zhenben congkan*, vols. 369–70. Haikou: Hainan chubanshe.

BCS Liu Ruojin 劉若金. *Bencao shu* 本草述. N.p., Huandu shanfang, 1810. Reprint, *Siku wei shou shu jikan*, ser. 5, vols. 11–12. Beijing: Beijing chubanshe, 2000.

BCSYBJ Lu Zhiyi 盧之頤, *Bencao shengya banji* 本草乘雅半偈. Edited by Leng Fangnan and Wang Qinan. Beijing: Renmin weisheng chubanshe, 1986.

BCTJ Su Song 蘇頌et al. *Bencao tujing* 本草圖經. Collated and edited by Shang Zhijun. Hefei: Anhui kexue jishu chubanshe, 1994.

BCYS Li Zhongli 李中立. *Bencao yuanshi* 本草原始. 1st edition. Qi County, Henan: 1612. Reprint, XXSKQS, vol. 992.

BCYS-1638 Li Zhongli. *Bencao yuanshi*. Edited by Ge Nai. Kunshan: Yonghuaitang, 1638.

BCYY-1879 Kou Zongshi 寇宗奭. *Bencao yanyi* 本草衍義. Southern Song edition. Edited by Lu Xinyuan. Reprinted in *Shiwanjuan lou congshu*, vols. 18–19. Gui'an: Lu family, Guangxu 5 [1879].

BJFY Zhang Lu 張璐. *Benjing fengyuan* 本經逢原. Suzhou: c. 1690. Reprint, XXSKQS, vol. 994.

JYBC Zhang Yuxi 掌禹錫 et al. *Jiayou bencao jifu ben* 嘉祐本草輯復本. Collated and edited by Shang Zhijun. Beijing: Zhongyi guji chubanshe, 2009.

SWBC-1643 Yao Kecheng 姚可成, ed. *Shiwu bencao* 食物本草. Beijing: Renmin weisheng chubanshe, 1994.

XXBC Su Jing 蘇敬 et al. *Tang xinxiu bencao* 唐新修本草. Collated and edited by Shang Zhijun. Hefei: Anhui kexue jishu chubanshe, 1981.

ZLBC Tang Shenwei 唐慎微. *Zhenglei bencao* 證類本草. Edited by Shang Zhijun et al. Beijing: Huaxia chubanshe, 1993.

ZLBC-1249 Tang Shenwei. *Chongxiu Zhenghe jingshi zhenglei beiyong bencao* 重修政和經史證

類備用本草. Pingyang: Huiming xuan, 1249. Edited by Zhang Cunhui 張存惠. Reprint, Beijing: Renmin weisheng chubanshe, 1957.

ZWBC Wu Jizhi [Go Keishi] 吳繼志. *Zhiwen bencao / Shitsumon Honzō* 質問本草. Reproduction of the 1837 Satsuma edition. In *Liuqiu wangguo hanwen wenxian jicheng*, edited by Gao Jinxiao and Chen Jie, vol. 22. Shanghai: Fudan daxue chubanshe, 2013.

Local Gazetteers (*Difangzhi*)

Translations for provincial gazetteers (*tong zhi*), prefectures (*fu*), subprefectures (*zhou*, also translated as "departments"), and county (*xian*) gazetteers are omitted for the sake of brevity. Given the uncertainty of locating the precise year of printing, I provide the names of the reign during which the gazetteer was compiled. Unless otherwise noted, titles are accessed through the *Airusheng Zhongguo fangzhi ku* database but marked by original pagination in this book's notes. When the original pagination is illegible, numbering from *Airusheng*'s pagination is used.

Anqing fu zhi 安慶府志 (Jiajing). Li Xun et al.

Bamin tongzhi 八閩通志 (Hongzhi). Huang Cuzhao.

Changsha fu zhi 長沙府志 (Jiajing). Yang Lin.

Changxing xian zhi 長興縣志 (Tongzhi). Zhou Xuejun.

Chaoyi xian zhi 朝邑縣志 (Zhengde). Han Bangjing et al.

[*Chongxiu*] *Taiping fu zhi* 太平府志 (Jiajing). Zhu Luan.

[*Chongxiu*] *Wuyuan xian zhi* 婺源縣志 (Republican). Jiang Fengqing.

Chunhua zhi 淳化志 (Longqing). Luo Tingxiu.

Dengzhou zhi 鄧州志 (Jiajing). Pan Tingnan.

Dinghai xian zhi 定海縣志 (Jiajing). He Yu et al.

Dongxiang xian zhi 東鄉縣志 (Jiajing). Rao Wenbi.

Gaocheng xian zhi 藁城縣志 (Jiajing). Li Zhengru.

Gusu zhi 姑蘇志 (Zhengde). Wang Ao.

Haizhou zhi 海州志 (Longqing). Zhang Feng.

Hangzhou fu zhi (Qianlong). Shao Jinhan.

Huizhou fu zhi 徽州府志 (Hongzhi). Wang Shunmin.

Huizhou fu zhi (Jiajing). Wang Shangning.

Jiading xian zhi 嘉定縣志 (Kangxi). Su Yuan.

Jiangnan tongzhi 江南通志. Yinjishan et al. SKQS edition.

Jiangyin xian zhi 江陰縣志 (Chongzhen). Feng Shiren.

Kuaiji xian zhi 會稽縣志 (Kangxi). Dong Qinde.

Laiwu xian zhi 萊蕪縣志 (jiajing). Chen Ganyu.

Lin'an zhi 臨安志 (Xianchun). Qian Shuoyou.

Linjiang fu zhi 臨江府志 (Longqing). Liu Song.

Linjiang fu zhi (Tongzhi). Zhu Sunyi.

Liuhe xian zhi 六合縣志 (Jiajing). Huang Shaowen.

Longqing zhi 隆慶志 (Jiajing). Xie Tinggui.

Nanling xian zhi 南陵縣志 (Jiaqing). Xu Xintian.

Pengxi xian zhi (Kangxi). Pan Zhibiao.

Qi xian zhi 杞縣志 (Qianlong). Zhou Ji.

Qiantang xian zhi 錢塘縣志 (Kangxi). Qiu Lian et al.

Qingjiang xian zhi 清江縣志 (Chongzhen). Qin Yong.

Qingjiang xian zhi (Qianlong). Xiong Weilin.

Qingjiang xian zhi (Tongzhi). Zhu Sunyi.

Renhe xian zhi 仁和縣志 (Kangxi). Shao Yuanping.

Shanxi tong zhi 山西通志 (Chenghua). Hu Mi.

Shanghai xian zhi 上海縣志 (Qianlong). Ye Cheng.

Shunchang yi zhi 順昌邑志 (Zhengde). Ma Xinglu.

Songjiang fu zhi (Chongzhen). Chen Jiru.

Songjiang fu zhi 松江府志 (Zhengde). Gu Qing.

Songjiang fu zhi (Jiaqing). Song Rulin.

Suzhou fu zhi 蘇州府志 (Tongzhi). Feng Guifen.

Wangjiang xian zhi 望江縣志 (Wanli). Long Zijia et al.

Weinan xian zhi 渭南縣志 (Jiajing). Nan Daji.

Wugong xian zhi 武功縣志 (Zhengde). Kang Hai.

Wujiang xian xuzhi 吳江縣續志 (Guangxu). Jin Fuzeng.

Wujiang xian zhi 吳江縣志 (Qianlong). Ni Shimeng.

Wuxian zhi 吳縣志 (Kangxi). Sun Ming'an.

Xuancheng xian zhi 宣城縣志 (Jiaqing). Zhang Tao.

Yingjing xian zhi 榮經縣志 (1745). Lao Shiyuan. Harvard-Yenching Library Rare Books
    Collection.

Yingshan xian zhi 營山縣志 (Wanli). Li Pengnian.

Yizhen xian zhi 儀真縣志 (Longqing). Li Wen.

Yongfeng xian zhi 永豐縣志 (Jiajing). Guan Jing.

Zhangqiu xian zhi 章邱縣志 (Jiajing). Yang Xunji.

Zhangzhou fu zhi 漳州府志 (Wanli). Luo Qingxiao.

Zhaowen xian zhi 昭文縣志 (Yongzheng). Chen Zufan.

Zhejiang tong zhi 浙江通志 (Jiajing). Xue Yingqi.

Other Works Cited

Akçetin, Elif. "Consumption as Knowledge: Pawnbrokers in Qing China Appraise Furs." In
    Living the Good Life: Consumption in the Qing and Ottoman Empires of the Eighteenth Century,
    edited by Elif Akçetin and Suraiya Faroqhi, 357–83. Leiden: Brill, 2018.

Allen, Barry. *Vanishing into Things: Knowledge in Chinese Tradition.* Cambridge, MA: Harvard
    University Press, 2015.

Allsen, Thomas T. *Culture and Conquest in Mongol Eurasia.* Cambridge: Cambridge University
    Press, 2001.

Anderson, Stuart. *Making Medicines: A Brief History of Pharmacy and Pharmaceuticals.* London:
    Pharmaceutical Press, 2005.

Andrews, Bridie. *The Making of Modern Chinese Medicine: 1850–1960.* Vancouver: UBC Press,
    2014.

Anonymous. *Buyi Leigong paozhi bianlan* 補遺雷公炮製便覽 [Complete synopsis of Master Thunder's pharmaceutical preparations]. Illustrated manuscript, 1591. Edited by Zheng Jinsheng. Reprint, Shanghai: Shanghai cishu chubanshe, 2012.

Anonymous. Zhe hai chaoguan zhengshou shuiyin zeli 浙海鈔關徵收稅銀則例 [Regulations on customs duty collection, Zhejiang Maritime Customs House]. In *Gugong zhenben congkan*, vol. 317–18. Haikou: Hainan chubanshe, 2000.

Appardurai, Arjun, ed. *The Social Life of Things: Commodities in Cultural Perspective.* Cambridge: Cambridge University Press, 1986.

Arber, Agnes Robertson. *Herbals, Their Origin and Evolution: A Chapter in the History of Botany, 1470–1670.* Cambridge: Cambridge University Press, 1912.

Aricanli, Sare. "Diversifying the Center: Authority and Representation within the Context of Multiplicity in Eighteenth Century Qing Imperial Medicine." PhD diss., Princeton University, 2016.

Atwell, William. "International Bullion Flows and the Chinese Economy, circa 1530–1650." *Past and Present* 95 (1982): 68–90.

Barnes, Linda L. *Needles, Herbs, Gods, and Ghosts: China, Healing, and the West to 1848.* Cambridge, MA: Harvard University Press, 2005.

Barzansky, Barbara M., and Norman Gevitz, eds. *Beyond Flexner: Medical Education in the Twentieth Century.* New York: Greenwood Press, 1992.

Benedict, Carol. *Golden-Silk Smoke: A History of Tobacco in China, 1550–2010.* Berkeley: University of California Press, 2011.

Bentancor, Orlando. *The Matter of Empire: Metaphysics and Mining in Colonial Peru.* Pittsburgh: University of Pittsburgh Press, 2017.

Berg, Daria. *Women and the Literary World in Early Modern China, 1580–1700.* Abingdon, Oxon: Routledge, 2013.

Bian, He. "Re-Collecting the Glorious Age: Yang Fuji and the Disciplining of *Zhaodai congshu*." *Late Imperial China* 40, no. 1 (June 2019): 1–41.

———. "Documenting Medications: Patients' Demand, Physicians' Virtuosity, and Genre-Mixing of Prescription-Cases (Fang'an) in Seventeenth-Century China." *Early Science and Medicine* 22 (2017): 103–23.

———. "An Ever-Expanding Pharmacy: Zhao Xuemin and the Conditions for New Knowledge in Eighteenth-Century China." *Harvard Journal of Asiatic Studies* 77, no. 2 (December 2017): 287–319.

———. "Shui zhu yao shi: Zhongguo gudai yiyao fenye licheng de zai tantao" 谁主药室：中国古代医药分业历程的再探讨 [Who is in charge of pharmaceutical chambers: Rethinking the division of labor between physicians and pharmacists in premodern China]. In *Xinshixue 9: Yiliao shi xin de tansuo,* edited by Yu Xinzhong, 38–69. Beijing: Zhonghua shuju, 2017.

Blair, Ann. *The Theater of Nature: Jean Bodin and Renaissance Science.* Princeton, NJ: Princeton University Press, 1997.

Bloch, Ernst. *Avicenna and the Aristotelian Left.* Translated by Loren Goldman and Peter Thompson. New York: Columbia University Press, 2019.

Bloom, Irene. *Knowledge Painfully Acquired: The K'un-chih chi.* New York: Columbia University Press, 1987.

BnF Chinois 2216. *Tizou shijian* [Court gazettes]. Beijing: Gongshentang, 1778–79. Bibliothèque nationale de France, Paris, France.

Bol, Peter K. *Neo-Confucianism in History.* Cambridge, MA: Harvard University Asia Center, distributed by Harvard University Press, 2008.

———. "The 'Localist Turn' and 'Local Identity' in Later Imperial China." *Late Imperial China* 24, no. 2 (2003): 1–50.

Boyanton, Stephen. "The Treatise on Cold Damage and the Birth of Literati Medicine: Social, Epidemiological, and Medical Change in China 1000–1400." PhD diss., Columbia University, 2015.

Bray, Francesca. "Chinese Literati and the Transmission of Technological Knowledge: The Case of Agriculture." In *Cultures of Knowledge: Technology in Chinese History*, edited by Dagmar Schäfer, 299–325. Leiden: Brill, 2012.

———. "Essence and Utility: The Classification of Crop Plants in China." *Chinese Science* 9 (1989): 1–13.

Bretschneider, Emil. *History of European Botanical Discoveries in China.* London: Sampson Low, Marston, 1898.

———. *Botanicon Sinicum: Notes on Chinese Botany from Native and Western Sources.* London: Trübner, 1882.

———. *On the Study and Value of Chinese Botanical Works, with Notes on the History of Plants and Geographical Botany from Chinese Sources.* Foochow, China: Rozario, Marcal, c. 1870.

Brokaw, Cynthia. *Commerce in Culture: The Sibao Book Trade in the Qing and Republican Periods.* Cambridge, MA: Harvard University Asia Center, distributed by Harvard University Press, 2007.

———. *The Ledgers of Merit and Demerit: Social Change and Moral Order in Late Imperial China.* Princeton, NJ: Princeton University Press, 1991.

Brook, Timothy. *Mr. Selden's Map of China: Decoding the Secrets of a Vanished Cartographer.* London: Bloomsbury, 2013.

———. *The Troubled Empire: China in the Yuan and Ming Dynasties.* Cambridge, MA: Harvard University Press, 2013.

———. *Vermeer's Hat: The Seventeenth Century and the Dawn of the Global World.* New York: Bloomsbury, 2008.

———. *Geographical Sources of Ming-Qing History.* Ann Arbor: Center for Chinese Studies, University of Michigan, 2002.

———. *The Confusions of Pleasure: Commerce and Culture in Ming China.* Berkeley: University of California Press, 1998.

———. "Rethinking Syncretism: The Unity of the Three Teachings and Their Joint Worship in Late-Imperial China." *Journal of Chinese Religions* 21, no. 1 (1993): 13–44.

Brown, Miranda. *The Art of Medicine in Early China: The Ancient and Medieval Origins of a Modern Archive.* Cambridge: Cambridge University Press, 2015.

Buell, Paul and Eugene Anderson. *A Soup for the Qan: Chinese Dietary Medicine of the Mongol Era as Seen in Hu Szu-Hui's Yin-shan cheng-yao: Introduction, Translation, Commentary and Chinese Text.* London: Kegan Paul International, 2000.

Burke, Peter. *Popular Culture in Early Modern Europe.* Ashgate, 3rd. revised edition, 2009.

Bussotti, Michele. "Woodcut Illustration: A General Outline." In *Graphics and Text in the Produc-*

tion of Technical Knowledge in China: The Warp and the Weft, edited by Francesca Bray, Vera Dorofeeva-Lichtmann, and Georges Métailié, 461–83. Leiden: Brill, 2007.

Cahill, James. *Pictures for Use and Pleasure: Vernacular Painting in High Qing China*. Berkeley: University of California Press, 2010.

———. *The Painter's Practice: How Artists Lived and Worked in Traditional China*. New York: Columbia University Press, 1994.

Cai Tao 蔡絛. *Tieweishan cong tan* 鐵圍山叢談 [Assorted conversations in Tiewei Mountain]. SKQS edition.

Cams, Mario. *Companions in Geography: East-West Collaboration in the Mapping of Qing China (c. 1685–1735)*. Leiden: Brill, 2017.

Chang Che-chia 張哲嘉, "Dahuang misi: Qingdai zhicai xiyang jinyun dahuang de celüe siwei yu wenhua yihan" 大黃迷思: 清代制裁西洋禁運大黃的策略思維與文化意涵 [The myth of rhubarb: Strategic rational and cultural meanings of the Qing embargo on rhubarb to the West]. *Bulletin of the Institute of Modern History* (Academia Sinica) 47 (2005): 43–100.

Chang, Hsien-che. "The *Pen-Ts'ao Pei-Yao*: A Modern Interpretation of Its Terminology and Contents." In *Approaches to Traditional Medical Literature*, edited by Paul U. Unschuld, 41–51. Dordrecht: Kluwer, 1989.

Chao, Yüan-ling. *Medicine and Society in Late Imperial China: A Study of Physicians in Suzhou, 1600–1850*. New York: Peter Lang, 2009.

Chemla, Karine, and Evelyn Fox Keller, eds. *Cultures without Culturalism: The Making of Scientific Knowledge*. Durham, NC: Duke University Press, 2017.

Chen Hao. *Shenfen xushi yu zhishi biaoshu zhijian de yizhe zhi yi* [The meaning of medical identity between identity narrative and knowledge expression]. Shanghai: Shanghai guji chubanshe, 2019.

Chen Hsiu-Fen 陳秀芬. *Yangsheng yu xiushen: Wan Ming wenren de shenti shuxie yu shesheng jishu* 養生與修身: 晚明文人的身體書寫與攝生技術 [Nourishing life and cultivating the body: Writing the literati's body and techniques for preserving health in the late Ming]. Taipei: Daoxiang chubanshe, 2009.

Chen, Kaijun. "Craft in *Six Records of A Life Adrift*." *Chinese Literature: Essays, Articles, Reviews* 39 (2017): 95–117.

Chen Li 陳櫟. *Shangshu jizhuan zuanshu* 尚書集傳纂疏 [Collected exegesis of commentaries on the Book of Documents]. SKQS edition.

Chen Menglei 陳夢雷 et al. *Qinding Gujin tushu jicheng* 欽定古今圖書集成 [Imperial encyclopedia of images and books in ancient and modern times]. Wuying dian: 1720. Accessed via the *Biaodian Gujin tushu jicheng* database, United Digital Publications (UDP), Taipei.

Chen Nianzu 陳念祖. *Chen Xiuyuan yixue quanshu* 陳修園醫學全書 [Complete medical works by Chen Nianzu]. Edited by Lin Huiguang et al. Beijing: Zhongguo zhongyiyao chubanshe, 1999.

Chen Yuanpeng 陳元朋. *Liang Song de "Shangyi shiren" yu "ruyi"* 兩宋的「尚醫士人」與「儒醫」 [The "medical amateurs" and "Confucian physicians" of Song China]. Taipei: National Taiwan University, 1997.

Chen Zilong陳子龍 et al. *Ming jingshi wenbian* 明經世文編 [Anthology of statecraft writings of the Ming]. Pinglutang: 1628–44.

Chia, Lucille. "The Uses of Print in Early Quanzhen Daoist Texts." In *Knowledge and Text Production in an Age of Print: China, 900–1400*, edited by Hilde de Weerdt and Lucille Chia, 167–203. Leiden: Brill, 2011.

———. "Of Three Mountain Street: The Commercial Publishers of Ming Nanjing." In *Printing and Book Culture in Late Imperial China*, edited by Cynthia Brokaw and Kai-wing Chow, 107–51. Berkeley: University of California Press, 2005.

———. *Printing for Profit: The Commercial Publishers of Jianyang, Fujian (11th-17th Centuries)*. Cambridge, MA: Harvard University Asia Center, 2002.

Chittick, Andrew. "The Development of Local Writing in Early Medieval China." *Early Medieval China* 9 (2004): 35–70.

Chow, Kai-wing. *Publishing, Culture, and Power in Early Modern China*. Stanford, CA: Stanford University Press, 2004.

Cipolla, Carlo M. *Public Health and the Medical Profession in the Renaissance*. Cambridge; New York: Cambridge University Press, 1976.

Clunas, Craig. *Screen of Kings: Royal Art and Power in Ming China*. Honolulu: University of Hawai'i Press, 2013.

———. *Superfluous Things: Material Culture and Social Status in Early Modern China*. Honolulu: University of Hawai'i Press, 2004.

———. "Modernity Global and Local: Consumption and the Rise of the West." *American Historical Review* 104, no. 5 (December 1999), 1497–511.

Cochran, Sherman. *Chinese Medicine Men: Consumer Culture in China and Southeast Asia*. Cambridge, MA: Harvard University Press, 2006.

Cook, Harold. *Matters of Exchange: Commerce, Medicine, and Science in the Dutch Golden Age*. New Haven, CT: Yale University Press, 2007.

———. *The Decline of the Old Medical Regime in Stuart London*. Ithaca, NY: Cornell University Press, 1986.

Craig, Sienna R. *Healing Elements: Efficacy and the Social Ecologies of Tibetan Medicine*. Berkeley: University of California Press, 2012.

Crossley, Pamela. *What Is Global History?* Cambridge: Polity, 2008.

Cullen, Christopher. "Patients and Healers in Late Imperial China: Evidence from the 'Jinpingmei.'" *History of Science* 31, no. 2 (June 1993): 99–150.

Daozang [The Daoist canon]. Shanghai: Han fen lou, 1923–26.

Dardess, John W. *Blood and History in China: The Donglin Faction and Its Repression, 1620–1627*. Honolulu: University of Hawai'i Press, 2002.

De Bary, William Theodore. *Neo-Confucian Orthodoxy and the Learning of the Mind-and-Heart*. New York: Columbia University Press, 1981.

Deng Yuanxi 鄧元錫. *Han shi* 函史 [History in a casket]. N.p. 1681. Harvard-Yenching Library Rare Book (https://listview.lib.harvard.edu/lists/drs-23975535).

Dennis, Joseph. *Writing, Publishing, and Reading Local Gazetteers in Imperial China, 1100–1700*. Cambridge, MA: Harvard University Asia Center, 2015.

———. "Financial Aspects of Ming Gazetteers." *Princeton East Asian Library Journal* 14, no. 1 (2010): 158–244.

Despeux, Catherine. "The System of the Five Circulatory Phases and the Six Seasonal Influences (*wuyun liuqi*): A Source of Innovation in Medicine under the Song (960–1279)." In *Innova-*

tion in Chinese Medicine, edited by Elisabeth Hsu, 121–66. Cambridge: Cambridge University Press, 2001.

Ding Yizhuang 定宜庄. *Geren xushu zhong de Tongrentang lishi* 个人叙述中的同仁堂历史 [The history of Tongrentang in individual narratives]. Beijing: Beijing chubanshe, 2015.

Ditmanson, Peter. "Imperial History and Broadening Historical Consciousness in Late Ming China." *Ming Studies* 71 (2015): 23–40.

Dong Qichang 董其昌. *Rong tai ji* 容臺集. N.p. 1629. Accessed through *Airusheng jiben guji ku*.

Du You 杜佑. *Tongdian* 通典 [Comprehensive statutes]. Academia Sinica, *Hanji quanwen ziliaoku* (Scripta Sinica) database.

Dunstan, Helen. *State or Merchant?: Political Economy and Political Process in 1740s China*. Cambridge, MA: Harvard University Asia Center, 2006.

Eamon, William. *Professor of Secrets: Mystery, Medicine and Alchemy in Renaissance Italy*. Washington, DC: National Geographic, 2010.

Ebrey, Patricia Buckley. *Emperor Huizong*. Cambridge, MA: Harvard University Press, 2014.

Elman, Benjamin A. *Civil Examinations and Meritocracy in Late Imperial China*. Cambridge, MA: Harvard University Press, 2013.

———. "Early Modern or Late Imperial Philology? The Crisis of Classical Learning in Eighteenth Century China." *Frontiers of History in China* 6, no. 1 (March 2011): 3–25.

———. "Collecting and Classifying: Ming Dynasty Compendia and Encyclopedias (*Leishu*)." *Extrême-Orient, Extrême-Occident* 1, no. 1 (2007): 131–57.

———. *On Their Own Terms: Science in China, 1550–1900*. Cambridge, MA: Harvard University Press, 2005.

———. *From Philosophy to Philology: Intellectual and Social Aspects of Change in Late Imperial China*. Revised edition. Los Angeles: UCLA Asian Pacific Monograph Series, 2001.

———. *A Cultural History of Civil Examinations in Late Imperial China*. Berkeley: University of California Press, 2000.

———. *Classicism, Politics, and Kinship: The Ch'ang-chou School of New Text Confucianism in Late Imperial China*. Berkeley, CA: University of California Press, 2000.

Elvin, Mark. *The Pattern of the Chinese Past*. Stanford, CA: Stanford University Press, 1990.

Engelhardt, Ute. "Dietetics in Tang China and the First Extant Works of *Materia Dietetica*." In *Innovation in Chinese Medicine*, edited by Elisabeth Hsu, 173–91. Cambridge: Cambridge University Press, 2001.

Fan, Fa-ti. *British Naturalists in Qing China: Science, Empire, and Cultural Encounter*. Cambridge, MA: Harvard University Press, 2004.

Fan, I-Chun, "Long Distance Trade and Market Integration in the Ming-Ch'ing Period 1400–1850." PhD Diss., Stanford University, 1992.

Fang Yizhi 方以智. *Wuli xiaoshi* 物理小識 [Notes on the principle of things]. SKQS edition.

———. *Tongya* 通雅 [Comprehensive refinement]. SKQS edition.

Fan Jiawei [Ka Wai] 范家偉. *Bei Song jiaozheng yishuju xintan* 北宋校正醫書局新探. Hong Kong: Zhonghua shuju, 2014.

———. *Liuchao Sui Tang yixue zhi chuancheng yu zhenghe* 六朝隋唐醫學之傳承與整合. Hong Kong: Zhongwen daxue chubanshe, 2004.

Farquhar, Judith. *Knowing Practice: The Clinical Encounter of Chinese Medicine*. Boulder, CO: Westview Press, 1994.

Faure, David. *Emperor and Ancestor: State and Lineage in South China.* Stanford, CA: Stanford University Press, 2007.

Fei, Siyen. *Negotiating Urban Space: Urbanization and Late Ming Nanjing.* Cambridge, MA: Harvard University Asia Center, 2009.

Feng Menglong 馮夢龍. *Xingshi hengyan* 醒世恆言 [Enduring discourses to awaken the world]. Vol. 3 in *Feng Menglong quanji.* Nanjing: Fenghuang chubanshe, 2007.

Findlen, Paula, ed. *Early Modern Things.* New York: Routledge, 2013.

———. *Possessing Nature: Museums, Collecting, and Scientific Culture in Early Modern Italy.* Berkeley: University of California Press, 1994.

Finnane, Antonia. "Furnishing the Home in Qing Yangzhou: A Case for Rethinking 'Consumer Restraint.'" In *Living the Good Life: Consumption in the Qing and Ottoman Empires of the Eighteenth Century,* edited by Elif Akçetin and Suraiya Faroqhi, 163–85. Leiden: Brill, 2018.

Fisher, Carney. *The Chosen One: Succession and Adoption in the Court of Ming Shizong.* Sydney: Allen & Unwin, 1990.

Fors, Hjalmar. *The Limits of Matter: Chemistry, Mining, and Enlightenment.* Chicago: University of Chicago Press, 2015.

Foucault, Michel. *The Order of Things: An Archaeology of the Human Sciences.* New York: Vintage, 1994.

———. *The Birth of the Clinic: An Archaeology of Medical Perception.* New York: Vintage, 1994.

Fox, Ariel. "Southern Capital: Staging Commerce in Seventeenth-Century Suzhou." PhD diss., Harvard University, 2015.

Furth, Charlotte. "The Physician as Philosopher of the Way: Zhu Zhenheng (1282–1358)," *Harvard Journal of Asiatic Studies* 66, no. 2 (2006): 423–59.

———. *A Flourishing Yin: Gender in China's Medical History, 960–1665.* Berkeley: University of California Press, 1998.

Furth, Charlotte, Judith T. Zeitlin, and Ping-chen Hsiung, eds., *Thinking with Cases: Specialist Knowledge in Chinese Cultural History.* Honolulu: University of Hawai'i Press, 2007.

Fu Yiling. *Ming Qing shehui jingji shi lunwen ji* [Collection of essays on Ming-Qing socioeconomic history]. Beijing: Renmin chubanshe, 1982.

Gao Lian 高濂. *Zunsheng bajian* 尊生八箋. Chengdu: Bashu shushe, 1988.

Gerritsen, Anne, and Giorgio Riello, eds. *The Global Lives of Things: The Material Culture of Connections in the First Global Age.* London: Routledge, 2016.

Giles, Lionel. *An Alphabetical Index to the Chinese Encyclopaedia . . . Qin ding gu jin tu shu ji cheng.* London: Trustees of the British Museum, 1911.

Goldschmidt, Asaf. *The Evolution of Chinese Medicine: Song Dynasty, 960–1200.* London: Routledge, 2009.

———. "Huizong's Impact on Medicine and on Public Health." In *Emperor Huizong and Late Northern Song China: The Politics of Culture and the Culture of Politics,* edited by Patricia Buckley Ebrey and Maggie Bickford, 275–323. Cambridge, MA: Harvard University Asia Center, 2006.

Grafton, Anthony, with April Shelford and Nancy Siraisi. *New Worlds, Ancient Texts: The Power of Tradition and the Shock of Discovery.* Cambridge, MA: Harvard University Press, 1992.

Grant, Joanna. *A Chinese Physician: Wang Ji and the "Stone Mountain Medical Case Histories."* London: Routledge Curzon, 2003.

Grass, Noa. "Imperial Silver Laundering: The Official Narrative on Gold Floral Silver and the Silverization of Ming State Finance." *Ming Studies* 76 (2017): 7–31.

Greene, Jeremy A. *Generic: The Unbranding of Modern Medicine.* Baltimore: Johns Hopkins University Press, 2014.

Guan Xueling 关雪玲. *Qingdai gongting yixue yu yixue wenwu* 清代宫廷医学与医学文物 [Court medicine and medicinal artifacts in Qing China]. Beijing: Zijincheng chubanshe, 2008.

Guy, R. Kent. *The Emperor's Four Treasuries: Scholars and the State in the Late Ch'ien-lung Era.* Cambridge, MA: Council on East Asian Studies, 1987.

Habu Kazuko 羽生和子. *Edo jidai kanpōyaku no rekishi* 江戸時代, 漢方薬の歴史 [History of Chinese medicine during the Edo Period]. Osaka: Seibundō, 2010.

Hamashita, Takeshi. *China, East Asia and the Global Economy: Regional and Historical Perspectives.* Edited by Linda Grove and Mark Selden. London: Routledge, 2008.

Hammond, Kenneth. "Wang Shizhen and Li Shizhen: Archaism and Early Scientific Thought in Sixteenth-Century China." In *Antiquarianism and Intellectual Life in Europe and China, 1500–1800,* edited by Peter N. Miller and François Louis, 234–49. Ann Arbor: University of Michigan Press, 2011.

Handler-Spitz, Rivi. *Symptoms of an Unruly Age: Li Zhi and Cultures of Early Modernity.* Seattle: University of Washington Press, 2017.

Handlin Smith, Joanna. *The Art of Doing Good: Charity in Late Ming China.* Berkeley: University of California Press, 2009.

Hang Shijun 杭世骏. *Daogu tang wenji* 道古堂文集 [Anthology of Daogu tang]. N.p., 1776. Reprinted in *Qingdai shiwenji huibian,* vol. 282. Shanghai: Shanghai guji chubanshe, 2010.

Han Qi. *Zhongguo kexue jishu de xichuan jiqi yingxiang, 1582–1793* 中国科学技术的西传及其影响 [The transmission of Chinese science and technology to the West and its influence]. Shijiazhuang: Hebei renmin chubanshe, 1999.

Hansen, Valerie. *Changing Gods in Medieval China, 1127–1276.* Princeton, NJ: Princeton University Press, 1990.

Hanson, Marta. "The Golden Mirror in the Imperial Court of the Qianlong Emperor, 1739–1742." *Early Science and Medicine* 8, no. 2 (2003): 111–47.

Harkness, Deborah. *The Jewel House: Elizabethan London and the Scientific Revolution.* New Haven, CT: Yale University Press, 2007.

Harper, Donald J. *Early Chinese Medical Literature: The Mawangdui Medical Manuscript.* New York: Kegan Paul International, 1998.

Hart, Roger. *Imagined Civilizations: China, the West, and Their First Encounter.* Baltimore: Johns Hopkins University Press, 2013.

He Daren 何大任. *Taiyiyuan zhuke chengwenge* 太醫院諸科程文格 [Examination standards to the various specialties of Imperial Academy of Medicine]. SKQS edition.

He Qiaoyuan 何喬遠. *Mingshan cang* 名山藏 [Depositories in famous mountains]. N.p. 1628–1644. Reprinted in XXSKQS, vols. 425–427.

He Xinhua 何新华. *Qingdai gongwu zhidu yanjiu* 清代贡物制度研究 [A study on the tributes and its system in Qing Dynasty]. Beijing: Shehui kexue wenxian chubanshe, 2012.

He, Yuming. *Home and the World: Editing the "Glorious Ming" in Woodblock-Printed Books of the Sixteenth and Seventeenth Centuries.* Cambridge, MA: Harvard University Asia Center, 2012.

Hegel, Robert. *Reading Illustrated Fiction in Late Imperial China.* Stanford, CA: Stanford University Press, 1998.

Heijdra, Martin. "The Socio-economic Development of Rural China during the Ming." In *The Cambridge History of China,* vol. 8, *The Ming Dynasty,* part 2, edited by Denis C. Twitchett and Frederick W. Mote, 417–578. Cambridge: Cambridge University Press, 1998.

Henderson, John. *The Development and Decline of Chinese Cosmology.* New York: Columbia University Press, 1984.

Heniantang zhiyao mulu 鶴年堂製藥目錄 [Pharmacy catalogue of Heniantang]. In *Qifen shi cang zhongyi dianji jingxuan,* edited by Niu Yahua, ser. 2. Beijing: Beijing kexue jishu chubanshe, 2017.

Higashionna Kanjun 東恩納寬惇. "*Shitsumon Honzō* to sono chūsha 質問本草とその著者." In *Yakuchū Shitsumon Honzō* 訳注質問本草, edited by Harada Nobuo, 586–604. Ginowan-shi: Yōju Shorin, 2002.

Hinrichs, TJ. "Governance through Medical Texts and the Role of Print." In *Knowledge and Text Production in an Age of Print: China, 900–1400,* edited by Lucille Chia and Hilde de Weerdt, 217–38. Leiden: Brill, 2011.

Hong Mai 洪邁. *Rongzhai suibi* 容齋隨筆 [Casual jottings of Rongzhai]. Beijing: Zhonghua shuju, 2005.

———. *Yi jian zhi* 夷堅志 [Record of the listener]. SKQS edition.

Hoshi Ayao 星斌夫. *Min Shin jidai shakai keizaishi no kenkyū* 明清時代社会経済史の研究 [Studies in Ming-Qing socioeconomic history]. Tokyo: Kokusho Kankōkai, 1989.

Hsia, Florence C. *Sojourners in a Strange Land: Jesuits and Their Scientific Missions in Late Imperial China.* Chicago: University of Chicago Press, 2009.

Hsia, Florence C., and Dagmar Schäfer. "History of Science, Technology, and Medicine: A Second Look at Joseph Needham." *Isis* 110, no. 1 (2019): 94–99.

Hsu, Ginger. *A Bushel of Pearls: Painting for Sale in Eighteenth-Century Yangchow.* Stanford, CA: Stanford University Press, 2001.

Hu, Shiu-ying. *An Enumeration of Chinese Materia Medica.* Hong Kong: Chinese University Press, 1980.

Huang, Ray. *1587, A Year of No Significance: The Ming Dynasty in Decline.* New Haven, CT: Yale University Press, 1981.

———. *Taxation and Governmental Finance in Sixteenth-Century Ming China.* London: Cambridge University Press, 1974.

Huangfu Lu 皇甫錄. *Huang Ming jilüe* 皇明紀略. In *Lidai xiaoshi,* vol. 85. Shanghai: Commercial Press, Minguo 29 [1940]. Reprint, XXSKQS, vol. 1167.

Huang Zongxi 黃宗羲. *Mingru xue'an* 明儒學案 [Cases of study for Ming Confucians]. Vols. 8–9 in *Huang Zongxi quanji* [Complete works of Huang Zongxi]. Taipei: Liren shuju, 1987.

Hu Baoguo 胡宝国. *Han Tang jian shixue de fazhan* 汉唐间史学的发展 [The development of historiography from Han to Tang]. Beijing: Commercial Press, 2003.

Hucker, Charles O. *The Censorial System of Ming China.* Stanford, CA: Stanford University Press, 1966.

Hukazawa, Akihito 深澤秋人. *Kinsei Ryūkyū Chūgoku kōryūshi no kenkyū* 近世琉球中国交流史の研究. Okinawa-ken Ginowan-shi: Yōju Shorin, 2011.

Hunan Manshi 湖南漫士. *Shuibian linxia* 水邊林下 [By the water and in the forest]. In *Beijing tushuguan guji zhenben congkan*, vol. 78. Beijing: Shumu wenxian chubanshe, 1988.

Hymes, Robert P. "Not Quite Gentlemen? Doctors in Sung and Yuan." *Chinese Science* 8 (1987): 9–76.

Jami, Catherine. *The Emperor's New Mathematics: Western Learning and Imperial Authority during the Kangxi Reign (1662–1722).* Oxford: Oxford University Press, 2012.

Janik, Erika. *Marketplace of the Marvelous: The Strange Origins of Modern Medicine.* Boston: Beacon Press, 2014.

Jiang, Lijing. "Retouching the Past with Living Things: Indigenous Species, Tradition, and Biological Research in Republican China, 1918–1937." *Historical Studies in the Natural Sciences* 46, no. 2 (2016): 154–206.

Jia Zhizhong 贾建中 and Yang Yanfei 杨燕飞. *Qingdai yaoxing ju* 清代药性剧 [Pharmaceutical dramas of the Qing dynasty]. Beijing: Xueyuan chubanshe, 2013.

Jiang Zhushan 蔣竹山 [Chiang Chu-shan]. *Renshen diguo: Qingdai renshen de shengchan, xiaofei yu yiliao* 人參帝国：清代人參的生产、消费与医疗 [Ginseng empire: The production, consumption, and medicinal use of ginseng in Qing China]. Hangzhou: Zhejiang daxue chubanshe, 2015.

Ji Yun 紀昀 et al. *Qinding Siku quanshu zongmu* 欽定四庫全書總目 [General catalog of the imperially commissioned Complete Library of Four Sections]. Vols. 1–5, SKQS.

Johnson, David, Andrew J. Nathan, and Evelyn S. Rawski, eds. *Popular Culture in Late Imperial China.* Berkeley, CA: University of California Press, 1985.

Kawakatsu Mamoru 川勝守. *Min Shin kōnōsei to kyodai toshi rensa: Chōkō to Daiunga* 明清貢納制と巨大都市連鎖：長江と大運河 [The tribute system of the Ming-Qing period and the giant chain of metropolitan cities: Yangzi River and the Grand Canal]. Tokyo: Kyūko Shoin, 2009.

Kerlouégan, Jérôme. "Printing for Prestige? Publishing and Publications by Ming Princes." *East Asian Publishing and Society* 1, no. 1 (2011): 39–73; 1, no. 2 (2011): 105–44; 2, no. 1 (2012): 3–75.

Kern, Martin, and Dirk Meyer, eds. *Origins of Chinese Political Philosophy: Studies in the Composition and Thought of the Shangshu (Classic of Documents).* Leiden: Brill, 2017.

Kim, Seonmin. *Ginseng and Borderland: Territorial Boundaries and Political Relations between Qing China and Choson Korea, 1636–1912.* Berkeley: University of California Press, 2017.

Kim, Yung Sik. *The Natural Philosophy of Chu Hsi (1130–1200).* Philadelphia: American Philosophical Society, 2000.

Kindō Tatsuo 近藤龍雄. *Kita Shina no busshi yakubutsu kenkyū* 北支那之物資藥物研究 [A study of material resources and pharmaceuticals in North China]. Qingdao [Chintao]: Shina Igaku Kenkyūkai, 1922.

Ko, Dorothy. *The Social Life of Inkstones: Artisans and Scholars in Early Qing China.* Seattle: University of Washington Press, 2017.

———. *Teachers of the Inner Chambers: Women and Culture in Seventeenth-Century China.* Stanford, CA: Stanford University Press, 1994.

Kremer, Edward, and George Urdang. *Kremer and Urdang's History of Pharmacy.* Philadelphia, PA: Lippincott, 1976.

Kuhn, Philip A. *Soulstealers: The Chinese Sorcery Scare of 1768.* Harvard: Harvard University Press, 1990.

Kuriyama, Shigehisa. *The Expressiveness of the Body and the Divergence of Greek and Chinese Medicine*. New York: Zone Books, 1999.

Lai Huimin 賴惠敏. *Qianlong huangdi de hebao* 乾隆皇帝的荷包 [Qianlong Emperor's private purse]. Taipei: Academia Sinica, Institute of Modern History, 2016.

Laing, Ellen Johnston. "*Suzhou Pian* and Other Dubious Paintings in the Received Oeuvre of Qiu Ying," *Artibus Asiae* 59, no. 3–4 (2000): 265–95.

Lei, Sean Hsiang-Lin. *Neither Donkey nor Horse: Medicine and the Struggle over China's Modernity*. Chicago: University of Chicago Press, 2014.

Leong, Elaine. *Recipes and Everyday Knowledge: Medicine, Science, and the Household in Early Modern England*. Chicago: University of Chicago Press, 2018.

Leung, Angela Ki Che. "Medical Instruction and Popularization in Ming Qing China," *Late Imperial China* 24, no. 1 (2003): 130–52.

———. "Medical Learning from the Song to the Ming." In *The Song-Yuan-Ming Transition in Chinese History*, edited by Paul Jakov Smith and Richard von Glahn, 374–98. Cambridge, MA: Harvard University Asia Center, 2003.

———. "Organized Medicine in Ming-Qing China: State and Private Medical Institutions in the Lower Yangzi Region." *Late Imperial China* 8, no. 1 (June 1987): 134–66.

Levenson, Joseph R. *Confucian China and its Modern Fate: A Trilogy*. Berkeley: University of California Press, 1968.

Li Chunxing 李春興. *Zhongyao paozhi fazhan shi* 中藥炮製發展史 [A history of development in Chinese pharmaceutical processes]. Taipei: Guoli Zhongguo yiyao yanjiusuo, 2000.

Liebenau, Jonathan. *Medical Science and Medical Industry: The Formation of the American Pharmaceutical Industry*. Baltimore: Johns Hopkins University Press, 1987.

Li Fang 李昉 et al. *Taiping yulan* 太平御覽 [Imperial reader of the Taiping era]. Academia Sinica: Hanji quanwen ziliaoku (Scripta Sinica) database.

Li Jianmin 李建民. *Lüxingzhe de shixue: Zhongguo yixueshi de lüxing* 旅行者的史學: 中國醫學史的旅行 [Out of place: Travels throughout Chinese medical history]. Taipei: Yunchen wenhua, 2009.

Lin, Fan. "The Local in the Imperial Vision: Landscape, Topography, and Geography in Southern Song Map Guides and Gazetteers." *Cross-Currents: East Asian History and Culture Review* 6, no. 2 (2017): 333–64.

Liscomb, Kathlyn Maurean. *Learning from Mount Hua: A Chinese Physician's Illustrated Travel Record and Painting Theory*. Cambridge: Cambridge University Press, 1993.

Liu, Lydia H. *The Clash of Empires: The Invention of China in Modern World Making*. Cambridge, MA: Harvard University Press, 2004.

Liu, Yan. "Toxic Cures: Poisons and Medicines in Medieval China." PhD diss., Harvard University, 2015.

Liu Chun 劉純. *Liu Chun yixue quanshu* 劉純醫學全書 [Complete medical works of Liu Chun]. Beijing: Zhongguo zhongyiyao chubanshe, 1999.

Liu Ruoyu 劉若愚. *Zhuo zhong zhi* 酌中志 [An account for deliberation]. Beijing: Beijing guji chubanshe, 1994.

Liu Shiji 刘石吉. *Ming Qing shidai Jiangnan shizhen yanjiu* 明清时代江南市镇研究 [A study of market towns in Ming-Qing Jiangnan]. Beijing: Zhongguo shehui kexue chubanshe, 1987.

Liu Wenpeng 刘文鹏. *Shengshi beihou: Qianlong shidai de weigao an yanjiu* 盛世背后: 乾隆时

代的伪稿案研究 [Behind the prosperous age: A study of the "Bogus Memorial" case in the Qianlong era]. Beijing: Renmin chubanshe: 2014.

Liu Yongcheng 刘永成 and He Zhiqing 赫志清. "Wanquan tang de youlai yu fazhan" 万全堂的由来与发展 [The origin and development of Wanquan Tang pharmacy]. *Zhongguo shehui jingjishi yanjiu* [Chinese Socioeconomic Historical Review], no. 1 (1983): 1–16.

Liu Zhiwei 刘志伟. *Zai guojia yu shehui zhijian: Ming Qing Guangdong lijia fuyi zhidu yanjiu* 在国家与社会之间: 明清广东里甲赋役制度研究 [Between state and society: An institutional study of Ming-Qing household registry and taxation]. Guangzhou: Zhongshan daxue chubanshe, 1997.

Liu Zongyuan 柳宗元. *Liu Hedong ji* 柳河東集 [Anthology of Liu Zongyuan]. Beijing: Zhonghua shuju, 1958.

Li Xian 李賢 et al. *Da Ming yitong zhi* 大明一統志 [Universal gazetteer of the great Ming]. 1461.

Li Zhongzi 李中梓. *Li Zhongzi yixue quanshu* 李中梓醫學全書 [Complete medical works of Li Zhongzi]. Edited by Bao Laifa. Beijing: Zhongguo zhongyiyao chubanshe, 1999.

Lo, Vivienne, ed. *Medieval Chinese Medicine: The Dunhuang Medical Manuscripts*. London: Routledge Curzon, 2006.

———. "Pleasure, Prohibition, and Pain: Food and Medicine in Traditional China." In *Of Tripod and Palate: Food, Politics, and Religion in Traditional China*, edited by Roel Sterckx, 163–85. New York: Palgrave Macmillan, 2005.

Lufrano, Richard John. *Honorable Merchants: Commerce and Self-Cultivation in Late Imperial China*. Honolulu: University of Hawai'i Press, 1997.

Lun yu [The Analects]. Translated by James Legge. https://ctext.org/analects. Accessed June 30, 2019.

Lu You 陸遊. *Laoxue an biji* 老學庵筆記 [Miscellany of Laoxue an]. SKQS edition.

Ma Duanlin 馬端臨. *Wenxian tongkao* 文獻通考 [Comprehensive study of documents and sources]. Academia Sinica, *Hanji quanwen ziliaoku* (Scripta Sinica) database.

Mao Jin 毛晉. *Yewai shi* 野外詩 [Poems from the outfield]. Changshu: Ding family, 1916. Reprinted in *Qingdai shiwenji huibian* [Collected anthologies of poetry and prose during the Qing Dynasty], vol. 12. Shanghai: Shanghai guji chubanshe, 2009–10.

Marcon, Federico. *The Knowledge of Nature and the Nature of Knowledge in Early Modern Japan*. Chicago: University of Chicago Press, 2015.

Marks, Robert B. *China: Its Environment and History*. Lanham, MD: Rowman and Littlefield, 2012.

———. *Tigers, Rice, Silk, and Silt: Environment and Economy in Late Imperial South China*. Cambridge: Cambridge University Press, 1998.

McDermott, Joseph P. *A Social History of the Chinese Book: Books and Literati Culture in Late Imperial China*. Hong Kong: Hong Kong University Press, 2006.

Medick, Hans. "Plebeian Culture in the Transition to Capitalism." In *Culture, Ideology and Politics: Essays for Eric Hobsbawm*, edited by Raphael Samuel and Gareth Stedman Jones, 84–112. London: Routledge, 1982.

Meng Yuanlao 孟元老. *Dongjing menghua lu jianzhu* 東京夢華錄箋註 [Annotated memoirs of the eastern capital]. Edited by Yi Yongwen. Beijing: Zhonghua shuju, 2006.

Métailié, Georges. "Concepts of Nature in Traditional Chinese *Materia Medica* and Botany

(16–17th century)." In *Concepts of Nature: A Chinese-European Cross-Cultural Perspective*, edited by Hans Ulrich Vogel and Günter Dux, 345–67. Leiden: Brill, 2010.

Métailié, Georges. "The *Bencao gangmu* of Li Shizhen: An Innovation in Natural History?" In *Innovation in Chinese Medicine*, edited Elisabeth Hsu, 221–61. Cambridge: Cambridge University Press, 2001.

Meyer-Fong, Tobie. "Conference Note: Early Modern China in the Late Imperial World." *Late Imperial China* 36, no. 2 (December 2015): 126–29.

———. *What Remains: Coming to Terms with Civil War in 19th-Century China*. Stanford, CA: Stanford University Press, 2013.

———. *Building Culture in Early Qing Yangzhou*. Stanford, CA: Stanford University Press, 2003.

Miao Xiyong. *Xianxingzhai guang biji* 先醒齋廣筆記. SKQS edition.

Miller, Peter N., and François Louis, eds. *Antiquarianism and Intellectual Life in Europe and China, 1500–1800*. Ann Arbor: University of Michigan Press, 2012.

Moran, Bruce. *Distilling Knowledge: Alchemy, Chemistry, and the Scientific Revolution*. Cambridge, MA: Harvard University Press, 2005.

Morton, Timothy. *The Poetics of Spice: Romantic Consumerism and the Exotic*. Cambridge: Cambridge University Press, 2000.

Munro, Donald J. *Images of Human Nature: A Sung Portrait*. Princeton, NJ: Princeton University Press, 1988.

Murdoch, John. "The Analytic Character of Late Medieval Learning: Natural Philosophy without Nature." In *Approaches to Nature in the Middle Ages*, edited by Lawrence D. Roberts, 171–213. Binghamton, NY: Center for Medieval and Early Renaissance Studies, 1982.

Nakagawa Tadahide [Chūei] 中川忠英. *Shinzoku kibun* 清俗紀聞 [An account of Qing customs]. Tōkyō: Heibonsha, 1966.

Nappi, Carla. "Surface Tension: Objectifying Ginseng in Chinese Early Modernity." In *Early Modern Things: Objects and Their Histories, 1500–1800*, edited by Paula Findlen, 31–52. New York: Routledge, 2012.

———. *The Monkey and the Inkpot: Natural History and Its Transformations in Early Modern China*. Cambridge, MA: Harvard University Press, 2009.

Naquin, Susan, and Evelyn S. Rawski. *Chinese Society in the Eighteenth Century*. New Haven, CT: Yale University Press, 1987.

Needham, Joseph. *The Grand Titration: Science and Society in East and West*. Toronto: University of Toronto Press, 1969.

Newman, William. *Atoms and Alchemy: Chymistry and the Experimental Origins of the Scientific Revolution*. Chicago: University of Chicago Press, 2006.

Ng, On Cho. *Cheng-Zhu Confucianism in the Early Qing: Li Guangdi (1642–1718) and Qing Learning*. Albany: State University of New York Press, 2001.

Ni, Yuping. *Customs Duties in the Qing Dynasty, ca. 1644–1911*. Leiden: Brill, 2017.

Nimick, Thomas. *Local Administration in Ming China: The Changing Roles of Magistrates, Prefects, and Provincial Officials*. Minneapolis: Society for Ming Studies, 2008.

Okanishi Tameto 岡西為人. *Chugoku isho honzō kō* 中国医書本草考 [A study of Chinese medical books and bencao literature]. Ōsaka: Maeda Shoten, 1974.

Ong, Chang Woei. "The Principles Are Many: Wang Tingxiang and Intellectual Transition in Mid-Ming China." *Harvard Journal of Asiatic Studies* 66, no. 2 (2006): 461–93.

Park, Katharine. "Natural Particulars: Medical Epistemology, Practice, and the Literature of Healing Springs." In *Natural Particulars: Nature and the Disciplines in Renaissance Europe*, edited by Anthony Grafton and Nancy Siraisi, 347–68. Cambridge, MA: MIT Press, 1999.

———. *Doctors and Medicine in Early Renaissance Florence.* Princeton, NJ: Princeton University Press, 1985.

Park, Katharine, and Lorraine Daston, eds. *The Cambridge History of Science. Vol. 3. Early Modern Science.* Cambridge: Cambridge University Press, 2006.

Pei Qin 裴芹. *Gujin tushu jicheng yanjiu* 古今图书集成研究 [A study of complete collection of illustrations and writings from ancient and modern Times]. Beijing: Beijing tushuguan chubanshe, 2001.

Perdue, Peter. "The Tenacious Tributary System." *Journal of Contemporary China* 24, no. 96 (2015): 1002–14.

———. *Exhausting the Earth: State and Peasant in Hunan.* Cambridge, MA: Harvard University Council of East Asian Studies, 1987.

Peterson, Willard J. "Advancement of Learning in Early Ch'ing: Three Cases." In *The Cambridge History of China, Vol. 9: The Ch'ing Dynasty to 1800*, part 2, edited by Willard J. Peterson, 513–70. Cambridge: Cambridge University Press, 2016.

———. "Dominating Learning from Above during the K'ang-hsi Period." In *The Cambridge History of China, Vol. 9: The Ch'ing Dynasty to 1800*, part 2, edited by Willard J. Peterson, 571–605. Cambridge: Cambridge University Press, 2016.

———. "Another Look at Li," *Bulletin of Sung and Yüan Studies* 18 (1986): 13–31.

———. *Bitter Gourd: Fang I-Chih and the Impetus for Intellectual Change.* New Haven, CT: Yale University Press, 1979.

Pickering, Andrew. *Science as Practice and Culture.* Chicago: University of Chicago Press, 1992.

Pomeranz, Kenneth. "Areas, Networks, and the Search for 'Early Modern' East Asia." In *Comparative Early Modernities: 1100–1800*, edited by David L. Porter, 245–69. London: Palgrave, 2012.

———. *The Great Divergence: China, Europe, and the Making of the Modern World Economy.* Princeton, NJ: Princeton University Press, 2000.

Pu Shizhen 浦世臣. *Xi'an du bencao kuai bian* 夕庵讀本草快編 [Quick reading notes on bencao by Mr. Xi'an]. In *Haiwai huigui zhongyi shanben guji congshu* [Collectanea of rare Chinese medical texts discovered overseas], vol. 10, edited by Zheng Jinsheng. Beijing: Renmin weisheng chubanshe, 2002–03.

Qian Dacheng 錢大成. "Mao Zijin nianpu gao" 毛子晉年譜稿 [Draft annalistic biography of Mao Jin]. *Guoli zhongyang tushuguan guankan* 1, no. 4 (1947): 9–23.

Qian Qianyi 錢謙益. *Qian Muzhai quanji* 錢牧齋全集 [Complete works of Qian Qianyi]. 8 vols. Shanghai: Shanghai guji chubanshe, 2003.

Qian Shutian 錢樹田. *Jingxiutang yaoshuo* 敬修堂藥說. Canton: c. 1800. In *Gugong zhenben congkan*, vol. 375. Haikou: Hainan chubanshe, 2000.

Qian Yuanming 钱远铭 et al. *Li Shizhen shi shi kao* 李时珍史实考. Guangzhou: Guangdong keji chubanshe, 1988.

Qiu Jun 丘濬. *Daxue yanyi bu* 大學衍義補 [Supplement to the abundant meanings of the Great Learning]. SKQS edition.

Qiu Ying 仇英. *Qiu Ying fang Qingming shanghe tu* 仇英仿清明上河图 [Qiu Ying's imitation of *Along the River during the Qingming Festival*]. Beijing: Wenwu chubanshe, 2007.

Rankin, Alisha M. *Panaceia's Daughters: Noblewomen as Healers in Early Modern Germany*. Chicago: University of Chicago Press, 2013.

Rawski, Evelyn S. "The Qing Formation and the Early Modern Period." In *The Qing Formation in World-Historical Time*, edited by Lynn Struve, 207–41. Cambridge, MA: Harvard University Asia Center, 2004.

Read, Bernard E., and Liu Ju-ch'iang, *Bibliography of Chinese Medicinal Plants from the Pen Ts'ao Kang Mu* (1596), Peking, Dept. of pharmacology, Peking union medical college, in collaboration with the Peking laboratory of natural history, 1927.

Ren Fang 任放. *Ming Qing Changjiang zhongyou shizhen jingji yanjiu* 明清长江中游市镇经济研究 [A study of market town economy in Mid-Yangzi during Ming-Qing times]. Wuchang: Wuhan daxue chubanshe, 2003.

Robinson, David M. *Martial Spectacles of the Ming Court*. Cambridge, MA: Harvard University Asia Center, 2013.

Rogaski, Ruth. *Hygienic Modernity: Meanings of Health and Disease in Treaty-Port China*. Berkeley: University of California Press, 2004.

Rong, Xinjiang. *Eighteen Lectures on Dunhuang*. Leiden: Brill, 2013.

Roos, Anna Marie. *The Salt of the Earth: Natural Philosophy, Medicine, and Chymistry in England, 1650–1750*. Leiden, Boston: Brill, 2007.

Rosenberg, Charles E. "The Therapeutic Revolution: Medicine, Meaning, and Social Change in Nineteenth-Century America." *Perspectives in Biology and Medicine* 20 (1977): 485–506.

Rowe, William T. "Political, Social, and Economic Factors Affecting the Transmission of Technical Knowledge in Early Modern China." In *Cultures of Knowledge: Technology in Chinese History*, edited by Dagmar Schäfer, 25–44. Leiden: Brill, 2012.

———. *Saving the World: Chen Hongmou and Elite Consciousness in Eighteenth-Century China*. Stanford, CA: Stanford University Press, 2001.

———. *Hankow: Commerce and Society in a Chinese City, 1796-1889*. Stanford, CA: Stanford University Press, 1984.

Roy, David Tod, trans. *The Plum in the Golden Vase, or, Chin P'ing Mei*. Princeton, NJ: Princeton University Press, 1993–2013.

Sakade Yoshinobu 坂出祥伸. *Chūgoku kindai no shisō to kagaku* 中国近代の思想と科学 [Science and thoughts in modern China]. Kyōto: Hōyū Shoten, 2001.

Salguero, C. Pierce. *Translating Buddhist Medicine in Medieval China*. Philadelphia: University of Pennsylvania Press, 2014.

Saxer, Martin. *Manufacturing Tibetan Medicine: The Creation of an Industry and the Moral Economy of Tibetanness*. New York: Berghahn Books, 2013.

Schäfer, Dagmar. *The Crafting of the 10,000 Things: Knowledge and Technology in Seventeenth-Century China*. Chicago: University of Chicago Press, 2011.

Schäfer, Dagmar, and Dieter Kuhn. *Weaving an Economic Pattern in Ming Times (1368–1644): The Production of Silk Weaves in the State-Owned Silk Workshops*. Heidelberg: Edition Forum, 2002.

Schafer, Edward H. *The Golden Peaches of Samarkand*. Berkeley: University of California Press, 1963.

Scheid, Volker. *Currents of Tradition in Chinese Medicine 1626–2006*. Seattle, WA: Eastland Press, 2007.

———. *Chinese Medicine in Contemporary China*. Durham, NC: Duke University Press, 2002.

Schipper, Kristoffer, and Franciscus Verellen, eds. *The Taoist Canon: A Historical Companion to the Daozang*, 3 vols. Chicago: University of Chicago Press, 2004.

Schlesinger, Jonathan. *A World Trimmed with Fur: Wild Things, Pristine Places, and the Natural Fringes of Qing*. Stanford, CA: Stanford University Press, 2017.

Schneewind, Sarah. *Shrines to Living Men in the Ming Political Cosmos*. Cambridge, MA: Harvard University Asia Center, 2018.

Schonebaum, Andrew. *Novel Medicine: Healing, Literature, and Popular Knowledge in Early Modern China*. Seattle: University of Washington Press, 2016.

Semedo, Alvaro. *The History of That Great and Renowned Monarchy of China*. London: E. Tyler, 1655.

Shang, Wei. "The Making of the Everyday World: Jin Ping Mei Cihua and Encyclopedias for Daily Use." In *Dynastic Crisis and Cultural Innovation: From the Late Ming to the Late Qing and Beyond*, edited by David Wang and Wei Shang, 63–92. Cambridge, MA: Harvard University Asia Center, 2006.

Shang Shu [The classic of documents]. Translated by James Legge. In https://ctext.org/shang-shu. Accessed June 30, 2019.

Shang Zhijun et al. *Lidai zhongyao wenxian jinghua* 历代中药文献精华. Beijing: Kexue jishu wenxian chubanshe, 1989.

Shapin, Steven and Simon Schaffer. *Leviathan and the Air-Pump: Hobbes, Boyle, and the Experimental Life*. Princeton, NJ: Princeton University Press, 1985.

Shen Defu 沈德符. *Wanli yehuo bian* 萬曆野獲編 [Anecdotes gleaned during the Wanli reign]. Beijing: Zhonghua shuju, 1980.

Shen Kuo 沈括. *Mengxi bitan* 夢溪筆談 [Brush talks of dream brooks]. Beijing: Zhonghua shuju, 2015.

Shiba, Yoshinobu. *Commerce and Society in Sung China*. Translated by Mark Elvin. Ann Arbor: Center for Chinese Studies, University of Michigan, 1970.

Shinno, Reiko. *The Politics of Chinese Medicine under Mongol Rule*. New York: Routledge, 2016.

Shinoda Osamu 篠田統. *Chūgoku shokumotsushi no kenkyū* 中国食物史の研究. Tokyo: Yasaka Shobō, 1978.

Siebert, Martina. "Animals as Text: Producing and Consuming 'Text-Animals.'" In *Animals through Chinese History: Earliest Times to 1911*, edited by Roel Sterxck, Martina Siebert, and Dagmar Schäfer, 139–59. Cambridge: Cambridge University Press, 2018.

———. "Making Technology History." In *Cultures of Knowledge: Technology in Chinese History*, edited by Dagmar Schäfer, 253–81. Leiden: Brill, 2012.

———. *Pulu: "Abhandlungen und Auflistungen" zu materieller Kultur und Naturkunde im traditionellen China* [Pulu: "Treatises and lists" of material culture and natural history in traditional China]. Opera Sinologica 17. Wiesbaden: Harrassowitz Verlag, 2006.

Sivin, Nathan. *Health Care in Eleventh-Century China*. New York: Springer, 2015.

———. "A Multi-Dimensional Approach to Research on Ancient Science." *EASTM* 23 (2005): 10–25.

Sivin, Nathan. *Traditional Medicine in Contemporary China: A Partial Translation of Revised Outline of Chinese Medicine.* Ann Arbor: Center for Chinese Studies, University of Michigan, 1987.

———. "Why the Scientific Revolution Did Not Take Place in China—or Didn't It?" *Chinese Science* 5 (1982): 45–66.

Skinner, G. William, ed. *The City in Late Imperial China.* Stanford, CA: Stanford University Press, 1977.

———. "Marketing and Social Structure in Rural China," parts 1–3, *Journal of Asian Studies* 24, no. 1–3 (1964).

Smith, Pamela H. *The Body of the Artisan: Art and Experience in the Scientific Revolution.* Chicago: University of Chicago Press, 2004.

Snyder-Reinke, Jeff. "Afterlives of the Dead: Uncovering Graves and Mishandling Corpses in Nineteenth-Century China." *Frontier of History in China* 11, no. 1 (2016): 1–20.

So, Billy K. L., ed. *The Economy of Lower Yangzi Delta in Late Imperial China: Connecting Money, Markets, and Institutions.* New York: Routledge, 2013.

Spence, Jonathan. *Treason by the Book.* New York: Viking, 2001.

———. *Ts'ao Yin and the K'ang-Hsi Emperor: Bondservant and Master.* 2nd ed. New Haven, CT: Yale University Press, 1988.

———. "Ch'ing." In *Food in Chinese Culture,* edited by C. K. Chang, 259–94. New Haven, CT: Yale University Press, 1977.

Stanley-Baker, Michael. "Drugs, Destiny and Disease in Medieval China: Situating Knowledge in Context." *Daoism: Religion, History and Society* 6 (2014): 113–156.

Stannard, Jerry. *Herbs and Herbalism in the Middle Ages and Renaissance.* Aldershot, VT: Ashgate, 1999.

Stuart, G. A. *Chinese Materia Medica: Vegetable Kingdom.* Revised from F. Porter Smith's work. Shanghai: American Presbyterian Mission Press, 1911.

Struve, Lynn, ed. *Time and Temporality in the Ming-Qing Transition: East Asia from Ming to Qing.* Honolulu: Association for Asian Studies and University of Hawai'i Press, 2005.

———. *The Qing Formation in World-Historical Time.* Cambridge, MA: Harvard University Asia Center, 2004.

Sugg, Richard. *Mummies, Cannibals and Vampires: The History of Corpse Medicine from the Renaissance to the Victorians.* London: Routledge, 2016.

Suh, Soyoung. *Naming the Local: Medicine, Language, and Identity in Korea since the Fifteenth Century.* Cambridge, MA: Harvard University Asia Center, 2017.

Sun Guoru 孙国如 and Huang Wenhong 黄文鸿. *Zhangshu zhongyiyao fazhan jianshi* 樟树中医药发展简史 [A concise history of pharmaceuticals in Zhangshu]. Nanchang: Jiangxi kexue jishu chubanshe, 2011.

Sun Simiao 孫思邈. *Qianjin yi fang jiaoshi* 千金翼方校释. Edited by Li Jingrong et al. Beijing: Renmin weisheng chubanshe, 1998.

Szonyi, Michael. *The Art of Being Governed: Everyday Politics in Imperial China.* Princeton, NJ: Princeton University Press, 2017.

Tang Tingyou 唐廷猷. *Zhongguo yaoye shi* 中国药业史 [A history of the Chinese pharmaceutical industry]. Beijing: Zhongguo yiyao keji chubanshe, 2013.

Tang Xianzu 湯顯祖. *Mudan ting* 牡丹亭 [The peony pavillon]. Beijing: Renmin wenxue chubanshe, 1978.

————. *Yuming tang quan ji* 玉茗堂全集 [Complete anthology of Yuming tang]. N.p. 1621–27. In XXSKQS, vol. 1363.

Tao Gu 陶穀. *Qing yi lu* 清異錄 [Records of the pure and unusual]. SKQS edition.

Thompson, E. P. *Customs in Common*. London: Merlin Press, 1991.

Tongrentang yaomu 同仁堂藥目. [A catalog of Tongrentang pharmacy]. Beijing: 1889.

Tong Yuejian 童岳薦. *Tiao ding ji* 調鼎集 [On the art of regulating cauldrons]. Zhengzhou: Zhongzhou guji chubanshe, 1988.

Totelin, Laurence. *Hippocratic Recipes: Oral and Written Transmission of Pharmacological Knowledge in Fifth- and Fourth-Century Greece*. Leiden: Brill, 2009.

Tuotuo et al., eds. *Jin shi* 金史. Accessed through *Hanji quanwen ziliaoku* (Scripta Sinica), Academia Sinica.

————. *Song shi* 宋史. Accessed through *Hanji quanwen ziliaoku* (Scripta Sinica), Academia Sinica.

Unschuld, Paul U. *What Is Medicine?: Western and Eastern Approaches to Healing*. Translated by Karen Reimers. Berkeley: University of California Press, 2009.

————. *Huang Di nei jing su wen: Nature, Knowledge, Imagery in an Ancient Chinese Medical Text*. Berkeley,: University of California Press, 2003.

————. *Medicine in China: A History of Pharmaceuticals*. Berkeley: University of California Press, 1986.

————. *Yü-chih pen-ts'ao p'in-hui ching-yao: ein Arzneibuch aus dem China des 16. Jahrhunderts*. Munich: Heinz Moos Verlag, 1973.

Unschuld, Paul U., and Zheng Jinsheng. *Chinese Traditional Healing: The Berlin Collections of Manuscript Volumes from the 16th through the Early 20th Century*. Leiden: Brill, 2012.

Unschuld, Ulrike. "Traditional Chinese Pharmacology: An Analysis of Its Development in the Thirteenth Century," *Isis* 68, no. 2 (June 1977), 224–28

Van Dyke, Paul A. *The Canton Trade: Life and Enterprise on the China Coast, 1700–1845*. Hong Kong: Hong Kong University Press, 2005.

Vedal, Nathan. "New Scripts for All Sounds: Cosmology and Universal Phonetic Notation Systems in Late Imperial China." *Harvard Journal of Asiatic Studies* 78, no. 1 (2018): 1–46.

Volkmar, Barbara. "The Physician and the Plagiarists: The Fate of the Legacy of Wan Quan." *Princeton East Asian Library Journal* 9, no. 1 (Spring 2000): 1–77.

Von Glahn, Richard. *An Economic History of China: From Antiquity to the Nineteenth Century*. Cambridge: Cambridge University Press, 2015.

————. *Fountain of Fortune: Money and Monetary Policy in China, 1000–1700*. Berkeley: University of California Press, 1996.

————. "The Enchantment of Wealth: The God Wutong in the Social History of Jiangnan." *Harvard Journal of Asiatic Studies* 51, no. 2 (December 1991): 651–714.

Waley-Cohen, Joanna. "Food and China's World of Goods in the Long Eighteenth Century." In *Living the Good Life: Consumption in the Qing and Ottoman Empires of the Eighteenth Century*, edited by Elif Akçetin and Suraiya Faroqhi, 283–306. Leiden: Brill, 2018.

Wang Bing 王冰 ed. Chongguang buzhu Huangdi neijing suwen 重廣補註黃帝內經素問 [Expanded Yellow Emperor's inner canon, plain questions, with new commentaries]. In *Sibu congkan*, facsimile of Northern Song edition. Shanghai: Commercial Press, 1936.

Wang Cheng-hua. "Guoyan fanhua: Wan Ming chengshi tu, chengshi guan yu wenhua xiaofei de yanjiu." In *Qingming shanghe tu xin lun*, edited by The Palace Museum, 281–302. Beijing: Gugong chubanshe, 2011.

Wang Kentang 王肯堂. *Yugang zhai bi zhu* 鬱岡齋筆塵 [Written chatters of Yugang Studio]. Vol. 4. N.p., 1602. Reprint, XXSKQS, v. 1130.

———. *Zhengzhi zhunsheng* 證治準繩 [Standard measure for symptoms and treatments]. SKQS edition.

Wang Lü 王履. *Su hui ji* 溯洄集 [Anthology of repeated searching]. SKQS edition.

Wang Shixing 王士性. *Guang zhi yi* 廣志繹 [Interpretive gazetteer of the provinces]. Beijing: Zhonghua shuju, 1981.

Wang Shizhen 王世貞. *Yanzhou shiliao* 弇州史料 [Historical sources of Yanzhou]. Vol. 100. N.p. Wanli 42[1614], Airusheng jiben guji database.

———. *Yanzhou xu gao* 弇州續稿 [Supplementary manuscript of Yanzhou]. Vol. 207. SKQS edition.

———. *Yanshantang bie ji* 弇山堂別集 [Alternative anthology of Yanshan tang]. Vol. 100. Taipei: Taiwan xuesheng shuju, 1965.

Wang Tao 王燾. *Waitai miyao* 外臺秘要 [Secret essential recipes from the outer offices]. SKQS edition.

Wang Wenjie 王文潔. *Taiyi xianzhi bencao yaoxing daquan* 太乙仙製本草藥性大全. [Complete collection of materia medica, the nature of drugs, and divine pharmaceutical processing by Master Thunder]. Jianyang: Jishantang, 1582. Vol. 8. Reprint, *Zhongyi guji guben daquan*, edited by Zheng Jinsheng. Beijing: Zhongyi guji chubanshe, 2008.

Wang Yingkui 王應奎. *Liunan suibi* 柳南隨筆 [Random jottings at the south of the willows]. Beijing: Zhonghua shuju, 1983.

Welch, Evelyn, and James Shaw. *Making and Marketing Renaissance Medicine: The Speziale al Giglio in Florence, 1493–1494*. Wellcome Trust History of Medicine Clio Medica series, Rodopi, Amsterdam, 2011.

Wen, Xin. "The Road to Literary Culture: Revisiting the Jurchen Language Examination System." *T'oung pao* 101, no. 1–3 (2015): 130–167.

White, Katharine. *Onward and Upward in the Garden*. New York: NYRB Classics, 2015.

Widmer, Ellen. "The Huanduzhai of Hangzhou and Suzhou: A Study in Seventeenth-Century Publishing." *Harvard Journal of Asiatic Studies* 56, no. 1 (June 1996), 77–122.

Will, Pierre-Etienne. *Bureaucracy and Famine in Eighteenth-Century China*. Translated by Elborg Forster. Stanford, CA: Stanford University Press, 1990.

Wilms, Sabine. *The Divine Farmer's Classic of Materia Medica: Shén nóng běncǎo jīng*. Corbett, OR: Happy Goat Productions, 2017.

Wong, R. Bin. *China Transformed: Historical Change and the Limits of European Experience*. Ithaca, NY: Cornell University Press, 1997.

Wu, Jiang. *Enlightenment in Dispute: The Reinvention of Chan Buddhism in Seventeenth-Century China*. Oxford: Oxford University Press, 2008.

Wu, Yi-Li. *Reproducing Women: Medicine, Metaphor, and Childbirth in Late Imperial China*. Berkeley: University of California Press, 2010.

Wu, Yulian. *Luxurious Networks: Salt Merchants, Status, and Statecraft in Eighteenth-Century China*. Stanford, CA: Stanford University Press, 2017.

Wu Han 吴晗. *Jiangzhe cangshu jia shilüe* 江浙藏书家史略. Beijing: Zhonghua shuju, 1981.

Wu Qian 吳謙 et al., eds. *Yuzuan Yizong jinjian* 御纂醫宗金鑑 [The imperially commissioned golden mirror of medical orthodoxy]. SKQS edition.

Wu Zun 吳遵. *Chu shi lu* 初仕錄 [Notes for beginners of office-holding]. Jinling: 1640.

Xiao Fang 蕭放. "Ming Qing shidai Zhangshu yaoye fazhan chutan" 明清时代樟树药业发展初探 [An initial study of pharmaceutical enterprises in Ming-Qing Zhangshu]. *Zhongguo shehui jingji shi yanjiu* 1 (1990): 65–70.

Xiaoxiaosheng 笑笑生. *Jin Ping Mei: Huiping huijiao ben* 金瓶梅会评会校本 [The plum in the golden vase: Collected commentaries]. Edited by Qin Xiurong. Beijing: Zhonghua shuju, 1998.

Xie Guozhen 谢国桢. *Ming Qing zhi ji dang she yundong kao* 明清之际党社运动考 [A study of literati parties and associations during the Ming-Qing transition]. Beijing: Zhonghua shuju, 1982.

Xie Zhaozhe 謝肇淛. *Wu za zu* 五雜組 [Five miscellanies]. Ruweiguan, Wanli 44. In XXSKQS, vol. 1130.

Xing Yihai 邢益海. *Fang Yizhi Zhuangxue yanjiu* 方以智庄学研究 [A study of Fang Yizhi's Zhuangzi scholarship]. Beijing: Beijing Normal University Press, 2015.

Xu Chunfu 徐春甫. *Gujin yitong daquan* 古今醫統大全 [Complete encyclopedia of ancient and modern medical traditions]. Edited by Cui Zhongping Cui and Yaoting Wang. Beijing: Renmin weisheng chubanshe, 1991.

Xu Dachun 徐大椿. *Yixue yuanliu lun* 醫學源流論 [On the origins and traditions of medical learning]. SKQS edition.

———. *Shennong bencaojing baizhong lu* 神農本草經百種錄 [A hundred varieties from the Divine Farmer's classic of materia medica]. SKQS edition.

———. *Shen ji chu yan* 慎疾芻言 [Humble opinions on discretion over illnesses]. Changzhou: Xie Jiafu, Daoguang 28 [48]. In XXSKQS, vol. 1028.

———. *Forgotten Traditions of Ancient Chinese Medicine: A Chinese View from the Eighteenth Century*. Translated by Paul U. Unschuld. Brookline, MA: Paradigm Publications, 1990.

Xu Menghong 許夢閎. *Beixin guan zhi* 北新關志 [Gazetteer of the Beixin customs house]. In *Hangzhou yunhe wenxian jicheng* [Collected sources on the canals of Hangzhou], vol. 1. Hangzhou: Hangzhou chubanshe, 2009.

Xu Sanzhong 徐三重. *Cai qin lu* 採芹錄 [Records of picking local vegetables]. SKQS edition.

Xu Tan 许檀. "Qingdai qianqi liutong geju de bianhua" 清代前期流通格局的变化 [Changing configurations in commodity circulation during early Qing]. *Qingshi yanjiu no. 3* (1999).

Xu Yang 徐揚. *Gusu fanhua tu* 姑蘇繁華圖 [Prosperous Suzhou]. Tianjin: Tianjin renmin meishu chubanshe, 2007.

Yamada Keiji 山田慶児. *Chūgoku igaku no kigen* 中国医学の起源 [The origin of Chinese medicine]. Tokyo: Iwanami Shōten, 1999.

———. *Mono no imēji: Honzō to hakubutsugaku e no shōtai* 物のイメージ: 本草と博物学への招待 [The image of things: An invitation to bencao and natural history]. Tokyo: Asahi Shinbunsha, 1994.

———. *Shushi no shizengaku* 朱子の自然学 [The natural studies of Zhu Xi]. Tokyo: Iwanami Shoten, 1978.

Yamamoto Susumu 山本進. *Min Shin jidai no shōnin to kokka* 明清時代の商人と国家 [Merchants and the state in Ming-Qing China]. Tokyo: Kenbun shuppan, 2002.

Yamane Yukio 山根幸夫. *Min Shin Kahoku teikishi no kenkyū* 明清華北定期市の研究 [A study of regular market fairs in Ming-Qing North China]. Tokyo: Kyūko Shoin, 1995.

Yang, Xiong. *Exemplary Figures = Fayan*. Translated by Michael Nylan. Seattle: University of Washington Press, 2013.

Yang Shoujing 楊守敬. *Riben fang shu zhi* 日本訪書志 [An account of book hunting in Japan]. Shenyang: Liaoning jiaoyu chubanshe, 2003.

Yang Tianhui 楊天惠. "Zhangming fuzi ji" 彰明附子記 [An account of aconite in Zhangming]. In *Shuo fu* [Discourses of the outer precinct], edited by Tao Zongyi, vol. 106. Shanghai: Shanghai guji chubanshe, 1988.

Yang Yuliang 杨玉良. "Wuying dian xiushu chu ji Neifu xiushu ge guan" 武英殿修书处及内府修书各馆 [The publishing office of Wuying Place and the various editorial offices in the imperial household]. *Gugong bowuyuan yuankan* 1 (1990): 28–40.

Yang Zhengtai 杨正泰. *Mingdai yizhankao* 明代驿站考 [A study of relay and post stations in Ming China]. Expanded ed. Shanghai: Shanghai guji chubanshe, 2006.

Yan Ruyu 嚴如煜. *Sansheng bianfang beilan* 三省邊防備覽 [Memorandum for border defense in the tri-provincial region]. N.p., 1822.

Yan Yu 嚴羽. *Canglang shihua jiaoshi* 滄浪詩話校釋 [Poetry criticism of Canglang] Beijing: Renmin wenxue chubanshe, 1961.

Yao Silian 姚思廉. *Liang shu* 梁書 [A history of the Liang Dynasty]. Beijing: Zhonghua shuju, 1973.

Ye Dehui 葉德輝. *Shulin qinghua* 書林清話 [Pure discourses in the forest of books]. Beijing: Zhonghua shuju, 1957 (1987 printing).

Young, James Harvey. *The Toadstool Millionaires: A Social History of Patent Medicines in America before Federal Regulation*. Princeton, NJ: Princeton University Press, 1961.

Yuan Liangyi 袁良义. *Qing yitiaobian fa* 清一条鞭法 [The single-whip law in the Qing Dynasty]. Beijing: Beijing daxue chubanshe, 1995.

Yuan shi 元史 [A History of the Yuan Dynasty]. Academia Sinica, *Hanji quanwen shujuku* (Scripta Sinica) database.

Yu Chang 喻昌. *Yuyi cao* 寓意草 [Meaningful scribbles]. SKQS edition.

———. *Yimen falü* 醫門法律 [Laws and rules of the medical profession]. SKQS edition.

Yue Chonghui jushi fangtan lu 樂崇暉居士訪談錄 [An interview with Mr. Yue Chonghui]. Taipei: Guoshi guan, 2013.

Yue Chongxi 樂崇熙. *Bainian Tongrentang* 百年同仁堂 [Tongrentang pharmacy's hundred years]. Taipei: Sixing wenhua, 2013.

Yu Hui 余輝. "Cong Qingming jie dao xiqing ri: sanfu *Qingming shanghe tu* zhi bijiao" 從清明節到喜慶日：三幅《清明上河圖》之比較. In *Qingming shanghe tu xin lun*, edited by The Palace Museum, 257–80. Beijing: Gugong chubanshe, 2011.

Yu Ruxi 俞汝溪. *Xinkan Leigong paozhi bianlan* 新刊雷公炮製便覽. N.p., Ming dynasty edition, no later than 1591, vol. 5. Reproduced in the series *Zhongyi guji guben daquan*, edited by Zheng Jinsheng. Beijing: Zhongyi guji chubanshe, 2008.

Yu Yingkui 余應奎. *Taiyiyuan buyi bencao gejue Leigong paozhi* 太醫院補遺本草歌訣雷公炮製 [Imperial Academy of Medicine's complete guide to materia medica rhymes and Master

Thunder's pharmaceuticals]. Jinling [Nanjing]: Zhou Yuejiao, 1587. https://iiif.lib.harvard.edu/manifests/view/drs:8486919$1i

Yu Ying-shih 余英時. *Fang Yizhi wanjie kao* 方以智晚節考 [A study of Fang Yizhi's late life]. Expanded ed. Taipei: Yunchen wenhua, 2011.

Yvan, Melchior-Honoré. *Lettre sur la Pharmacie en Chine.* Paris: Labé, 1847.

———. "Extrait d'un travail sur Singapore." *Journal de Chemie Médicale* 1 (1845): 148–55.

Zeitlin, Judith. "The Literary Fashioning of Medical Authority: A Study of Sun Yikui's Case Histories." In *Thinking with Cases: Specialist Knowledge in Chinese Cultural History,* edited by Charlotte Furth et al., 169–202. Honolulu: University of Hawai'i Press, 2007.

Zelin, Madeleine. *The Merchants of Zigong: Industrial Entrepreneurship in Early Modern China.* New York: Columbia University Press, 2005.

Zhan, Mei. *Other-Worldly: Making Chinese Medicine through Transnational Frames.* Durham, NC: Duke University Press, 2009.

Zhang, Meng. "Timber Trade along the Yangzi River: State, Market, Environment, and Frontier, 1750–1911," PhD Diss., University of California, Los Angeles, 2017.

Zhang, Qiong. *Making the New World Their Own: Chinese Encounters with Jesuit Science in the Age of Discovery.* Leiden: Brill, 2015.

Zhang, Ying. *Confucian Image Politics: Masculine Morality in Seventeenth-Century China.* Seattle: University of Washington Press, 2016.

Zhang Guangdou 張光斗. *Zengbu Leigong yaoxing paozhi* 增補雷公藥性炮製. Jixiutang, 1714. In Digital Collection of Die Staatsbibliothek zu Berlin—Preußischer Kulturbesitz. http://resolver.staatsbibliothek-berlin.de/SBB00002FCA00000000.

Zhang Ji 張籍. *Zhang Siye ji* 張司業集. SKQS edition.

Zhang Jiebin. *Zhang Jingyue yixue quanshu.* Beijing: Zhongguo zhongyiyao chubanshe, 1999.

Zhang Lu 張璐. *Zhang Luyu yixue quanshu* 張路玉醫學全書 [Complete medical works of Zhang Lu]. Zhang Minqing et al., eds. Beijing: Beijing zhongyiyao chubanshe, 1999.

Zhang Peiyu et al. *Beijing Tongrentang shi* 北京同仁堂史 [A history of Tongrentang Pharmacy in Beijing]. Beijing: Renmin ribao chubanshe, 1993.

Zhang Rui 張叡. *Xiushi zhinan* 修事指南. N.p., n.d. Reprint in *Gugong zhenben congkan,* vol. 374. Haikou: Hainan chubanshe, 2000.

Zhang Shichen and Guan Huai. "Leigong paozhi lun chengshu niandai xin tan" [New inquiries on the date of composition of *Master Thunder's Pharmaceuticals*]. *Zhongguo zhongyao zazhi (China Journal of Chinese Materia Medica)* 25, no. 3 (2000): 179–83.

Zhang Wei and Zhang Ruixian. "Bencao yuanshi banben kaocha" [A study of different editions of *Bencao yuanshi*]. *Zhongyi wenxian zazhi,* no. 1 (2010): 2–5.

Zhang Yingyu 張應俞. *Dupian xinshu* 杜騙新書 [A new book for foiling swindlers]. Cunren tang Chen Huaixuan, 1465–1620. https://iiif.lib.harvard.edu/manifests/view/drs:53917507$1i.

Zhang Zhibin 張志斌. "Ming 'Shiwu bencao' zuozhe ji chengshu kao" [A study of authorship and compilation of *Dietetic Materia Medica* during the Ming]. *Zhongyi zazhi* 53.18 (2012): 1588–91.

Zhang Zhicong 張志聰. *Lüshantang leibian* 侶山堂類編 [Assorted discourses of Lüshan tang]. Nanjing: Jiangsu kexue jishu chubanshe, 1981.

Zhan Ruoshui 湛若水. *Gewu tong* 格物通 [Compendium for the investigation of things]. SKQS edition.

Zhao, Gang. *Qing Opening to the Ocean: Chinese Maritime Policies, 1684–1757.* Honolulu: University of Hawai'i Press, 2013.

Zhao Erxun et al. *Qing shi gao* [Draft history of the Qing Dynasty]. Beijing: Zhonghua shuju, 2015.

Zhao Nanxing 趙南星. *Shangyi bencao* 上醫本草 [Materia medica of the Supreme Physician]. N.p: 1620. Reproduced in *Zhongguo Zhongyi yanjiuyuan tushuguan cang shanben congshu* [Collectanea of rare books held at the library of the Chinese Academy for the Study of Chinese Medicine]. Beijing: Zhongyi guji chubanshe, 1996.

Zhao Yuhuang 趙燏黃. *Qizhou yaozhi* 祁州藥志 [A study of pharmaceuticals at the Qizhou market fair]. Fuzhou: Fujian kexue jishu chubanshe, 2004.

Zhao Yushi 趙與時. *Bin tui lu* 賓退錄 [Records after the guest retired]. SKQS edition.

Zhen Xueyan and Zheng Jinsheng. "Shi Zhenduo *Bencao bu* yanjiu" [A Study of Pedro Piñuela's *Bencao bu*]. *Zhonghua yishi zazhi* 32, no. 4 (2002): 205–7.

Zheng Jinsheng. *Yaolin waishi* 药林外史 [External history of pharmacy in China]. Guilin: Guangxi shifan daxue chubanshe, 2007.

———. *Song dai bencao shi* 宋代本草史 [History of materia medica during the Song dynasty]. MA thesis, Chinese Academy of Traditional Medicine, Institute of Medical History and Philology, 1981.

Zhonghua renmin gongheguo yaodian 中华人民共和国药典 [Pharmacopeia of the People's Republic of China]. Beijing: Renmin weisheng chubanshe, 1963.

Zhonghua yaodian 中華藥典 [Pharmacopeia of China]. Nanjing: Neizheng bu weisheng shu, 1930.

Zhongyong [Doctrine of the mean]. Translated by James Legge, at https://ctext.org/liji/zhongyong. Accessed June 14, 2019.

Zhou Hongzu 周弘祖. *Gujin shuke* 古今書刻 [Printed books and inscriptions in ancient and modern times]. Ming edition, mid-sixteenth century. Reprint, *Lilou congshu*, edited by Ye Dehui. Changsha: Ye Family, 1907.

Zhou Mi 周密. *Wulin jiushi* 武林舊事. *Zhibuzu zhai congshu* edition.

Zhu Guozhen 朱國楨. *Yongchuang xiaopin* 湧幢小品 [Short essays under the pavillon of mirages]. Shanghai: Zhonghua shuju, 1959.

Zhu Su 朱橚. *Jiuhuang bencao* 救荒本草 [Materia medica for famine relief]. SKQS edition.

Zhu Xi 朱熹. *Zhuzi yulei* 朱子語類 [Assorted quotes from Master Zhu Xi]. Vol. 140, n.p., Chen Wei, 1473. Airusheng.

Zhu Yizun 朱彝尊. *Pushuting ji* 曝書亭集. In *Sibu congkan*, facsimile of Kangxi edition. Shanghai: Commercial Press, 1936.

Zhuang Chuo 莊綽. *Jilei bian* 雞肋編 [Useless jottings]. SKQS edition.

Zhuang Jifa 莊吉發. *Zhenkong jiaxiang: Qingdai minjian mimi zongjiao shi yanjiu* 真空家鄉: 清代民間秘密宗教史研究 [A study of the history of secret popular religious sects in Qing China]. Taipei: Wenshizhe chubanshe, 2002.

Zimmermann, Francis. *The Jungle and the Aroma of Meats: An Ecological Theme in Hindu Medicine.* Berkeley: University of California Press, 1987.

Zuo, Leah Ya. *Shen Gua's Empiricism.* Cambridge, MA: Harvard University Asia Center, 2018.

INDEX

Page numbers in *italics* refer to illustrations.

A NOTE ON THE TYPE

This book has been composed in Arno, an Old-style serif typeface in the classic Venetian tradition, designed by Robert Slimbach at Adobe.